The Quiet Revolution in American Psychoanalysis

This book brings together for the first time in one volume selected papers by one of the leading contemporary intellectual figures in the field of psychoanalysis, Arnold M. Cooper.

Cooper has addressed every aspect of American psychoanalytic life: theory, clinical work, education, research, the interface with neighboring disciplines, and the institutional life of the profession. In these papers, he both documents and critiques what he calls a 'Quiet Revolution,' following the death of Freud, in the way psychoanalysis is conceived: as a science, as a theory of mental life, as a treatment, as a profession.

Throughout his professional life, the process of change has fascinated Cooper. His own contributions to psychoanalytic clinical theory have changed our understanding of work with patients to include a greater appreciation of narcissistic and pre-Oedipal themes in development and of the human encounter embedded in the psychoanalytic situation. His progressive leadership in our educational and professional organizations has done much to promote change toward greater self-examination and tolerance of new ideas, and, indeed, to create the conditions that make change possible.

Above all, Cooper's unique ability to observe and reflect upon the process of change, recorded here in papers selected from over 150 written in the 50-plus years between 1947 and 2002, has helped make him the guide to whom psychoanalysts repeatedly turn to understand not only where, but even what, psychoanalysis is.

Arnold M. Cooper is the Stephen P. Tobin and Dr Arnold M. Cooper Emeritus Professor in Consultation–Liaison Psychiatry at the Joan and Sanford I. Weill Medical College of Cornell University, and Training and Supervising Psychoanalyst at Columbia University Center for Psychoanalytic Training and Research.

Elizabeth L. Auchincloss is Vice Chair for Graduate Medical Education and Professor of Clinical Psychiatry at the New York Weill Cornell Medical Center and Associate Director and Training and Supervising Psychoanalyst at the Columbia University Center for Psychoanalytic Training and Research.

THE NEW LIBRARY OF PSYCHOANALYSIS
General Editor Dana Birksted-Breen

The New Library of Psychoanalysis was launched in 1987 in association with the Institute of Psychoanalysis, London. It took over from the International Psychoanalytical Library, which published many of the early translations of the works of Freud and the writings of most of the leading British and Continental psychoanalysts.

The purpose of the New Library of Psychoanalysis is to facilitate a greater and more widespread appreciation of psychoanalysis and to provide a forum for increasing mutual understanding between psychoanalysts and those working in other disciplines such as the social sciences, medicine, philosophy, history, linguistics, literature and the arts. It aims to represent different trends both in British psychoanalysis and in psychoanalysis generally. The New Library of Psychoanalysis is well placed to make available to the English-speaking world psychoanalytic writings from other European countries and to increase the interchange of ideas between British and American psychoanalysts.

The Institute, together with the British Psychoanalytical Society, runs a low-fee psychoanalytic clinic, organizes lectures and scientific events concerned with psychoanalysis and publishes the *International Journal of Psychoanalysis*. It also runs the only UK training course in psychoanalysis that leads to membership of the International Psychoanalytical Association – the body which preserves internationally agreed standards of training, of professional entry, and of professional ethics and practice for psychoanalysis as initiated and developed by Sigmund Freud. Distinguished members of the Institute have included Michael Balint, Wilfred Bion, Ronald Fairbairn, Anna Freud, Ernest Jones, Melanie Klein, John Rickman and Donald Winnicott.

Previous General Editors include David Tuckett, Elizabeth Spillius and Susan Budd. Previous and current Members of the Advisory Board include Christopher Bollas, Ronald Britton, Donald Campbell, Stephen Grosz, John Keene, Eglé Laufer, Juliet Mitchell, Michael Parsons, Rosine Jozef Perelberg, David Taylor, Mary Target, Catalina Bronstein, Sara Flanders and Richard Rusbridger.

ALSO IN THIS SERIES

Impasse and Interpretation Herbert Rosenfeld
Psychoanalysis and Discourse Patrick Mahony
The Suppressed Madness of Sane Men Marion Milner
The Riddle of Freud Estelle Roith
Thinking, Feeling, and Being Ignacio Matte-Blanco
The Theatre of the Dream Salomon Resnik
Melanie Klein Today: Volume 1, Mainly Theory Edited by Elizabeth Bott Spillius
Melanie Klein Today: Volume 2, Mainly Practice Edited by Elizabeth Bott Spillius
Psychic Equilibrium and Psychic Change: Selected Papers of Betty Joseph Edited by
    Michael Feldman and Elizabeth Bott Spillius
About Children and Children-No-Longer: Collected Papers 1942–80 Paula
    Heimann. Edited by Margret Tonnesmann
The Freud–Klein Controversies 1941–45 Edited by Pearl King and Riccardo
    Steiner
Dream, Phantasy and Art Hanna Segal
Psychic Experience and Problems of Technique Harold Stewart
Clinical Lectures on Klein and Bion Edited by Robin Anderson
From Fetus to Child Alessandra Piontelli
A Psychoanalytic Theory of Infantile Experience: Conceptual and Clinical Reflections
    E Gaddini. Edited by Adam Limentani
The Dream Discourse Today Edited and introduced by Sara Flanders
*The Gender Conundrum: Contemporary Psychoanalytic Perspectives on Femininity
    and Masculinity* Edited and introduced by Dana Breen
Psychic Retreats John Steiner
The Taming of Solitude: Separation Anxiety in Psychoanalysis Jean-Michel
    Quinodoz
Unconscious Logic: An Introduction to Matte-Blanco's Bi-logic and Its Uses Eric
    Rayner
Understanding Mental Objects Meir Perlow
Life, Sex and Death: Selected Writings of William Gillespie Edited and introduced
    by Michael Sinason
What Do Psychoanalysts Want? The Problem of Aims in Psychoanalytic Therapy
    Joseph Sandler and Anna Ursula Dreher
Michael Balint: Object Relations, Pure and Applied Harold Stewart
Hope: A Shield in the Economy of Borderline States Anna Potamianou
Psychoanalysis, Literature and War: Papers 1972–1995 Hanna Segal
Emotional Vertigo: Between Anxiety and Pleasure Danielle Quinodoz
Early Freud and Late Freud Ilse Grubrich-Simitis
A History of Child Psychoanalysis Claudine and Pierre Geissmann
Belief and Imagination: Explorations in Psychoanalysis Ronald Britton

THE NEW LIBRARY OF PSYCHOANALYSIS

General Editor: Dana Birksted–Breen

The Quiet Revolution in American Psychoanalysis

Selected Papers of Arnold M. Cooper

Arnold M. Cooper

Edited and introduced by
Elizabeth L. Auchincloss

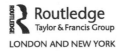

Routledge
Taylor & Francis Group

LONDON AND NEW YORK

First published 2005
by Brunner-Routledge

This edition published by Routledge 2013
27 Church Road, Hove, East Sussex BN3 2FA

Simultaneously published in the USA and Canada
by Routledge
711 Third Avenue, New York NY 10017

Routledge is an imprint of the Taylor & Francis Group

Typeset in Bembo by Keystroke, Jacaranda Lodge, Wolverhampton
Paperback cover design by Sandra Heath

British Library Cataloguing in Publication Data
A catalogue record for this book is available from the British Library

Library of Congress Cataloging-in-Publication Data
Cooper, Arnold M.
The quiet revolution in American psychoanalysis : selected papers of Arnold M. Cooper /
Arnold M. Cooper; introduced and edited by Elizabeth L. Auchincloss.
p. cm. – (The new library of psychoanalysis)
Includes bibliographical references and index.
ISBN 1-58391-891-4 (hardback : alk. paper) – ISBN 1-58391-892-2 (pbk. : alk. paper)
1. Psychoanalysis. 2. Psychotherapy. I. Auchincloss, Elizabeth L., 1951– II. Title.
III. Series: New library of psychoanalysis (Unnumbered)

RC501.2.C66 2004
616.89′17′0973–dc22   2004009620

ISBN 978-1-58391-891-3 (hbk)
ISBN 978-1-58391-892-2 (pbk)

CONTENTS

Contents

FOREWORD

This book owes its existence to two people: Elizabeth Bott Spillius and Elizabeth Auchincloss. More than a dozen years ago, out of the blue, I received from Dr Spillius a detailed summary and brilliant critique of my then extant writings and the suggestion that they be compiled into a volume for publication. I had never had such a thought, although I probably did have such dreams. I responded with my usual reaction – feeling enormously flattered, feeling it didn't apply to me, and putting aside the whole idea. Liz Spillius was persistent and eventually I began to consider the possibility seriously. Succeeding editors Susan Budd and Dana Birksted-Breen at the New Library of Psychoanalysis continued to show interest in my work and eventually I thought I should take myself seriously.

Betsy Auchincloss has given me more of her time and intelligence than any human being deserves to receive of another and it is her devotion to the project that has finally created this book in spite of my dilatoriness, vagueness, self-doubts and hesitation. My publication doubts, fears and reluctance have been longstanding and many of the chapters of this book originally appeared as requested talks for symposia and were written to order, providing me the opportunity to express deeply held views which I might not otherwise have written down.

The encouragement of dear friends, most importantly the late Joseph Sandler, has been critical in my being able to commit any of my ideas to paper. This book also would not exist without the dedicated help of my wife Katherine Addleman and my extraordinarily able and cheerful assistants, Linda Pilgrim and Emily Tucker as well as Anna Weiss and Judy Mars. Dana Birksted-Breen and dedicated anonymous readers at the New American Library provided invaluable editorial advice.

I also wish to express a debt of gratitude to my many colleagues at Columbia Psychoanalytic Center, the Payne-Whitney Clinic, the American Psychoanalytic

Association, the International Psychoanalytic Association, and the *International Journal of Psychoanalysis*, who have nurtured and encouraged me throughout my career.

Arnold M. Cooper, MD
October 3, 2003

INTRODUCTION

The aim of this book is to bring together for the first time in one volume selected papers by one of the leading intellectual figures in the field of psychoanalysis in the last quarter of the twentieth century, Arnold M. Cooper. Cooper has addressed every aspect of American psychoanalytic life including theory, clinical work, education, research, the relationship between psychoanalysis and neighboring disciplines, and the institutional life of the profession. It is my hope that all readers, young and old, familiar and unfamiliar with Cooper's work, will find in this collection a thoughtful chronicle of where psychoanalysis has been as well as an inspiring vision of where it might be heading.

In his 1986 paper, 'Psychoanalysis Today: New Wine in Old Bottles or The Hidden Revolution in Psychoanalysis,' presented as the Distinguished Psychiatrist Lecture of the American Psychiatric Association, Cooper suggested that in the half century following the death of Freud there had been 'quiet, largely unadvertised revolution in the way psychoanalysis is conceived.' This revolution, he argued in the mid-1980s, was still only partly acknowledged in the 'ordinary discourse of psychoanalysis.' In his view, evidence of revolutionary change could be found in every aspect of the psychoanalytic enterprise including our understanding of psychoanalysis as a science, our theories about mental life, our conduct in the treatment setting, and our organizational politics (Cooper 1986i).* While in many ways American psychoanalysis was a field mired in complacent adherence to a 'party line' handed down by self-appointed heirs to the father, it was quietly, without an open challenge to authority, being reinvigorated through critical review of its basic assumptions, reconsideration of the factors at work in psychoanalytic treatment, and, above all, greater tolerance of multiple and competing points of view.

---

* Cited publications of which Cooper was author or coauthor are listed in the Bibliography; other publications are listed in the References.

Throughout his professional life, the process of change has fascinated Cooper. His own contributions to psychoanalytic clinical theory have changed our understanding of work with patients to include a greater appreciation of narcissistic and pre-Oedipal themes in development and of the human encounter embedded in the psychoanalytic situation. His progressive leadership in our educational and professional organizations has done much to promote change toward greater self-examination and tolerance of new ideas, and, indeed, to create the conditions that make change possible. Above all, his unique ability to observe and reflect upon the process of change, recorded here in papers selected from over 150 written in the 50-plus years between 1947 and 2002, has helped make Cooper the guide to whom the profession has repeatedly turned to understand not only where, but even what, psychoanalysis is.

Arnold Michael Cooper was born on March 9, 1923, in Brooklyn, New York. His father, Morris Cooper (né Coopervogh), and his mother, Clara Aronow, met on Manhattan's Lower East Side; they had been born in villages within 50 miles of each other in Russian-ruled Ukraine. Arnold was the second of four sons.

When Cooper was less than one year old, his father quit his job as a cutter in a textile factory and moved the family to New Jersey, where he ran a grocery store in Jersey City and later a shirt factory in Elizabeth. The family settled for good in Roselle, New Jersey. This town was important in helping to shape Cooper's attitudes toward divisions and injustices that later carried into his professional and political life.

In 1930, Roselle, New Jersey was a small semi-rural pre-Revolutionary War town, with a population of fewer than 4,000. The town was sharply divided into a white, upper middle-class section of beautiful old houses with carefully tended gardens, and a mostly black, extremely poor area with a few immigrant Poles and Italians. The black population had been lured North during World War I as labor for a munitions factory in Elizabeth and now served as the house-maids, gardeners, etc. for the middle-class whites. Cooper recalls that his family was one of only two Jewish families in town. The sense of extreme distance between 'ins' and 'outs' was vivid in Roselle, providing a kind of sociology lesson made more meaningful by young Cooper's uncertainty as to where exactly he fit in. As a middle-class white boy, he belonged on one side of the fence; as a Jew, he was excluded like the blacks. His confusion was made more profound by his father's deep ambivalence toward their religion.

Morris Cooper was a talented and imaginative businessman who rapidly went on to build an extremely successful shirt-manufacturing business (later in partnership with his oldest son, Donald). As the shirt business prospered, Morris supported his own extended immigrant family as well as that of his wife. Later, in the mid-1950s, he started to buy orange groves and ranch land in Florida, and in 1959, having retired from the shirt business, he founded the municipal corporation of Cooper City, Florida, near Fort Lauderdale. While Cooper City is now a thriving community, its development proved to be an economic disaster for the Cooper family as Morris wiped out the family fortune shortly before his death, paying off creditors to keep Cooper City alive.

By all accounts, Morris Cooper, though physically diminutive, was a larger-than-life figure given to unpredictable rages that terrorized his wife and children, as well as to effusive affection, often directed at his favorite son, Arnold. If these contradictory moods were hard for his son to understand, so was the choice of Roselle, New Jersey, as a place to make a home. It was difficult for Arnold to reconcile his father's wish to raise his children in a non-Jewish community with his demand that the family keep up strict religious observance, a demand that caused his children considerable distress in their school and social lives. It gradually became apparent to Cooper that while the family maintained ultra-orthodox religious practice in accord with the wishes of his maternal grandparents, his father was rather anti-Semitic and quite ashamed of his Jewishness. Shortly after Arnold's Bar Mitzvah, Morris Cooper announced that the family was leaving the poor orthodox synagogue to which they walked every Friday evening and Saturday morning, to join a new, more elegant reform temple in Elizabeth. Suddenly, it was all right to drive on the Sabbath. In response to this decision, and in keeping with a growing skepticism toward religion in any form, the 13-year-old Arnold immediately and permanently abandoned all religious observance.

While it is not hard to picture a young Arnold Cooper thriving in a struggle to make sense of his father's contradictory attitudes toward religion, it is harder to imagine him surviving a childhood that he describes as profoundly non-intellectual. In the absence of books or any exchange of ideas, Cooper immersed himself in playing the clarinet, sometimes up to four or five hours a day. He led the school marching and concert bands and later played first chair in the New Jersey All-State Orchestra. Weekend visits with his charismatic maternal Uncle Sut (Edward I. Aronow), who took young Cooper with him to explore New York City and the bohemian life of Greenwich Village, provided the first hints of a larger, more interesting world.

Cooper followed his older brother, Donald, to Columbia University where he began undergraduate study in 1940, partly supported by a music scholarship. Columbia University changed his life. While describing himself as too shy to talk to the professors, Cooper quickly found new friends among the native New York City boys, many of whom became lifelong friends. For the first time, Cooper began to feel that being Jewish need not mean being an outsider. He also began to feel that reading books and thinking seriously about ideas need not be 'sequestered activities engaged in by the odd few.' 'It had a profound effect on me,' he reflected later, 'that these guys were interested in literature, jazz, art, philosophy, sports *and* having a good time. It was the first sense I had of how many kinds of things there are in the world to be interested in' (Cooper 2002, in conversation with author). Being in college during wartime meant that

3

everyone was also interested in politics. A deepening friendship with his Uncle Sut, who among other things was the personal attorney for Earl Browder, the head of the American Communist Party, brought Cooper into even more conflict with his father, whose politics ran sharply towards the right. The experience of negotiating divided family loyalties in which emotional ties are complicated by ideology would resonate with later challenges. In the midst of it all, a friend suggested that Cooper read Freud.

Writing later about this first reading, Cooper wrote, 'I experienced a sense of instant revelation into myself and my adolescent miseries, into my friends, and into my world of politics and literature . . . Things seemed clearer than they ever had before' (Cooper 1998c). Abandoning half-formed plans to become an English teacher or to go to law school, Cooper decided to go to medical school with the goal of becoming a psychoanalyst. After graduating from Columbia in 1943 and spending seven months in the Army Special Training Program that sent young men to medical school, he began study at the University of Utah School of Medicine.

In the early 1940s, the School of Medicine at the University of Utah was a new four-year medical school with no department of psychiatry! While this might have seemed like an unlikely place for a future psychoanalyst to find himself, this young, relatively small school with the feel of the frontier provided Cooper with new opportunities both for independence and for collaboration with faculty, many of whom were only recently recruited from the East. They included Louis Goodman, chairman of pharmacology and physiology, and the hematologist, Maxwell Wintrobe, who was chairman of the Department of Medicine. Cooper immersed himself in the study of physiology under the direction of Mark Nickerson, publishing his first paper on the 'Effect of anti-reticular cytotoxic serum (ACS) on the healing of experimental wounds in rats' (Nickerson *et al*. 1946).

After receiving his MD in 1947, still focused on physiology and less sure of his earlier choice to become a psychiatrist, Cooper continued his training as a research fellow at Harvard University, studying liver physiology under the supervision of Charles Davidson at the Thorndike Memorial Laboratory at Boston City Hospital. Cooper published four papers with Davidson's group on Wilson's disease, amino acid metabolism, and the treatment of cirrhosis of the liver (Eckhardt *et al*. 1948; Faloon *et al*. 1949a, 1949b; Cooper *et al*. 1950). 'I was interested in amino acid metabolites that I thought might affect the sensorium in Wilson's disease,' Cooper said, looking back. 'Of course I was wrong; we knew nothing yet about the role of copper. However, my experience in the laboratory was terrific preparation for clinical training' (Cooper 2002, in conversation with author). Between 1948 and 1950, Cooper did a two-year internship in Internal Medicine at the Columbia-Presbyterian Hospital in New York City. In 1950, returning to his original interest in the mind, he began three years of psychiatric residency training at Bellevue Hospital in New York City.

His third year of residency training was spent as night admissions physician at Bellevue.

In 1952, Cooper began psychoanalytic training at the Columbia University Center for Psychoanalytic Training and Research, from which he graduated in 1956. Since 1954, he has maintained a private practice as a psychiatrist and psychoanalyst in New York City, while developing an academic career. By 1971, he had advanced to the position of Clinical Professor of Psychiatry at Columbia College of Physicians and Surgeons, and Adjunct Professor of English in Columbia College where he originated and ran The Program for Psychoanalytic Studies for undergraduates. In 1974, he joined the full-time faculty of Cornell Medical College as Professor and Associate Chairman for Education. In 1992, he became the Stephen P. Tobin and Dr Arnold M. Cooper Emeritus Professor in Consultation–Liaison Psychiatry at the Joan and Sanford I. Weill Medical College of Cornell University. This chair was endowed by the father of an adolescent boy who died of a malignant melanoma while in analysis with Cooper. The professorship was created by the boy's father to honor the relationship of the young patient and his doctor.

Cooper returned to New York City in 1948 in time to enjoy the post-war explosion in the cultural life of the city. New friends included poets, painters, musicians, and scientists in addition to many future psychoanalysts. In contrast to the upheavals going on in the arts, however, American psychoanalysis in the 1950s was characterized by its growing rigidity. The most powerful psychoanalytic institutions were controlled by an autocratic elite that sought to perpetuate itself by encouraging orthodoxy rather than creativity and by punishing 'dissident' thinkers. The 'official' position of psychoanalysis in America during the 1950s included a version of scientific/psychoanalytic positivism which asserted that psychoanalysis was the basis for a 'general psychology' and that the psychoanalytic situation alone provided sufficient scientific proof to establish the validity of its theory. Theories of the mind had become codified in the scientistic vocabulary of American ego-psychology, which spoke with confidence about distributions of drive energy and the nature of instinct. Theories of technique had become codified in a mechanistic vocabulary that described analysis as consisting of a single technique characterized by interpretation of clearly definable resistances and transference 'distortions.' While revolutionary forces were at work, they were operating behind the scenes.

Cooper quickly established a reputation as an outstanding clinician from whom other clinicians sought consultation for their own work and help for their friends, family, and often themselves. Immersion in clinical practice formed the basis from which all his other professional and academic activities emerged and to which he demanded that all other activities ultimately contribute. Simultaneously, and in line with his undergraduate realization of 'how many things there are in the world to be interested in,' Cooper's involvement in non-clinical activities has been intense. Throughout his professional life, his career has been characterized by immersion in scholarship, education, and organizational work and by a demand that all aspects of professional life support the pursuit of new knowledge. He also led a diverse intellectual life outside of his work, which included passionate engagement in literature and the arts, and playing the clarinet in a variety of groups. Cooper's wide range of interests supported his demand that psychoanalysis maintain strong connections with the larger world of ideas.

Against this background, Cooper's career as a psychoanalyst was shaped by his lifelong involvement with his home base, the Columbia University Center for Psychoanalytic Training and Research. The Columbia Center was founded in 1942 when the maverick Hungarian psychoanalyst, Sandor Rado, led a splinter group away from the New York Psychoanalytic Institute with a mission that included the reform of psychoanalytic theory, the forging of closer ties to the university, and the development of psychoanalytic research. All aspects of the original Columbia mandate had a profound effect on the development of Cooper's career. In his written reflections on 'The impact on clinical work of the analyst's idealizations and identifications' (Cooper 1998c), published as the first paper in this collection, Cooper discusses the emotional and intellectual influence of his attachment to Columbia and its founders (including Abram Kardiner, George Daniels, Aaron Karush, David Levy and Lionel Ovesey), who were on the one hand revolutionary from the point of view of mainstream American psychoanalysis, and on the other hand intensely autocratic in their own right. Training in psychoanalysis at Columbia created unresolvable tensions around questions that lie at the heart of Cooper's work, such as the scientific status and the language of psychoanalysis, the role of research in psychoanalytic inquiry, the proper setting for psychoanalytic education, orthodoxy versus heresy and nihilism, and the implications of 'insider' versus 'outsider' status in professional organizations.

From the outset, Cooper involved himself in the efforts of the Columbia faculty 'to restore psychoanalysis to the more important findings of Freud concerning the core of psychic life' (Cooper 1998c). The goal was to delineate essential psychoanalytic concepts in a language free from the mechanistic, pseudo-scientific, and clinically irrelevant superstructure of classical Freudian metapsychology as codified in American ego-psychology. His first psychoanalytic publications (Karush *et al*. 1964; Cooper *et al*. 1966) described his efforts with Aaron Karush, Ruth Easser and Bluma Swerdloff to develop the Adaptive Balance Profile, an instrument designed to standardize the information gathered in initial interviews of patients with the aims of both clarifying concepts and conducting research in psychoanalytic process and outcome. While the project ultimately collapsed as the questions raised by the investigators outstripped the research methods and funding available to them, it was evidence of the lasting impact of Cooper's early research training and it marked the beginning of his lifelong commitment to the idea that psychoanalysis can progress only if it includes systematic study of its theory and technique. Later, during the 1980s and 1990s,

Cooper conducted research with Barbara Milrod, Fred Busch and Theodore Shapiro on the study of psychodynamic psychotherapy in patients with panic disorder, which resulted in the publication of one of the first ever manuals of psychoanalytic psychotherapy suitable for research (Milrod *et al.* 1997).

Shortly after completing psychoanalytic training, Cooper joined the faculty of the Columbia Center where he has taught and supervised continuously since 1956. His first teaching assignment was to design a seminar on the work of psychoanalytic 'dissidents' who, at the time, included Jung, Horney, Adler, Reich, Klein, Sullivan, and others. His initial reading of these authors evoked an airy dismissal of their ideas, but as Cooper studied them more seriously, he began to take an interest in ideas that did not appear in the versions of psychoanalysis with which he was familiar – neither the prevailing orthodox analysis of ego-psychology nor the 'adaptational analysis' of Columbia's founding group. Preparation for the course on dissidents ignited his longstanding interest in the boundaries as well as the politics of psychoanalytic theory-making. Cooper became a training analyst at Columbia in 1961. From 1970 to 1977, he was Chairman of the Curriculum Committee. The Cooper curriculum, as it was called, was organized around a set of core psychoanalytic concepts presented from the point of view of a contemporary critique. Reading of 'the dissidents' was encouraged; unthinking adherence to the canon was not.

Early in his psychoanalytic career, Cooper became interested in the work of Edmund Bergler, a brilliant intellectual figure whose abrasive personality and originality led to his being largely banished from official analytic publications. In Cooper's opinion, Bergler's emphases on pre-Oedipal development, the importance of narcissism in individual development, the role of the superego, and the broad use of various masochistic defenses, were significant precursors of Kohut, Kernberg, and other innovative psychoanalysts. Cooper's own development of these themes is a significant part of his work. His papers on the varieties of narcissistic–masochistic character and their many clinical presentations have had a major influence on young analysts.

Beginning immediately upon graduation from Columbia Psychoanalytic, his commitment to teaching and his concern with issues related to education have marked every aspect of Cooper's career. Cooper is known as a brilliant classroom teacher as well as a gifted supervisor. In the course of his long and varied career as an educator, his students have included undergraduates, graduate students, medical students, psychiatry residents, students of psychology and psychoanalytic candidates, among others. He has been invited to serve as a visiting professor or educational consultant to many universities and psychoanalytic institutes and has won many awards for teaching. Cooper's influence on his many individual students as well as on the institutions where he worked and over which he presided will be a huge part of his legacy. In one of his earliest papers on the subject, 'Some suggestions for the education of psychoanalysts' (Cooper 1983c), he stressed the point that psychoanalytic education has placed too much emphasis on training and not enough on education. This theme has dominated his thinking on the subject, as he has repeatedly stressed the importance of educating psychoanalysts capable of independent thinking, critical analysis, and the generation of new knowledge. Cooper has vigorously advocated a university model of psychoanalytic education where interdisciplinary study and opportunities for research are offered in addition to traditional training in clinical psychoanalysis (Cooper 1999).

The founders of the Columbia Center imagined that psychoanalysis would be enriched through maintaining ties with the university; Cooper has spent much of his professional life working to strengthen those ties. In 1957 he was invited to give a set of lectures entitled 'Twenty Years after Freud' as part of the prestigious Columbia University Lectures series. Having been planned for an auditorium that could seat 40 people, the lectures had to be moved to accommodate hundreds of students. In the 1960s, with the backing of Columbia professor and literary critic Lionel Trilling, Cooper founded the Program in Psychoanalytic Studies at Columbia University and later, with Columbia Professor of English Literature, Steven Marcus, the Seminar on Psychoanalytic Thought at Columbia University. The Columbia college program, one of the first such university-based programs in the world, was the spawning ground for many future psychoanalysts. From 1984 to 1994, Cooper chaired the Committee on University and Medical Education of the American Psychoanalytic Association, a committee he had formed when he was president to explore ways to deepen ties between psychoanalysis and the broader academic world. His own enduring interest in art, music, and literature added depth to his belief that psychoanalysis and the humanities have much to learn from each other. Throughout the 1980s and the 1990s, Cooper continued to co-teach a graduate seminar at Columbia on Psychoanalysis and Literature with Marcus. Over the years, he offered versions of this seminar to medical students, psychiatry residents, and psychoanalytic candidates. He has also worked continuously to find ways to offer in-depth psychoanalytic education to non-clinicians interested in applying psychoanalytic concepts to other disciplines.

Cooper has always believed in the special importance of the ties between psychoanalysis and psychiatry. While immersing himself in psychoanalysis, he never lost contact with the psychiatric world. His first jobs after residency had included serving as Assistant Attending on the inpatient Female Adolescent Service at Bellevue Hospital and director of the Vanderbilt Clinic Community Service at Columbia-Presbyterian Hospital. In 1974 he was appointed Professor of Psychiatry, Associate Chairman for Medical Education and Director of Residency Training at the New York Hospital–Payne Whitney Clinic of Cornell University Medical Center – a full-time academic position. The Cornell Department of Psychiatry in the late 1970s was undergoing a major renaissance under the Chairmanship of Robert Michels. Cooper's leadership in education from 1974 to 1988 established the Cornell program as one of the most prestigious centers for psychiatric residency training in the United States. Cooper demanded that his residents strive for the highest level of excellence in both brain-based and psychoanalytically oriented psychiatry, establishing Cornell as a center for balanced clinical training in an era of increasing biological reductionism in psychiatry. He also demanded that his residents develop their potential for scholarship, research, teaching, and leadership.

During the 1970s, American psychiatry underwent a complete revision of its nosological system sparked by the rise in biological psychiatry and the need of a growing research community for clearly defined diagnostic categories. This revision culminated in 1980 with the publication of the 3rd edition of the *Diagnostic and Statistical Manual of Mental Disorders* (DSM-III) by the American Psychiatric Association. The strategy behind the DSM-III was to use only observable phenomena in the construction of diagnostic categories with the aim of improved reliability necessary for research. In its effort to be 'theory-neutral,' the DSM-III specifically eliminated all psychoanalytic concepts (such as neurosis or conflict) from the new diagnostic system. From the vantage point of his position as an educator in psychiatry and a member of the DSM-III Ad Hoc Advisory Committee of the American Psychiatric Association as well as the Ad Hoc Committee on DSM-IV of the American Psychoanalytic Association, Cooper was in an ideal position to introduce psychoanalysts to the newly revised psychiatric nosology as well as to represent psychodynamic principles in the ongoing work of revision (Frances and Cooper 1980, 1981; Koenigsberg *et al.* 1985) As a preeminent psychoanalyst in the world of psychiatry during the explosion of brain science beginning in the 1970s, Cooper was led repeatedly to consider areas of overlapping interest such as the influence of neurobiology on psychoanalysis, the theoretical and clinical issues raised by combined medication and psychoanalytic therapies, and the question of how to integrate psychoanalytic and brain-based perspectives on such clinical phenomena as panic disorder (Shear *et al.* 1994; Busch *et al.* 1995; Milrod *et al.* 1997). In 1988 he served as President of the New York County District Branch of the American Psychiatric Association, and in 1992 he was appointed one of two Deputy Editors of the *American Journal of Psychiatry*, serving until 2003.

As Cooper became more involved in academic psychiatry, he also become more active in organized psychoanalysis. In 1974, he became the first psychoanalyst from Columbia to hold a major position at the American Psychoanalytic Association when he was appointed Chairman of the Program Committee. Cooper had had little involvement in the administrative workings of the 'American' prior to his chairmanship of the Program Committee – an appointment made by George Pollock, then President, in response to a challenge to end the freeze-out of Columbia graduates from significant positions in the organization. Between 1974 and 1978, he instituted changes in the national meetings which challenged the traditional boundaries of the organization. These changes included seminars on non-psychoanalytic research topics of interest to

Parts III and IV focus more on clinical aspects of psychoanalysis. Part III, 'Vicissitudes of narcissism,' includes five papers which explore a variety of clinical syndromes in relation to the problems of narcissism. Some of these papers present Cooper's view of what he calls the 'narcissistic–masochistic character,' described by him for the first time. Others offer a fresh look at syndromes with a long history in the psychoanalytic literature. Part IV, 'The analyst at work,' presents Cooper's views of changing theory and technique in psychoanalytic practice. Detailed case presentations provide a window into the clinical world and a glimpse of how 'the quiet revolution' has affected the patient–analyst pair at work.

Elizabeth L. Auchincloss
September 9, 2003

1

THE IMPACT ON CLINICAL WORK OF THE ANALYST'S IDEALIZATIONS AND IDENTIFICATIONS*

Psychoanalysis has been a profession in which overt idealization and identification have perhaps been more prominent and problematic than in any other profession. I thought that it might be of some interest in our time of theoretical plurality and, I hope, creative uncertainty, to give some account of my struggles to achieve some peace of mind as a working psychoanalyst. I never had difficulty over the question of whether I was a psychoanalyst, because if I wasn't an analyst then I wasn't anything, but I have had tremendous problems over whether I was the right kind of psychoanalyst or a good enough psychoanalyst.

It will help to give some background of my analytic education. It began when I was a student at Columbia University and someone suggested I should read Freud. I dutifully read through the then available Brill translation. Like so many others of my generation, I experienced a sense of instant revelation into myself and my adolescent miseries, into my friends, and into my world of politics and literature. This was a new way of seeing and understanding, an affirmation of my previously unvoiced conviction that more was going on than I was privy to, a primal scene fantasy, if you wish. Things seemed clearer than they ever had before. I asked a friend of mine what one had to do to become a psychoanalyst and he said you have to go to medical school. I had never thought of going to medical school. At times I had thought of law, sociology, or English literature, but I had no clear direction. With some difficulty I managed to go to medical school after the Army, thinking this would be the start of my analytic career, but it so happened that the medical school I went to had no department of psychiatry at that time. This turned out be something of a blessing, because I became

* This paper was presented as part of a panel with the same title at the 87th Annual Meeting of the American Psychoanalytic Association in Toronto, Canada in 1998.

involved in physiology and did a research fellowship before my internship. My ideals and convictions about the merits of empirical research crystallized at that time, and have been a core of my psychoanalytic being, as I never gave up on the idea that psychoanalysis could contain a truly scientific vision without sacrificing any of its humanist core.

My first attempt at analysis began shortly after graduation from medical school while I was doing a research fellowship in Boston. I knew I needed an analysis for personal reasons, and although psychoanalysis still fascinated me, I was uncertain that anyone as neurotic as I felt myself to be could help other people. I thought I would probably pursue a career in clinical research, which I enjoyed and seemed pretty good at, rather than risk an analytic career. I had no money or connections but eventually was directed to a recent graduate of the Boston Institute who was being supervised by Beatta Rank and he wanted a fourth supervised case. I was in analysis with him for eight months before moving to begin my internship in New York City. The experience was extraordinarily painful. Each session was excruciating. I found myself tongue-tied and he was entirely silent. I had read just enough to convince myself that this was how analysis had to be, and any lack of progress merely proved the depth of my pathology – a secret I already knew. The discomfort was compounded by my doing this analysis secretly – I didn't dare tell the directors of the Thorndike Lab that I was in analysis, convinced that they would throw me out. To this day I am not sure whether that was a paranoid fantasy, or sound realistic judgment. In later years I came to know my first analyst in the American Psychoanalytic Association and discovered that he was a nice, friendly person, rather rigidly bound to an orthodox view of analytic technique. During one meeting he came over to me to report that he had just successfully analyzed a schizophrenic patient 'using no parameters.' I was mildly stunned by his pride in such an unlikely venture but I better understood my first attempt at analysis. Almost two years after my first analytic effort, during a medical residency, again for personal reasons, I began another analysis, again without informing my medical chief; I began this time with a rather eminent New York analyst who had himself been a patient of Freud's. To my astonishment this man was responsive and talkative and I began to feel a new confidence blossoming in me. When I complained to my second analyst that he lacked the austerity of my first analyst, and that perhaps this was not authentic analysis, he told me of an incident that occurred during his analysis with Freud. During one session as he lay on the couch, he began to boast about his uncanny capacity to guess people's ages. Freud found this interesting, whereupon he rose from his chair, left the office to go into the family rooms and returned with the family photograph album. He sat down on the couch next to his analysand and began pointing to various photographs of his relatives in the album, asking 'How old is this one? How old is that one?' Clearly, Freud's curiosity took precedence over any rules of technique. I began to have some idea that perhaps psychoanalysis consisted of more than abstinence.

After three years in medicine I decided that my initial instinct was correct and I took a psych residency and applied to analytic school. I was accepted at both the New York and Columbia institutes, and was told that Columbia would accept my ongoing analysis as a training analysis, while New York told me I would have to begin again with a different training analyst. It tells you something of my state of mind that I made no attempt to investigate what the differences were between the institutes. I was aware that my interviewers at Columbia seemed interested in the fact that I had done physiology research and had published some papers, while my New York interviewers never broached the topic. I didn't know analysts or analytic candidates, except for one friend who was a candidate at New York, who told me they were all the same and I might as well go where I didn't have to start a new analysis. I took his advice. I had no idea that Columbia was considered somewhat renegade, tainted by culturalism, and lacking real analytic vigor, and that, in fact, Columbia was on a campaign to abolish the metapsychology that was dominant at the time.

I went through a period of great uncertainty during my years as a candidate at Columbia and for long afterwards. My first reaction to the teachings of Rado, Kardiner, Ovesey, and others at Columbia had been rather contemptuous, believing, since I had no difficulty understanding what they were saying, that they must be simplistic. That couldn't be psychoanalysis. Rado's use of everyday language in psychoanalysis was distressing to me. Words such as pride, hope, welfare emotions, and self-assertion (rather than aggression) led me to think I was back in literature or sociology rather than in the science of psychoanalysis. Although it made sense to me, how could family and couples therapy be a part of an analytic curriculum since 'real' analysts didn't do that? In contrast, the language of ego psychology held a fascination for me because it seemed as if it might be science, I found it difficult to understand, and it seemed to be the way all psychoanalysts spoke – except for those relative outsiders in my institute. At the same time libido economics seemed clearly a dead end and the language of instinct theory seemed hopelessly outdated biologically. I reflected the uncertainty of my entire institute as we wavered between trying to enjoy the comfort of being part of the mainstream as it was reflected in the American Psychoanalytic Association, or sustaining our courage to continue the battle that Rado, Kardiner, Daniels, Karush, and Ovesey had begun. In their view, they were fighting to restore psychoanalysis to the more important findings of Freud concerning the core of psychic life in the struggle to find an emotionally accept-able adaptation to inner conflicts within the constraints of biology, culture, and the experience of care-taking persons. Moreover, the interest of Columbia's founders tended to be more in present functioning than in the infantile past. For many years, I vacillated between feeling that I was not a real analyst because I could not comfortably adapt to mainstream ego psychology, and rather angrily feeling that the excitement of psychoanalysis was being strangled by the hold of the so-called classical analysts.

15

to me, it was also the beginning of my reeducation in learning anew to listen closely and carefully and collaboratively to my patients, it was an early lesson in the limits of analytic authority, and the real awakening of an intersubjectivist view of my work with my patients. My positivism died an early and painful death and another phase of my analytic career began, with a continuing appreciation for the importance of pre-Oedipal events but with a renewed openness to the vicissitudes and complexities of early experience and later development, and a new sense of the possible powers, abuses and limitations of analytic theory and knowledge.

Rather early in my career I had what was for me a highly traumatic experience. At the first regional meeting of the psychoanalytic societies of the New York area, I presented my first paper on the narcissistic–masochistic character, one of the first papers I ever gave in public. I was enjoying the friendly and ecumenical atmosphere of the vacation spot where the meeting was being held, and I was flattered that a number of the elder and revered New York analysts were welcoming and warm. In my paper I suggested that the core pathology in the patients I was describing was pre-Oedipal in origin and I was at some pains to indicate that this contradicted what Freud had referred to earlier in his writings as a shibboleth of psychoanalysis: that the Oedipus complex is the nucleus of neurosis. I was horrified and terrified when my discussant from the New York Psychoanalytic Institute, one of those revered elders, angrily and, I thought, viciously attacked me. I was accused of being totally anti-psychoanalytic and charged with accusing Freud of being unscientific since the word 'shibboleth' was not in the vocabulary of science. My discussant seemed unaware that the word 'shibboleth' was a quote from Freud himself. Although I was intellectually on solid ground, the personal effect on me was devastating. It was years before I attempted to write up any of this material or to present it again.

I think such an event can no longer occur in the analytic community. We are much more alert to the need to develop creative young colleagues and we no longer have an investment in the preservation of every thought of Freud's (or indeed of 'sanitizing' his thought). The positive side of the experience, however, was that it did lead me to think very carefully about the sociology of psychoanalysis and the power of group processes. I emerged with a slightly thicker hide – a requirement for anyone who wishes to engage in scientific discourse.

For by now obvious reasons, the issue of analytic identity has long been both puzzling and interesting to me. It seems to me a uniquely psychoanalytic issue, a guild issue rather than a genuinely professional one. I know of no other specialty in which one's professional identity is such a perplexing ongoing question. At the same time, it was many years before I developed real comfort with the idea that I was a psychoanalyst by any serious definition, even if I differed with the mainstream. It was of enormous importance that throughout my career I was a teacher as well as a practitioner. Teaching kept me on my toes, forced me to read the literature more diligently than I might have otherwise, and constantly confronted me with the deep and unanswerable questions that only naive students could ask. I also loved supervision – at both ends – and it did seem to me that I was able to help others see unconscious processes in their patients and that my students and I learned new things together.

Fascinated as I was with psychoanalysis, I always enjoyed psychotherapy, again something that at that time made me feel different from other analysts, and my practice always contained a fair number of psychotherapy patients. This, too, no doubt represents the workings of old idealizations. When I was a candidate, we all took psychotherapy cases from the clinic, supervised by the analytic faculty, before starting our first analytic care: a practice that has been discontinued. Those supervised psychotherapy cases were hugely important, indelible experiences for me. I have written elsewhere of my own lack of conviction concerning the clear boundary between these two modes of treatment. I had the not infrequent experience that some of my sitting-up so-called psychotherapy patients were experiencing an analytic process (however that is defined), and that some of my lying-down five-times-a-week psychoanalytic patients were at best having a psychotherapy, perhaps a less effective one than they would have had had I labeled their treatment psychotherapy.

In effect, I have throughout my psychoanalytic career rarely enjoyed the experience of feeling that I really knew how to do it right. My idealizations and identifications, while powerfully sustaining, were always also subject to great ambivalence, a trait that my analyses did not abolish. My early personal uncertainties concerning my analytic abilities were compounded by the sense that I was trained at a renegade institute, that I had attached myself to a theoretician who was in general disfavor, and that I rather masochistically enjoyed the notion of myself as an iconoclast. Of course in more recent years I became aware of the irony that I had become at least a partial member of the inner circle; a position, I confess, that I have hugely enjoyed. I also confess that I have experienced a certain amount of *schadenfreude* as I watched analysts previously contemptuous of anything other than strict ego psychological technique leap to join the bandwagon of newer ideas, describing that, of course, they too had always been warm, responsive, surely not authoritarian and eagerly open to the interplay of subjectivities. Perhaps that was, in fact, the case. The openness of the current era of theoretical plurality has for me been a godsend. At least some of my discomforts and uncertainties can now be acknowledged as themselves part of the analytic process, something I share with all analysts, an important aspect of authentic work with my patients and not solely a source of private discomfort. I think that most of my generation, at one level or another, has always known that the theory of technique was badly flawed and incomplete; with each new development we hoped we had now arrived at a method in which we could place greater assurance. While the conflicts I have described had highly individual aspects relating to my particular experience, in fact, to one degree or another, in one way or another, they were quite universal among analysts, and it is nice to know that we are all having a more interesting and more productive time today.

PART I

The quiet revolution

2

PSYCHOANALYTIC INQUIRY
AND NEW KNOWLEDGE*

I believe that this is one of the great periods in psychoanalysis. Our scientific discourse is livelier, more informed, more diverse, and less embittered than at any other time in my memory. We are discussing ideas that not so many years ago would not have been discussed seriously within mainstream psychoanalysis; and we are doing so, and I believe will continue to do so, without further danger of split or fragmentation. I think psychoanalysis in America has reached a point of scientific health and maturity that allows for stress and change without danger and loss of our self-cohesion. We owe much of this present excitement to the work of Dr Kohut and his followers.

The appearance of Heinz Kohut's book *The Analysis of the Self* in 1971 had an electrifying effect on our science and profession. Although there had been harbingers of what was to come in Kohut's work of the preceding decade, the book was greeted with an interest and enthusiasm previously reserved for the works of Anna Freud and Heinz Hartmann. Kohut's work was an instant topic of conversation within analytic circles. Candidates in analytic institutes were enormously excited. Because the work lay outside the curriculum, they pressed their instructors to join in their interest, an invitation that was sometimes accepted reluctantly or even declined. However, unlike the works of Anna Freud or Hartmann, Kohut's book stimulated an immediate controversy in the psychoanalytic literature. Opinions ranged from the enthusiastic belief that Kohut's ideas presented a needed and long-awaited opportunity to revitalize psychoanalysis to a view that echoed Samuel Johnson's criticism: The work is both good and original, but unfortunately what is original in it is not good and what is good is not original.

* A version of this paper was first presented as the keynote address at the grand banquet of the third annual symposium on self psychology sponsored by the Boston Psychoanalytic Institute in 1980, when Cooper was President of the American Psychoanalytic Association. It was later published as Cooper (1983b); reproduced with permission of The Analytic Press.

If we explore the reasons why Kohut's work has excited us, both positively and negatively, it might help us to understand the relationship of theory to the development of knowledge in psychoanalysis. Other theories, some equally sweeping, some not dissimilar in their intent, have been put forth over the years, but none has engaged us as have those of Kohut and his followers. Although this may represent the merit of the work, we know from the history of ideas that merit alone does not automatically lead to interest. *The Interpretation of Dreams* did not become an immediate bestseller.

Our attention to the factors that lead to acceptance and rejection of ideas in psychoanalysis, in particular Heinz Kohut's ideas, may also teach us something about the current state of psychoanalytic theory and technique and its historical development. It may also inform us about some aspects of the present state of psychoanalysis as a 'movement' – an organization of people sharing common goals, who wish to enlarge the acceptance and importance of these goals in our culture. I raise many more questions than I answer, but a consideration of these questions may provide a perspective on what is sure to be a longstanding, ongoing discussion of self psychology, a discussion which is also an opportunity to reexamine ourselves.

One way to view our present interest in the self is to say that it is simply and clearly an idea whose time has come – that the theoretical infrastructure it required was put in place during previous decades. In this view, the psychology of the self would be the capstone of several developmental lines in psychoanalytic theory. I would like briefly to describe some of these. First, one can trace the effort in psychoanalytic theorizing to arrive at propositions or concepts of increasingly comprehensive scope. We can follow the progression from the distinction between conscious and unconscious, through the elaboration of the drives and their vicissitudes, to an increasing focus on the ego and its adaptations, to the conceptualization of the self as a more ultimate organizer of behavior. The common theme in this developmental line is a quest for the unifying conception out of which all the elaborations of psychoanalysis would be secondary and derivative hypotheses. The concept of the self as the ultimate organizer of behavior presumably contains within it all of the concepts that previously were regarded as basic and definitional for psychoanalysis. In fact, I believe Kohut has made this claim, although not without some hesitations and extenuations. It is not entirely clear, therefore, whether Kohut regards the concept of the self as the supraordinate hypothesis from which all other hypotheses and data are derivative, or as one of several equally important concepts, with a principle of complementarity at work to define which concept is most useful for the exploration of which particular situation. Historically, the theories of the self advanced by Mead, Sullivan, Horney, and Rado show important relationships to the work of Kohut.

A second line of development assumes that psychoanalysis has explored the psyche archeologically from the surface down. Having originally discovered the extraordinary world of the Oedipal child, psychoanalysis has continued its laborious digging and has revealed a new civilization underlying the Oedipal that had never been imagined by the original discoverers. Freud used this metaphor in 1931 to describe his response to the finding of the important role of pre-Oedipal life for the development of the female. I think it is fair to say that Freud was both surprised and somewhat dismayed by his discovery. In his paper on 'Female sexuality,' he said:

> Our insight into this early pre-Oedipal phase in girls comes to us as a surprise, like the discovery, in another field, of the Minoan–Mycenean civilizations behind the civilization of Greece.
>
> Everything in the sphere of the first attachment to the mother seemed to me so difficult to grasp in analysis – so grey with age and shadowy and almost impossible to revivify – that it was as if it had succumbed to an especially inexorable repression.
>
> (Freud 1931: 226)

In this paper he also said:

> The pre-Oedipus phase in women gains an importance which we have not attributed to it hitherto . . . Since this phase allows room for all the fixations and repressions from which we must trace the origin of the neuroses, it would seem as though we must retract the universality of the thesis that the Oedipus complex is the nucleus of the neuroses. But if anyone feels reluctant about making this correction, there is no need for him to do so.
>
> (Freud 1931: 226)

Perhaps this is an indication of even Freud's difficulty in accepting the breadth of theoretical revision that data may require at times. He had maintained with consistency that the Oedipus complex was the nucleus of the neurosis, and now he had data suggesting that this idea should be abandoned. Rather than give up his position, he sought a compromise that would allow the old view to stand, although modified by new discoveries. Some would hold that this compromise was inadequate and that one of the tensions in psychoanalytic thinking during the past five decades has resulted from the extraordinary unfolding of our knowledge of earlier and earlier psychologically significant events in the lives of children and the attendant uncertainty concerning Freud's dictum of the centrality of the Oedipus complex.

Some British analysts, Edmund Bergler in America, and some infant researchers have pressed for the central role of pre-Oedipal events. Seen in this light, Kohut's work represents an organized and coherent statement concerning the importance and nature of the pre-Oedipal world, establishing its fatefulness for later development, prior to and overriding the Oedipus complex. The development of the self is seen as both the first and the most complex lifelong task of the child. The Oedipus complex involves another but secondary task, in that the shape of the Oedipus complex, its individual vicissitudes, and its outcome will be significantly or crucially predetermined by the nature of the self with which the child enters the Oedipal phase. In this perspective Kohut's view represents one culmination and overarching conceptualization of many years of effort and research on pre-Oedipal development.

A third way to view Kohut's significance is to discuss the oscillation within psychoanalysis between the roles of nature and nurture. One may see psychic development as proceeding mainly, or most importantly, for heuristic purposes from the nature of the biological equipment of the organism's instincts, which have a natural unfolding. Although the accidents of life create tensions that must be coped with, the natural flowering of maturation takes precedence, at least for purposes of understanding, over any social, interpersonal, or interactive events. The biology of infancy inevitably leads to frustration, to fantasy distortions due to defective reality testing, and to the emphasis on bodily experience as the defining source of ideation. The alternative view, briefly entertained by Freud but revived in more sophisticated form by the group of analysts who were then called culturalists, states that the instincts and the maturational schema have a degree of flexibility so great that the matters of interest to us involve individual difference stemming from experience, rather than the sameness conferred by instinct. Psychic development can be understood as a consequence of inter-personal impingements on the individual. From this point of view, the actual relationship with the actual mother is of greater psychoanalytic significance than the innate instinctual program of attachment. Adaptation and fitting together are of primary importance.

In this regard, Kohut would seem to have come part way around the circle of dispute. He gives the actual mother and her actual successes and failures in empathic rearing of her infant a central place in understanding the fate of the infant and the adult's later behavior in psychoanalytic treatment. The dispute over the primacy of nature or nurture, or maturation or development, actually involves the hypotheses we make concerning the sources of desire and of satis-faction and their innate or social qualities. Although Kohut's view is more comprehensive and sophisticated, it is nonetheless reminiscent of the work of both Sullivan and Kardiner.

A fourth longstanding debate concerns the model of discourse in psy-choanalysis. Freud was concerned that psychoanalysis be based on the model of biological science as he knew it. There has always been another trend among analysts who either are inclined to deny the claim of psychoanalysis to science or feel that Freud's scientific base is no longer appropriate. Such diverse figures as Sandor Rado, Sandler, Schafer, George Klein, and Gill have all in one way or another rejected classical metapsychology and its attendant concepts of energy and mechanism, have rejected the language of theory with its experience-remote phrasing, or have rejected the attempt at a science of cause rather than a science of meanings. Schafer has suggested that the concept of 'self' is itself a transitional idea in our continuing effort to rid ourselves of an outmoded metapsychology that significantly hampers our research and our perspective. Kohut, in his most recent work, seems to have joined those who have discarded traditional metapsychology in favor of a more existential, phenomenological approach that acknowledges the centrality and indivisibility of the self. The empathic introspective methodology enables the participant observer to share the patient's experience, which is itself ultimate and more fully describable. Kohut attempts to place the method of observation based on empathy and introspection at the center of our scientific position and to derive all the propositions of psychoanalysis from this method. Models from other sciences are of little help because the other sciences are inspectional, exteropathic. Critics of this holistic, nonmechanistic view will complain that the phenomenological method, although avoiding reductionism, reduces our capacity for theory formation – there are not enough parts to play with, which makes it difficult to explain complex processes. It is not clear to me where Kohut stands on the issue of hermeneutic science versus causal science, but my impression is that the empathic methodology forces a hermeneutic stance.

As self psychology has developed, in both its theoretical and clinical ambitions, we seem to be witnessing the construction of a new metapsychology. The original descriptions of self functions seemed experience-near, but the concepts of the supraordinate self, with its bipolar character and linking tension arc, and the increasing emphasis on developmentally significant self–selfobject relations throughout the lifespan, appear to me to be concepts of high abstraction, no longer simply phenomenological. We are, perhaps, witnessing the widening scope of self psychology. I have no quarrel with this development, but it does seem to be moving away from some of the earlier attempts to avoid high-level abstraction. Similarly, I believe that the connection of the concept of 'self' with sets of adjectives such as 'enfeebled,' 'firm,' or 'vigorous' is problematic. It may be that we are confusing levels of discourse – metapsychological and clinical – and I am not sure then of the referent of 'self,' 'I,' and 'person.' Just what is it that is feeble, and who is feeling feeble, and who knows about it?

These issues relate to a fifth tension in psychoanalysis – that between the traditional Freudian view of human beings as conflicted, neurotic, and guilty at the core, and the emphasis, explicit in Rado and implied in Hartmann, that unifying, synthesizing processes are central, and human beings are capable of self-actualization as creatures of joyous activity. Issues of the nature of psychopathology clearly follow from this – if the psyche is conflicted, pathology represents bad conflicts or poor defenses; if the psyche is a unit, pathology represents deficit or incapacity (a view suggested in the past by David Levy and Michael Balint, among others). There is also a historical tendency for those who are more phenomenological and holistic to be identified as 'humanistic,' as opposed to the reductionistic, conflictual, and 'scientific' view. This tension could be further broadened into one between an affective and a cognitive emphasis, or even between romantic and scientific world views. The very definition of analysis is involved. Kris and others saw psychoanalysis as the study of human beings in conflict, whereas Kohut sees psychoanalysis as the study of complex mental states.

Kohut is explicit in rejecting Freud's views on human nature and development from infancy to adulthood. When Kohut speaks of Tragic Man in contrast to Freud's Guilty Man, he rejects the human nature that Freud assumed. Kohut (1980), speaking of at least one group of classical analysts, refers to 'the conceptions of those who emphasize the primacy of hostility and destructiveness in human nature and, consequently, man's propensity to be beset by conflict, guilt, and guilt-depression' (p. 478). These terms contrast with the views of self psychology in which the entire course of development from infancy to adulthood is seen as the movement of an 'independent, assertive, strong' creature who is 'psychologically complete so long as it breathes the psychological oxygen provided by contact with empathically responsive selfobjects' (p. 481). This view of the infant as strong, assertive, and complete within its appropriate environment of selfobjects is in the strongest contrast to the view of classical analysis in which the baby is incomplete, symbiotically dependent, fearful of separation, and inevitably subject to anxiety because of its helplessness in both the real world and the inner world of its own libidinal and aggressive drives. What Freud saw as the inevitably fantastic mental content of an immature ego apparatus striving to cope with drive demands, Kohut views as an avoidable disintegration product of failures of self-cohesion. Kohut sees the joy of creative achievement as a clear human potential; Freud saw joy as always tempered by the reproaches of an insatiable superego.

On questions of such complexity as the nature of being human, we are usually unable to distinguish which portions of any psychoanalyst's views are determined by objective data and which reflect the personal apperceptive lens through which all clinical experience and data are filtered and altered. Infant research seems to demonstrate that the infant is born into a more comfortable world than Freud envisioned. Drives or affects are generally quantitatively and qualitatively attuned both to the average expectable environment and to the infant's developmental timetable. Affects, rather than requiring taming, grow in hierarchic complexity. The relation of mother and child is a two-way channel of intricate communication rather than a simple funneling of welfare handouts from a 'have' to a 'have-not.' None of these altered views of childhood, however, dictates Kohut's view of adult human nature. Moreover, Kohut may be doing Freud an injustice in contrasting Tragic with Guilty Man. Surely the Freudian baby's infantile omnipotence assures the human being's constant search for greatness and immortality as well as his tragic failure in the quest. In Freud's view, our misery and our greatness are inextricably interwoven, and guilt is only one index of the outcome.

28

Intrinsic to the views of all those depth psychologists who choose to see humanity's potential as open-ended is the notion of the human being as unified. Kohut's individual acts out of the inherent goals of its self, which is perceived as an 'independent center of initiative.'

> Once the self has crystallized in the interplay of inherited and environmental factors, it aims towards the realization of its own specific programme of action – a programme that is determined by the specific, intrinsic pattern of its constituent ambitions, goals, skills and talents, and by the tensions that arise between these constituents. The patterns of ambition, skills and goals; the tensions between them; the programme of action that they create; and the activities that strive towards the realization of this programme are all experienced as continuous in space and in time – they are the self, an independent centre of initiative, an independent recipient of impressions.
>
> (Kohut and Wolf 1978: 414)

It is clear that the self, the only psychological structure that Kohut describes, is in all its aspects an integrating, self-motivating force. Instincts do not lie behind it, pushing it on. The self aims to fulfill a future-oriented program, which it develops itself. While the psychic structures and functions that Freud described can be understood in widely disparate ways and through differing frames of reference, depending on how one chooses to interpret aspects of Freud's conceptual scheme, there is clearly a radical difference between Freud and Kohut.

Yet another longstanding and sometimes disguised issue that has come to the fore in the discussion of Kohut's work concerns the appropriate atmosphere of the analytic situation – the relationship between analyst and analysand. Posed against the so-called 'classical' view of the analytic situation, there has always been an alternate tendency suggesting less frustration of the patient, or more reality, or greater display of the analyst's human qualities. The classical view has been set forth most cogently by Kurt Eissler, who suggested that the proper activity of the psychoanalyst is mainly interpretation. Alternate views have been suggested at one time or another – Ferenczi's active technique, Alexander's flexible technique needed for the corrective emotional experience, Gitelson's stress on the nurturant role of the analyst, Winnicott's description of the holding function, and Greenson's and Zetzel's emphasis on the therapeutic alliance or real relationship. Freud, as many have now pointed out, seemed to describe this 'classical' technique in his major technical papers, but he often did other things in practice. Self psychologists themselves seem to be unsure about whether or not they adhere to classical technique (it is refreshing to see that self psychology is not a unified movement), though it has seemed to most of us from reading Kohut that the analytic climate he describes differs significantly, at least some of the time, from that of the traditional setting – the temperature is warmer and the weather is less stormy in Dr Kohut's office. Pathological sexual and aggressive fantasies and persistent negative transferences have lost their traditional significance and, in fact, are not, in and of themselves, of specific significance in clinical analysis; rather, they reflect defects of self-functioning or, in the case of the negative transference, failures of the analyst's empathy, which will correct themselves as the underlying self-pathology is repaired. It is my impression that Kohut is suggesting that *all* pathological manifestations of sexual and aggressive disintegration products, including those related to the Oedipal period, will repair themselves without requiring special analytic attention if one succeeds in repairing the disorders of the self–selfobject relationships. If this is the claim of self psychology, does it mean that sexual and aggressive distorted fantasy productions are of analytic interest only as cues to defects of the self? Is that the meaning of the concept of 'disintegration products?' Are there no defects of the self that originate in the terrors of infantile sexual and aggressive fantasy, regardless of how those bizarre and frightening products themselves originated? What are the criteria for concluding that only defects of the self–selfobject tie are pathogenic and require therapeutic attention? Perhaps Kohut's most radical idea is the suggestion that the developmental line of the self takes almost total precedence over any inherent developmental lines of sex and aggression; developmental disorders of sex and aggression are always and only disintegration products of self-disorder. It is clear, at any rate, that the presentation of self psychology has powerfully revived and influenced our discussions of technique and of the relationship between theory and practice. I would find it disturbing if theoretical revisions as sweeping as Kohut's did not have very significant implications for parallel technical innovations. Yet, as one reads the work of self psychologists, one has the impression that some say 'yea,' others 'nay.'

I have suggested six areas of longstanding tension in psychoanalysis concerning: (1) the scope of our concepts; (2) the role of pre-Oedipal events; (3) the role of the real environment of adaptation; (4) the nature of our inquiry – causal or hermeneutic; (5) the nature of human beings – conflicted or unified; and (6) the therapeutic action of the psychoanalytic treatment situation. One could describe other tensions in analytic theory and practice. It is a testament to the importance of Kohut's thought that so many of these currents of controversy are addressed in his formulations; and it is an index of the controversy now surrounding Kohut that his view regarding almost all these tensions would generally be considered nonclassical. I hope it is clear that my use of that phrase is in no way pejorative; in fact, an interesting discussion is just beginning on the role of the concept of 'classical' in psychoanalysis.

Self psychology, in this perspective, can be seen as the most advanced, best organized attempt to synthesize newer developments in psychoanalysis that have evolved over many decades, taking account of the accumulating scientific findings and increasing discontent with our older formulations. This is the perception of many psychoanalysts and might in itself be sufficient to explain the effect that Kohut has upon us. An alternate view is that self psychology is popular precisely because it represents a coherent organization of dissident or diluting elements in psychoanalysis – the abandonment of the difficult psychoanalytic ideas of sex, aggression, the Oedipus complex, and the negative transference. In either interpretation, however, I think the extraordinary interest in self psychology reflects its inclusion of so many of the long-simmering ideas in the psychoanalytic scientific cauldron.

The Nobel Prize winner Leon N. Cooper has said:

Forty years from now – not to speak of a century in the future – physics is unlikely to have the same shape or to be founded on the same assumptions we make now. We can reasonably expect that currently fashionable assumptions will be abandoned to be replaced by unexpected new ones. It is here that our problems with science arise, for there are many beliefs, concepts, or ideas dear to us that we wish to retain even though science does not need them to construct its theories. But science, like Laplace, is strict – it makes no assumptions unless they are necessary.

(L. N. Cooper 1980: 5)

What is true for physics is true for psychoanalysis. However distressing it may be to have to change assumptions, it would be even more distressing if our assumptions did not change.

As is always the case in the history of ideas, the immediacy of our interest in Dr Kohut did not stem only from the new synthesis he offered of some of our scientific dilemmas. Other historical factors also played a role. Psychoanalysts, beginning at least with Edward Glover, who discussed the analytic situation in Britain in the 1930s, have been claiming that there has been a change in the human condition. They say that the classical neurotic patient seen by Freud has gradually disappeared, to be replaced by types of severe character pathology, especially the narcissistic character, with a consequent diminution of analytic effectiveness and a lengthening of the analysis. Much of our literature since that time has concerned our need to understand that change, to reconcile it with our analytic theories, and to devise effective psychoanalytic treatment techniques in response to it. In recent years everyone from Spiro Agnew to Christopher Lasch has argued that we are living in an age of narcissism, surrounded by the characterologic fallout of postindustrial society and the cultural decline of the West. The capacity for love, work, and creativity allegedly has been damaged, with a loss of idealism and humanity. The period from the mid-1960s to the mid-1970s seemed to offer powerful corroboration of this view, as America went through the Vietnam War, the Johnson and Nixon years, the student riots, the near destruction of the universities, and a sense of general despair. This period of natural discouragement and dejection was paralleled in psychoanalysis, as we seemed to go through our own bleak phase. We were threatened with the

31

loss of the historical cultural climate required for the ideals of introspection to flourish; many had begun to feel a sense of repetitiousness about our teaching and literature; we saw the fountain of bright young candidates for analytic training drying up; some analysts were fearful of the rise of biological psychiatry with its astonishing triumphs; and some analysts felt discouraged over the prospect of carrying on long analyses with doubtful outcome while surrounded by joyous cries that psychoanalysis was dead and had been superseded by brilliant, quick therapies perfectly attuned to a hurry-up, 'gimme' culture.

In this climate the appearance of *The Analysis of the Self* in 1971 seemed to be the right remedy at the right moment. Kohut's work seemed fresh, new, and hopeful. He offered therapeutic optimism and a calm sense of confidence that we would prevail. His personal literary style illuminated his understanding and his mission, and we were able to feel a resonant sense of the analytic empathy he described and share some of his rich vision of the nature of humanity. The quality of his writing and his ideas conveyed an extraordinary optimism – not only about our immediate problems, but also about our capacity to transcend the ordinary boundaries of creativity and joy through the help of psychoanalysis. When reading Kohut one is always aware of the man whose interests are in the entire human condition rather than in psychoanalysis alone. There is an attractive quality, almost of ecstasy, in some of the writings of self psychologists. The plight of Tragic Man speaks to the existential core of the human condition and makes the problems of Guilty Man seem rather puny. Furthermore – and this was important in the 1970s – Kohut's Tragic Man could achieve joy and creativity, whereas Freud's Guilty Man was promised only ordinary human misery. These factors of cultural crisis, literary style, and personal attitude are, I believe, of great moment in helping to understand the intensity of our interest in Kohut's work at this time in the history of psychoanalysis. The history of science reveals many instances in which this confluence of theoretical issues, cultural need, and literary style was necessary for a scientific idea to come to notice.

I wish to bring up one more consideration to help us understand why Kohut has excited us, while many of his scientific antecedents left us cool. It is now four decades since Freud's death, and it may be only now that we begin to feel the strength to step out from under his massive, sheltering presence. In 1914, Freud was able to say: 'I regard myself as justified in maintaining that even today no one can know better than I what psychoanalysis is, how it differs from other ways of investigating the life of the mind, and precisely what should be called psychoanalysis and what would better be described by another name' (Freud 1914: 7). I think Freud always had that feeling, and probably justifiably so. It is striking that as Freud changed his views, it was often difficult for his followers to adapt; Anna Freud's *The Ego and the Mechanisms of Defense* (1946) is, in part, an exhortation to a generation of analysts to incorporate her father's more recent ideas about structural theory, the theory of anxiety, and the dual instinct theory. Today we must live without anyone who is able to tell us with complete assurance what psychoanalysis is and, perhaps more important, what it is not. Furthermore, Freud felt it was essential that a certain amount of freedom be sacrificed to the goal of retaining the identity of psychoanalysis; his poignant correspondence with Bleuler reveals the importance he attributed to psychoanalysis as a *movement* as well as a science. Today, largely because of the successes of that movement, psychoanalysis has been disseminated far too widely in the culture for any person or group to exert authority over its directions of interest and advance, and I believe that no one would want the authority that Freud could claim as the definer of psychoanalysis. This newer spirit of scientific and institutional maturity also contributes to the welcome Kohut's ideas have received and to the productivity of their discussion.

For the variety of reasons I have been suggesting and no doubt others as well, we now have powerful and competing ideas before us and grand occasions such as this one to try to adjudicate or at least to understand better the claims of the different points of view. Each theory and each theorist presents clinical evidence to support his or her position, although students cannot always agree on what has been presented. For example, Goldberg and his coauthors have presented a casebook to demonstrate self psychology in action, but readers of varying sympathies interpret it variously as proving its case, as not being different from any other analysis, or even as differing only in being bad analysis. Some discussants of the two analyses of Mr Z conclude that Mr Z did better in his second analysis because Dr Kohut had become a better analyst and more empathic, regardless of his theory, and that there are no detectable differences in the two analyses that are clearly attributable to theory. If the individual case report is not persuasive, what methods have we for judging theories and their clinical consequences?

We do have some old-fashioned guidelines to help our evaluation of theory. The classical rules indicate that a theory should be elegant (i.e. parsimonious, using the least number of propositions and constructs required for its subject); it should be consonant with knowledge and theory in other sciences (i.e. there would have to be compelling reasons to contradict established knowledge, and the theory is strengthened if it can draw on other sciences); and it should be useful (i.e. it should lead to further ideas and activities that will yield new knowledge). An old Bostonian, Henry Adams, had great difficulty coping with Poincaré's idea that theories were merely useful rather than true. Various attempts have been made to subject analytic theory to these tests, most prominently by Rappaport, who felt that only a few of our propositions were essential. This is another good time to subject our theories to this kind of philosophical scrutiny. We may be more willing now to alter conceptions that no longer stand up to such examination. The positivist philosophers of science have suggested that a good hypothesis would yield the disconfirming experiment, and we know that analytic hypotheses are not likely to yield that possibility. More modern philosophers of science, including Ricouer, Rubenstein, Simpson, Polanyi, and others, have demonstrated that many of the complex sciences cannot yield such methods of confirmation and must rely on the weight of evidence, on affirming predictions (which are available to psychoanalysis), and on postdiction. These are the methods with which we are familiar. There is clearly a need, however, for the planned experiment, for sophisticated outcome research, for the greater use of a shared data base through recorded analyses, and for bringing the knowledge of extra-analytic fields to bear in our psychoanalytic thinking. We do all these things, but too seldom, with insufficient intensity, and without the cadre of trained full-time researchers that psychoanalysis must eventually develop. Kohut's 1970 paper on 'Scientific activities of the American Psychoanalytic Association: An inquiry' urged that organized psychoanalysis assume the vital task of taking its research as seriously as it takes its educational and professional goals. We have not yet begun to realize this ideal, which I take as one of the important aims of organized psychoanalysis. I would be very happy with my tenure as president of the American Psychoanalytic Association if I thought I had advanced the research aim that Heinz Kohut so clearly outlined to even a small degree.

Whether or not self psychology represents a new paradigm in psychoanalysis as some have suggested, Kohut's work has led us to nothing less than a reassessment of our basic theories. The same historical processes that bring Kohut's work to the forefront also permit a new level of discussion of our scientific activities – more open and more tolerant of uncertainty than has sometimes been the case in the past. All science requires acts of faith. Arno Penzias, in his Nobel laureate address, described the development of the faith that certain conditions *must* obtain in the universe, although there were then no data for it. But with faith, the data were sought and eventually found. In psychoanalysis however, the faith of the inquirer has become the tradition of the conserver. A dialectic of these trends is necessary in science. It seems to me that the current climate of bolder reexamination of our present ideas and fearless exploration of new ideas can be a source of anxiety that should be respected. We should not lightly give up any tradition, and we should take full cognizance of the anxiety engendered by any change of belief – an issue that, as I mentioned earlier, even Freud confronted with his followers when he changed his views. However, it is the essence of our Freudian tradition that we have the courage to use the best of the scientific method of our era in the effort to add to our knowledge, to correct errors, and to improve our theories. Penzias quotes Eddington as saying: 'Never fully trust an observational result until you have at least one theory to explain it' (Penzias 1979). In psychoanalysis we rarely lack theories, but we rarely subject either our data or our assumptions to the most rigorous tests possible.

The issue of whether or not psychoanalysis is scientific is, I think, irrelevant in the light of our current views of science – that quivering, imaginative, uncertain enterprise of the human observer entwined with the observed in a pursuit of new knowledge that can be validated. I believe that Kohut, in developing self psychology as boldly as he has and in paying such close attention to methodological issues, has been a main source of energy invigorating psychoanalytic science. Whatever the ultimate fate of Kohut's psychology will be, the theory of the self has already fulfilled at least one of the criteria of a good theory: It has led to an explosion of scientific activity, new ideas, and new investigation. It will be a test of our scientific maturity to maintain our discourse as we look for still better ways to add to our knowledge, to test our theories, and to improve our clinical capacity. I am greatly encouraged concerning our ability to do just that by the knowledge that Kohut has attracted some of our most gifted and creative people and that self psychology is developing as a genuine field of inquiry, with questions and disagreements, rather than with a unified belief system.

3

PSYCHOANALYSIS AT ONE
HUNDRED

Beginnings of maturity*

One hundred years ago, in November 1882, Joseph Breuer gave to his young colleague, Sigmund Freud, a detailed account of his successful treatment of a case of hysteria. The treatment had lasted two years and had been completed in June of that year. The patient is known to us as Anna O. and in most histories of psychoanalysis, she is accorded the honor of being the first proto-psychoanalytic patient – the inventor of 'chimney sweeping' as she called it (Breuer and Freud 1893–1895: 30), or free association, as we call it. It was Breuer's genius to have recognized his patient's special gift, and, no doubt influenced by his own powerful countertransferences, he was able to use his observations and his emotional responses to adopt a technique unusual for physicians in that authoritarian age; that is, he decided to listen to what his patient had to tell him. Freud was deeply impressed by the case report, and it clearly informed his own early work with hysterics and his developing psychological interests. Exactly ninety years ago on this date, December 18, 1892, Freud wrote the following to Wilhelm Fliess: 'I am delighted to be able to tell you that our theory of hysteria (reminiscence, abreaction, etc.) is going to appear in the *Neurologisches Centralblatt* on January 1, 1893, in the form of a detailed preliminary communication' (Breuer and Freud 1893–1895: xiv). Freud was, of course, referring to the forthcoming publication of *Studies on Hysteria*. If anyone is interested in trying to date the birth of psychoanalysis, one might consider that conception occurred when Breuer planted the seed in Freud's mind one hundred years ago and that psychoanalysis was born after a ten-year gestation, an appropriately long pregnancy for such a

* A version of this paper was presented as the Presidential Address at the plenary session of the Fall meeting of the American Psychoanalytic Association, New York City in 1982. It was later published as Cooper (1984c) in *Journal of the American Psychoanalytic Association*. Reproduced with permission.

complex child. We have a choice today whether to celebrate the centennial of the conception or the ninetieth birthday.

Ninety or one hundred years is not a long time in the history of science, but neither is it a short time. It is the time it has taken for us to pass from our scientific and professional infancy, through the stormiest period of early development, to the beginnings of professional maturity. Some time during the past decade or so, when none of us was paying much attention, we began to be grown-up. As happens with our children and our patients, we often do not notice the early signs of change and are surprised to discover that maturational landmarks have been achieved. I believe that in the case of American psychoanalysis one striking sign of the beginnings of maturity was an event that at first glance seemed to be only another indication of immaturity – the raucous battle over Heinz Kohut's new theories. However, as that dialogue developed, something interestingly different occurred. Despite the more than gentle hints from some of our members that Kohut and his followers were nonanalytic or anti-analytic, the debate went on and still goes on. I believe that all parties involved in the battle have influenced each other, and that they will all continue to remain within psychoanalysis. As we all know, significant theoretical disagreements in psychoanalysis did not always evolve in this way in the past. This new way of handling our differences is a sign of our growing up. Furthermore, Kohut's was only the most prominent of a number of competing ideas that are now clamoring for analytic allegiance.

The thesis of my presentation is that the passing of our analytic childhood is reflected in a number of deep changes occurring in the nature of psychoanalytic inquiry, education, organization, and practice. We are changing from a special organization known as the psychoanalytic movement to a more typical organization of professionals dedicated to the basically scientific pursuit of increasing knowledge in our field and to the advancement of our specialty in society. The sad news of Anna Freud's death this past year further symbolizes that we are without living parents and must begin to behave as independent grown-ups.

I would like to digress briefly to emphasize how rapidly growth has occurred in psychoanalysis. It might provide a perspective for maturation in scientific fields to compare our time span with that of another branch of medicine. In 1628, William Harvey, after at least a dozen years of thought and experimentation, published *De Motu Cordis*, setting forth the evidence he had accumulated, and the arguments in support of, the concept of the circulation of the blood. This greatest of all physiological discoveries encountered violent opposition and resulted in the falling off of Harvey's personal practice. Interestingly, however, not all practitioners rejected his findings and two logical conclusions were drawn almost immediately from his work: the prospect of intravenous injection of medication, and of transfusion of blood. Because technique was clumsy and thrombi and emboli occurred with frequency, the techniques were abandoned after early experiments and were not really revived until 250 years later

(Ackerknecht, 1955). This, too, is perhaps part of a regular tendency in scientific development. Good ideas that derive from major discoveries often lead to early experiments that fail because of gaps in knowledge or technique, and that place the good ideas under a cloud for many years. Freud's early errors in regard to the seduction hypothesis and the subsequent excessive deemphasis of environmental influences are examples of this process in our field.

After Harvey's discovery, it took 150 years before the next great discovery by Priestley and Lavoisier that the purpose of the circulation was to distribute oxygen to the tissues. It took almost 300 years for the development of practical methods for measuring blood pressure, and the great advances in clinical cardiology – anticoagulants, diuretics, antihypertensives, cardiac surgery, and now the artificial heart have all occurred in the last half-century, and at an increasingly rapid pace.

This truncated account of 350 years of circulatory physiology illustrates commonalities of scientific development: the great discovery, often initially resisted, followed by slow, steady accumulation of basic knowledge, punctuated by epochal discoveries, and an enormous quickening of the pace of both knowledge acquisition and application as a field matures. In the light of 350 years of physiology, we have not done badly during 100 years of psychoanalysis – we are hardly fully mature, but we are no longer children. Furthermore, the maturational model for persons, which we conceive as proceeding from infantile turmoil to quiet latency to rebellious adolescence to the stable wisdom of maturity, seems not to be the maturational model for intellectual disciplines. Here, the growth is from the relative peace of early work around a unifying new idea, to the struggle to defeat the old idea, to a maturation that consists of a stable instability of endless challenge, competition of new ideas, and discarding of ideas whose usefulness has passed. It is a part of our beginning maturity that we must confront the possibility of abandoning ideas which are, indeed, very dear to us, but which we may no longer require. The alternative is stagnation.

I suspect that every past president preparing a plenary address did what I have done – read the plenary addresses of past presidents. My debt to them will become apparent as I proceed. With few exceptions, the theme has been the same – change and our resistance to it: organizational change, scientific change, social change. Past presidents take from the experience of the presidency an irresistible urge to warn the membership against excessive resistance to change. This seems to be the case regardless of the personal conservatism or liberalism of the individual. Francis McLaughlin (1978), for example, identifying himself as conservative, stated, 'To many, Freudian is synonymous with orthodoxy, but we need to remind ourselves that the essence of Freud's work and thinking was that, with very few exceptions, everything was open to change, and that he never hesitated to alter his own views in the light of his broader understanding of the human condition' (p. 4).

We know from studies in the sociology of science that resistance to change is a built-in characteristic of scientific thinking and has many desirable qualities. Ideas are to a science as mutations are to an evolving species. Most are detrimental or even lethal, and the organism requires a capacity to stifle them. A few, however, are adaptive and essential for long-range survival, and there must be mechanisms to assure their assimilation. For a science to grow and flourish it is necessary that it maintain a sense of historical continuity, a point emphasized by Kohut himself. Resistance to change assures that new ideas will be subject to sharp scrutiny, thus providing some safeguard against fads and cults, the lethal mutations. However, there have been special qualities to the resistance to change in psychoanalysis, and I would like to discuss some of them.

Oddly, the first source of our conservatism is the revolutionary figure of Freud himself. Understanding our relation to Freud is essential to understanding our relation to ideas in psychoanalysis. In 1953, Robert Knight said, 'Perhaps we are still standing too much in the shadow of that giant, Sigmund Freud, to permit ourselves to view psychoanalysis as a science of the mind rather than as the doctrine of a founder' (p. 211). I think that Knight was right and it has taken until the last few decades for us to develop the confidence and courage required to step out from under Freud's great shadow. This may have been the time necessary for grieving over the loss of a great leader, and the time required for our own group scientific ego to develop from imitation to a deeper identification with his essence as explorer of the unconscious. One could even suggest that our present fevered excitement of scientific activity represents a bit of hypomania as we recover from the loss of the father figure.

However, the history of the relation of Freud to his followers continues to influence us deeply. I shall refer to two aspects of that relation: first, the quality of discipleship, and second, the determination to establish a psychoanalytic movement. Discipleship was a characteristic of the early psychoanalytic era. As demonstrated in the letters between Freud and his followers (Roustang 1982), the nascent movement centered not only on the ideas, but also on the person of Freud himself. The relation of Freud to his followers was significantly different from, for example, the relation of Darwin or Einstein to their adherents. Freud's relations were characterized by an extraordinary intensity. His followers gave themselves to him completely or they did not remain in the movement. One might even say that a 'cult of personality' surrounded Freud and his followers. Probably only an individual who attracted transferences of such power and who could tolerate an unusual degree of transference love and hate could have been the person who would make the discovery of the immensity of the role of transference in mental life. It also seems likely that the quality of discipleship among the early adherents to psychoanalysis was a necessary consequence of the large psychological sacrifice required of them for their continuing acceptance of difficult psychoanalytic ideas and their compensatory need for an idealized father imago to whom they could give total allegiance and who could reward them for that sacrifice.

Freud's correspondence with Bleuler in 1910 (Alexander and Selesnick, 1965) illustrates both the meaning of discipleship and the importance Freud attached to creating a movement out of psychoanalysis. Bleuler was of great importance to Freud because he was one of the few international figures in psychiatry who had accepted Freud's ideas, and he also controlled Swiss psychiatry. Having originally joined the new International Psycho-Analytical Association, Bleuler resigned in disagreement over what he termed its scientific closed-door policy.

While trying to convince Bleuler to rejoin the Association, Freud wrote the following to him:

> The reasons for organizing a society were: first, the need to present to the public genuine psychoanalysis and protect it from imitations (counterfeits) which soon would arise, and second . . . that we must be ready now to answer our opponents and that it is not proper to leave the answers up to the whim of individuals. It is to the interest of our cause to bring a personal sacrifice and to relegate polemics to a central office.

In other words, we should not express individual views but should speak with one voice. Bleuler, unable to be a disciple, replied:

> There was a difference between us, which I decided I shall point out to you, although I am afraid that it will make it emotionally more difficult for you to come to an agreement. For you evidently it became the aim and interest of your whole life to establish firmly your theory and to secure its acceptance. I certainly do not underestimate your work. One compares it with that of Darwin, Copernicus and Semmelweis . . . For me, the theory is only one new truth among other truths. I stand up for it, for psychoanalysis, because I consider it valid and because I feel that I am able to judge it since I am working in a related field. But for me it is not a major issue, whether the validity of these views will be recognized a few years sooner or later. I am therefore less tempted than you to sacrifice my whole personality for the advancement of the cause of psychoanalysis.

In response, Freud attributed Bleuler's attitude to unanalyzed resistances, and developed a coldness toward him.

In retrospect, I think Freud was correct in his insistence on establishing psychoanalysis as a movement of adherents to his ideas, rather than allowing, as Bleuler wished, for free scientific interplay to determine, over time, the correctness of his views. The result was that psychoanalysis became a powerful force in our culture within decades rather than within centuries. The price, however, was relative isolation from the academic community and from the other sciences, a price Bleuler clearly foresaw.

One of the interesting consequences of our having seen ourselves as a movement rather than as an ordinary professional association has been our use of the terms 'classical' and 'orthodox.' These terms, especially 'classical,' remain in common usage, referring either to technique or theory. They are value-laden terms and more often than not carry a connotation of approval. The *Oxford Universal Dictionary* gives several definitions of 'classical': '1. Of the first rank or authority; standard, leading. 2. Of the standard Greek and Latin writers; belonging to the literature or art of Greek and Roman antiquity.' The illustrations given all refer to evidences of authority or antiquity. The word 'orthodox' is defined as: '1. Holding correct, i.e. currently accepted, opinions. 2. Of opinions or doctrines: Right, correct, true; in accordance with what is authoritatively established as the true view or right practice.' We know the good reasons why terms such as classical and orthodox arose in psychoanalytic thought and literature. They helped to regulate our growth and change during a more uncertain period of scientific childhood. But I suggest that at this time in our maturation, these terms should be considered as what, in fact, they are: references to a past time, perhaps idealized, when authority and correctness in doctrine could be or had to be asserted with assurance. When the Renaissance rediscovered classical Greece, its great artists used the classic models as a source of inspiration for new experiments in art and for the construction of new aesthetic ideals; they did not do classical sculpture. In the modern world of science, or even of philosophy, and surely in therapeutic practice, the terms are of use to a historian of the field but can no longer be carried proudly by the practitioner whose obligation is to be expert in current theory and technique as well as to know and use the past.

A second source of resistance to change, related to but separate from our relation to Freud, derives from our longstanding, and surprising, uncertainty regarding our professional identity. I believe this self-doubt is also a consequence of our history. Despite all the achievements of psychoanalysis, we retain a deep concern to define what analysis is and what a psychoanalyst is. Other scientists or intellectuals do not worry about their identity. Freud, however, as we have seen, had a deep desire to retain the purity of psychoanalysis, and he had no qualms about asserting that he was the person who could define it. Those who disagreed were invited to pursue their researches elsewhere under a different title.

On the other hand, Freud gave multiple definitions of psychoanalysis and the psychoanalyst, running the full scale from liberal and ecumenical to limiting and dogmatic. His most famous and most neutral definition was the tripartite one (Freud 1923b: 235), describing psychoanalysis as a method of investigation of unconscious mental processes, a method of treatment, and a theory of the mind. At the liberal end of the scale, Ernest Jones (1946) gave Freud's definition of psychoanalysis as 'simply the study of mental processes of which we are unaware, of what for the sake of brevity we call the unconscious. The psycho-analytic method of carrying out this study is that characterized by the free association technique of analysing the observable phenomena of transference and resistance

... anyone following this path is practising psycho-analysis' (p. 11). At the dogmatic end of the scale, Freud a number of times used the word 'shibboleth' in order to define psychoanalysis: once concerning the nuclear role of the Oedipus complex (1905b: 226), once with reference to the division of mental life into conscious and unconscious (1923a: 13), and twice alluding to the theory of dreams (1914: 57; 1933a: 7). On each occasion he asserted that these were 'shibboleths,' passwords which separate analysts from nonanalysts. We have continued Freud's effort at definition and have, over a considerable period, tried, with only limited success, to distinguish psychoanalysis from dynamic psychotherapy, or to define psychoanalysis as the study of mental conflict, or as a set of technical procedures such as the use of the couch and the number of hours a week – or even to define a psychoanalyst by the number of hours he devotes to the actual practice of psychoanalysis. Certainly one determinant of this need to define our identity so sharply stems from our fear that ever-present resistances to analysis and its disagreeable discoveries about self-deception, love, and hate, will lead to the loss of or dilution of those truths. But I believe that our concern with identity also represents our continued attempt at disciple-ship and isolation, although that mode no longer advances psychoanalysis. The legitimacy of Freud's need for definition of his new science may no longer apply in the current psychoanalytic situation.

Accustomed as we are to seeing ourselves as embattled, we may be a bit blinded to the realization that psychoanalysis is, in our culture, after 100 years, a basic point of view for the study of man as well as a basic science of psychiatry. Viewed that way, our boundaries cannot and ought not to be kept too sharply delineated. Just as scientists are no longer concerned to distinguish the boundaries between chemistry and physics or between physiology and anatomy, one aspect of our maturity is that there will be increasing difficulty defining the boundaries between psychoanalysis and other disciplines. It seems clear that, with increasing speed, psychoanalytic knowledge spills into other fields, and information not psychoanalytically derived, whether about the nature of infant attachment or the biological determinants of anxiety, will be important for the psychoanalyst. I believe that, in the future, the identity of the analyst will stem from the solidity of his analytic education and its pervasive influence on his professional life, rather than from a single uniform activity or belief. It would be folly to attempt to define psychoanalysis on the basis of a technique or practice. Techniques change over time and the essence of psychoanalysis lies in the nature of its inquiry and its views of man, not in its technical procedures. Where Freud's concern with analytic identity helped advance the early cause of analysis, an excessive concern with protection of its boundaries may retard our future development. At a time of rapid growth, and this is such a time, it is a good strategy to keep porous boundaries and to allow our discoveries to define our field rather than to risk that excessively sharp boundary-setting might inhibit discovery.

A third resistance to change, following our relation to Freud and our concern with self-definition, is, perhaps paradoxically, related to the fact that the core of our professional activity consists of assisting people to change themselves. It is an obvious suggestion that those of us who spend our professional lives immersed in uncertainties and powerful affects, rarely enjoying enormous confidence over our understanding of our patients, and always aware of how many elements in a dream or an action we cannot account for, would seek, both in our theories and in our organizational life, the certainty, predictability, and reassurance we cannot find in our daily professional activity.

Finally, of course, it is the nature of all organizational life to resist change and psychoanalytic organizational life is only a little better at it. I will not discuss the psychology of group life. However, I do want to note the importance of the sources of organizational reward in our discipline. As long as research is a relatively low priority, and as long as analysts lack recognition for systematic relations with other scientific or humanistic disciplines, then there is a natural tendency for reward to be sought in the organizational life of the profession; and we are no worse than other professions in the extent of our bureaucratization and the pull of the reward systems that bureaucracy establishes.

As psychoanalysts, we are dedicated to the study of history and the nature of continuities and discontinuities. I have presented this sketchy review of some of our resistances to change in order to provide a perspective for viewing the current situation of psychoanalysis at our ninetieth or hundredth birthday. Our past adaptations have been, in the main, enormously successful. But, continuing our metaphor of organismic maturation, we expect growth to proceed through epigenetic processes, with the emergent development of new capacities, creating new crises or challenges. The stimulus barriers we required to help regulate the early stages of our maturation may no longer be appropriate. At our present stage we require a greater range of curiosity and object seeking, new opportunities for identification and emulation, and the acquisition of new skills for the realization of our potential capacities and talents. In fact, our field has already undergone much greater change than our rhetoric acknowledges. Gertrude Stein (1935) once wrote an essay on 'contemporaneousness' in which she stated that individuals always live their lives in the culture that existed twenty years earlier. In her view, it was only the artist that had the ability to see the actual present. I think we will recognize Stein's characterization as generally true for organizations as well as individuals, but we can try our best to separate the 'realistic here-and-now' from the distorted misperceptions that are overladen with persistent images of our past. We know the difficulties of that task. Our resistances to change have not prevented change; rather, they have modified it and may have limited our accurate self-perception. New realities of psychoanalysis and its world require, with some urgency, that we initiate other changes that are not yet in process.

★ ★ ★

I would like now to speak of a few of the newer developments in American psychoanalysis. Most important is the change in our scientific life to which I have alluded before. More now than at any previous time in my memory, our journals and our scientific programs reflect a continuing clash of diverse and divergent ideas. Where once American psychoanalysis followed a single line of advance through ego psychology, largely as described by Hartmann, we are currently living with a *mélange* of points of view – ego psychology, self psychology, object-relations theory, revivals of interpersonal theory, Lacanian derivatives, Kleinian views, and more. As each group struggles to dominate our scientific life, we are reliving many of the enduring controversies in psychoanalysis that have been a motive force for our new ideas since our beginnings. Some of these disputes are more philosophical than scientific and will always be with us. Others are disputes that, one day, will be settled by scientific data. Embedded in the debates between schools or points of view are such fundamental controversies as: the relative importance of nature and nurture; the nucleus of neurosis – Oedipal or pre-Oedipal; the nature of man – tragic or guilty; the nature of our inquiry – scientific or hermeneutic; the appropriate language of our discourse – metapsychological or clinical; the origins of motivation; the intrinsic nature of the mind – unified or conflicted; the nature and source of therapeutic effectiveness; and of course the question of our identity and the limits of technique. One can add to the list. These kinds of questions have always been at the core of our field. What is different at the present time is that our questioning goes on with a new openness and with no possibility that the questions can be answered or thrown out of court, by appeal to authority.

Different strategies suit a particular science at different points in its development. Lumping and splitting are two different scientific strategies. The lumper finds underlying unity in superficially diverse phenomena. The splitter explores hidden differences among seemingly similar phenomena. Lumping was important early in our history. For example, it was important to demonstrate that the Oedipus complex was universal. I believe that at the present time, however, the splitters have a greater contribution to make. For example, it is important now to discover the differences in the Oedipus complex under different psychological circumstances. At a panel last spring on the relation between psychoanalytic theory and technique, I perceived a tendency for persons with enormously divergent theoretical views to insist that their psychoanalytic technique was the same as everyone else's (Richards 1984). It seems clear to me that if theoretical innovation does not lead to technical diversity, then the theories are trivial. We will benefit most from our current scientific debate if we pursue boldly the implications of our differences. It would be astonishing, and disturbing, if the psychoanalytic situation and the psychoanalytic technique we devised more than half a century ago were never to develop further. While we are appropriately suspicious of desires for quick cure during an age of narcissism, we should welcome any developments that speeded the achievement of analytic results and made the benefits of analysis available to larger numbers. This was clearly Freud's wish. We must also be prepared to face the fact that, in scientific debates, often one party is wrong, and compromise is not possible. As I indicated before, in contrast to philosophical debates, which can be endlessly enriching, scientific debates can often be settled with startling suddenness by new data.

This current style of scientific discourse in American psychoanalysis suggests that the remaining discipleship and movement characteristics that served psychoanalysis well during its early development will now fade rapidly. We shall never be able to return to the era where a small and devoted group shared, and fought for, a unified system of belief. It is implicit in my welcome of our current mode of scientific debate that some of the questions we are raising will be subjected to scientific research and that psychoanalysts will undertake to do that research. The challenge and opportunity before us is huge and daunting. As a 100-year-old discipline, it is essential that we find the ways to provide the cadre of dedicated researchers every serious discipline – be it history or molecular biology – requires, if it is to remain a serious force in science or humanities. Psychoanalytic ideas are too important for our research to remain a cottage industry, even recognizing how productive that has been in the past. Modern research methodology is required for our inquiry and we must create new structures for the education and support of those rare persons who have research passion. At the present time the scarcity of psychoanalytic researchers seriously threatens our continued psychoanalytic development. Our exciting debates will become arid if they are not sprinkled with new data. You have all heard many pleas for more research, but I believe I am saying something a bit different. We need a different quality of research, one that requires a special breed of researcher who requires a special education and support structure, and we have only just begun to face the problem. I cannot overemphasize its urgency. Even if we do not feel impelled by our scientific and theoretical curiosity, we might respond to the demands of a society that will not forever allow us to practice clinical psychoanalysis without evidence of its efficacy. Being more grown-up sometimes carries greater responsibilities, and this is one of them. I shall return shortly to a brief consideration of the educational institution that might begin to undertake this research task.

Another new fact of our maturing psychoanalytic life, the significance of which may have escaped us, pertains to the demography of our profession. Following decades of rapid growth, it is clear that in recent years membership in the American Psychoanalytic Association and applications for training are stable. Out of our active membership of roughly 1250, many of whom are not yet eligible for training analyst status, over 500 or one of every 2.5 is a training analyst. Even if there is a surge in the number of members or the number of candidates as a result of changes in our by-laws, in time we shall again reach a steady state and in that steady state simple mathematics indicates that if each training analyst analyzes only 10 candidates in his entire career, only 10 per cent of analysts can ever become training analysts. When the chances of becoming a training analyst change from more than one in 2.5 to one in 10, training analyst status can no longer be a meaningful career goal for the majority of serious analysts, as I believe it has been in the past. This is a radical change in our professional life. Other data from our recent survey of psychoanalytic practice are of interest in this regard (Shapiro 1981). About half of our active members now have salaries derived from academic or institutional work. The vast majority of our active members participate in the work of academic institutions. Only a minority of analysts devotes more than half of its time to the conduct of analysis. My earlier discussion about our concern with analytic identity is pertinent here. In this situation, a healthy profession must find ways of providing career satisfaction for the majority who cannot attain training analyst status and who do not, out of choice or necessity, devote the greater part of their time to the actual practice of psychoanalysis.

In some of our institutes, the student dropout rate approximates the entry rate of new students, and the graduation rate is very low. Educators long ago learned that high dropout rates are neither necessary nor desirable for excellence in education. Some of these dropouts may be failed candidates who, perhaps, could have been screened before entry. But a number of them are candidates who feel they have received the training they want and have not been inspired to go on to complete the curriculum. We may be looking at the signs of a budding educational crisis. Solving this problem will require a deep rethinking of some of our educational and professional goals and organization.

I shall discuss one more area where changes have occurred that signal a new phase of our profession. The psychoanalytic situation no longer involves only the therapist and the patient. Our recent survey of our members reveals the astonishing fact that the majority of analyses now involve a third-party payer (Shapiro 1981). While some of us may wish this were not true, without third-party assistance, either psychoanalysis would be available to very few patients or psychoanalysts would cease to be members of the middle class. With our acceptance of the third-party payer, we have also accepted inevitable intrusions on our cherished autonomy. In sixteenth-century Japan, a wealthy noble approached the great landscape architect of the time and asked him to construct his palace garden. The architect agreed to undertake the task if three conditions were met: first, no limit on the available funds; second, no limit to the time he required; and third, no inspection of the work until it was entirely completed. Those are attractive terms and many of us have enjoyed the practice of psychoanalysis under somewhat similar circumstances. However, as professionals now functioning as part of the social fabric, we know that money, time, and freedom from scrutiny are no longer privileges, but are matters of negotiation with governmental and financial agencies. Our Association and our component societies have been increasingly vigorous in fighting to protect our patients and our own professional and financial welfare. We have lost our political virginity and such losses are irreversible.

Actually, we have undertaken a new social responsibility. Believing deeply in the value of psychoanalysis, we must prove that value to those from whom we require assistance to bring the best care to our patients and to carry out our research. We must develop the political sophistication necessary to win our battles to protect the quality of our patients' treatment and their confidentiality, and we must be prepared to *demonstrate* our quality, integrity, and capacity for professional self-regulation. Others will not be satisfied with trust alone. Most of us shrink from the idea of crass political involvement, but it now seems clear that, as in almost every branch of medicine or science, we are inextricably involved in the political process. Our clinical obligation to our patients requires that we accept these political responsibilities.

I hope it is clear from what I have been saying that it is my view that psychoanalysis is, at the age of 100, in a process of epigenetic change. The conduct of our science, the nature of our clinical activity, and our role in society all seem radically different from the situation that obtained only a few decades ago. Cliché though it may be, we really are faced with new realities, new challenges, and new opportunities. Problem-solving modes that served so well at earlier stages will be inadequate to our newer developmental needs. We have to build a research establishment. We must establish closer ties to the intellectual and scientific communities. We have to find new values for guiding our professional lives and new ways to participate in the political process.

As someone who has spent most of his professional life as a practitioner and educator, it is natural for me to turn to education for solutions to our problems. I will close by suggesting that although our current educational institutes work well in providing rigorous training for analytic practitioners, we now require a broader educational enterprise. We must work toward achievement of the full-time analytic school, about which we have dreamed for years. I think this is a favorable time for that development to begin. The new excitement in psychoanalysis has revived our standing among the other intellectual disciplines, and at present our welcome in the intellectual community is cordial and enthusiastic. Furthermore, in psychiatry, the rampant anti-analytic trends of a while ago have given way to serious efforts to find the ways to combine the basic science of psychodynamics with basic sciences of psychobiology. The either-or quality of biology or psychodynamics is no longer tenable for intelligent minds, and interesting new concepts will develop in this atmosphere. In this favorable intellectual and academic climate, we must seize the chance to build the broad-based psychoanalytic school that can serve our multiplicity of needs. We must educate psychoanalytic researchers and accept a new openness in the exchange of analytic data. We must, of course, continue to train analytic practitioners to the most rigorous standards, certifying, and re-certifying, ourselves. We must prepare analysts for gratifying *analytic* lives, while devoting major portions of their time to psychotherapy, education, administration, social policy, and research. Anyone familiar with today's bright psychiatric residents knows that many of them are deeply interested in analysis because nothing else can provide them with the depth of human knowledge and the clinical skills they seek. But many of them will apply that knowledge and skill to tasks other than psychoanalytic treatment, and they will boldly engage in psychotherapeutic experiments and new applications of analytic points of view. We should welcome and assist this process. I am convinced there will always be a group of patients for whom psychoanalysis will be the treatment of choice. And I am confident that there will always be a group of therapists who derive the most satisfaction and best expression of their talents in administering this treatment. But the science and profession of psychoanalysis are clearly much more than psychoanalytic treatment. Some group of our educational institutions must take seriously our scientific and intellectual obligations and assure that psychoanalysis and the multiplicity of scientific and intellectual fields adjacent to it will continue to inform and enrich each other. Applied psychoanalysis has only begun to make its potential contribution, and the number of people able to make such contributions is still far too small. Agencies of government have renewed interest in psychotherapy research, and it will be exceedingly unfortunate if we lack the capacity to assume our proper role in that project. The contribution psychoanalysis can make to understanding ideology and group behavior, thus perhaps contributing to more intelligent social policy, has barely been explored. We should not forget that Freud, devoted as he was to his movement and jealous as he was of his discoveries, took the largest conceivable view of the contribution psychoanalysis had to make to society and human welfare.

We have no educational establishment at the present time that can help us realize these goals. If we consider what we have achieved in our first 100 years, we should not be modest in looking forward to what we may do in the future. One might say that psychoanalysis is far too important to be left only to psychoanalysts, and it is certainly too important to be confined solely to the conduct of psychoanalytic treatment. The enlightened spread of psychoanalysis in the culture is an obligation in the best psychoanalytic tradition and was a part of Freud's bold vision.

Old habits die hard. I cannot resist calling upon authority to support what I am saying. In 1966, Anna Freud quoted her father as saying the following in 1926:

> If – which may sound fantastic to-day – one had to found a college of psychoanalysis, much would have to be taught in it which is also taught by the medical faculty: alongside of depth-psychology, which would always remain the principal subject, there would be an introduction to biology, as much as possible of the science of sexual life, and familiarity with the symptomatology of psychiatry. On the other hand, analytic instruction would include branches

of knowledge which are remote from medicine and which the doctor does not come across in his practice: the history of civilization, mythology, the psychology of religion, and the science of literature. Unless he is well at home in these subjects, an analyst can make nothing of a large amount of his material.

(Freud 1926b: 246)

Anna Freud went on:

It goes without saying that it is tempting for me to pursue a plan of this kind and to enlarge on its implications. But as matters stand at present, I have to admit to myself that it is in truth a piece of 'fantastic' wishful thinking, and as such I have omitted it regretfully from the image of the Ideal Institute.

(A. Freud 1966: 75)

Her discussion of what is feasible in the ideal analytic institute includes the goals to which I have alluded and many more. She also made the following important statement, in referring to analytic training: 'The present *part-time* system [of education] seems as out of date to me as if church services were still conducted in catacombs since this is where the early Christians were obliged to meet' (p. 81; emphasis added). Of course, the pedagogic arrangement, which seemed so outlandish to her in 1966, is still the only one we have. We have not even addressed the issue. To carry my appeal to authority even further, let me quote from the report of the Commission on the Ideal Institute of the American Psychoanalytic Association:

The Commission members generally favored an increased effort by the psychoanalytic establishment to offer its knowledge broadly, and not only for specific professional purposes. Perhaps, if the traditional perspective were modified, such phrases as full training, partial training, and extension programs would become obsolete. The institutes might begin their own eventual transformation by reconstituting themselves as university-like structures, including both professional and nonprofessional schools.

(Goodman 1977: 157)

I fully concur. Again, as far as I know, this Association has given no resources to the attempt to realize this goal.

The prospect that seemed to Freud fantastic; to Anna Freud partly unrealistic; and to our COPER commission desirable, seems now necessary, urgent, and feasible. Our dedication to psychoanalysis at this stage of our development demands that we pursue the creation of a new educational institution and new educational alliances in which the traditional training of the practitioner will be one important pursuit embedded in our broadened research and scholarly tasks.

49

In fact, if we do not take the lead in developing this form of full-time educational enterprise for psychoanalysis, others, perhaps bolder than we, intellectually dedicated, but without our essential *clinical* background, will pursue the implications of psychoanalysis without us. The immediate difficulties of creating a new educational structure – lack of money, lack of time, lack of organization – may seem insuperable. But I believe the immediate difficulties are only that. The history of the American Psychoanalytic Association demonstrates its ability to bring extraordinary human resources of dedication, energy, and innovation to the pursuits it considers worthy. Those resources can be mobilized to make this task a realistic one. Furthermore, we have no choice. It must be done if psychoanalysis is to thrive in the future. The time is ripe.

We are celebrating a most significant birthday. Whether we reckon our age at 100 or 90, it is a time of professional maturation, an occasion for enormous pride in the achievement of psychoanalysis. That achievement was made under special circumstances, which have given a unique shape to our enterprise. But as we achieve maturity, we have begun to change in new and not entirely predictable ways, which call for new perceptions, the development of new attitudes, and the creation of new structures for our functioning. A new form of educational institution deserves our most urgent attention.

It is predictable that the pace of change will quicken. It is part of our psychoanalytic heritage that we show the courage to face new realities and to find new adaptations, which will insure the recruitment of bright young minds, the continuing advance of psychoanalysis, and our growing contribution to human welfare. I am optimistic for our future.

4

PSYCHOANALYSIS TODAY

New wine in old bottles or the hidden revolution in psychoanalysis[*]

In a recent article a literary critic, Harold Bloom (1986), detailed the extraordinary influence of Freud upon our culture. In this piece, generally unfriendly to psychoanalysis, Bloom attributed much of this influence to the power and cogency of Freud's writings, considering him 'the most persuasive of modern discursive writers . . . the most fascinating of all really tendentious writers in the Western intellectual tradition,' whose 'conceptions are so magnificent in their indefiniteness that they have begun to merge with our culture.' In this view, Freud's literary power, combined with the immense scope of his interest, has changed forever all the intellectual disciplines – sociology, anthropology, literature, history, as well as medicine. This extraordinary cultural effect, the Freudianization of our thought, has included the transfer into ordinary consciousness of a whole new terminology. It is part of everyday lingo to speak of the Freudian slip, the unconscious, defenses and defensiveness, transference, conflicts, the effects of early mothering on the adult's character, and so on.

It is easy to forget, as Bloom seems to, caught up in the beauty of Freud the writer, that while Freud was quite aware of his literary skill and the scope of his work, intending nothing less than to change the world, he derived his ideas and his language from his clinical work, changed his ideas on the basis of his clinical work, and constantly refreshed them from his clinical work. *Studies on Hysteria* (Breuer and Freud 1893–1895), the first proto-psychoanalytic work, already contains within it the core ideas of psychoanalysis and Freud vividly describes how his new terminology derived directly from his clinical experience and was

[*] A version of this paper was first presented as the Distinguished Psychiatrist Lecture at the annual meeting of the American Psychiatric Association, Washington, DC in 1986. This revised version includes some of what first appeared in Cooper (1987e).

invented to serve his clinical needs and observations. For example, Freud used the term 'transference' because he sensed that the patient literally transferred onto the doctor the feelings, thoughts, and representations that pertained to significant figures of the past. The terms 'resistance' and 'defense' referred, again literally, to Freud's sense of having to do work to overcome obstacles that the patient interposed to the free disclosure of his thoughts. Free association literally meant the instruction to the patient to speak 'freely,' without inhibition, concern, or judgment, so that the products of the mind could emerge uncontaminated by social reason. It is remarkable that so many of these original terms remain with us. The names for and descriptions of mental operations such as condensation, displacement, primary and secondary process, the mechanisms of defense and many more, described more than three-quarters of a century ago, are still a part of our active usage, and even in DSM-III, Freud's syndromal names and descriptions are alive. Furthermore, many of his later, more complex, metapsychological terms (for example, the systems of unconscious, pre-conscious, and conscious; or the structural scheme of ego, superego, and id; or the concept of drive; or the stages of psychosexual development; or the genetic point of view) are actively used, not only in the psychoanalytic literature but in psychiatric and popular literature as well. It is a tribute to Freud's literary and clinical genius that the words he gave us for thinking about the mind have remained so alive and so constant.

It is my view that this extraordinary endurance of the language of psychoanalysis has been a mixed blessing. The unchanging words, each of them clinical at root, have been screens hiding their constantly changing meanings and applications. In fact, a literary scholar like Bloom still assumes that psychoanalysis is coterminous with the early writings of Freud and, like most people outside the field, he is unaware that there has been a quiet, largely unadvertised, revolution in the way psychoanalysis is conceived. Basic ideas have changed radically in response to our vastly expanded clinical experience as well as to researches in ethology, infant observation, and psychoanalytic process, but little of this is reflected in the ordinary discourse of psychoanalysis. The changes in psychoanalysis are of a magnitude that most fields would consider a major paradigm shift. I shall discuss some of the reasons why this change has remained largely hidden, and describe some examples of the paradigm shift that has occurred. Psychoanalysis, a central source of ideas and information for psychiatry and branches of neuroscience as well as for social science and humanities, has a responsibility to communicate clearly.

Laplanche and Pontalis (1973) in their dictionary, aptly titled *The Language of Psychoanalysis*, describe the problem. Referring to 'transference' they say:

> The reason it is so difficult to propose a definition of transference is that for many authors the notion has taken on a very broad extension, even coming to connote all the phenomena which constitute the patient's relationship with

the psychoanalyst. As a result, the concept is burdened down more than any other with each analyst's particular views on the treatment – on its objective, dynamics, tactics, scope, etc. The question of the transference is thus beset by a whole series of difficulties which have been the subject of debate in classical psychoanalysis.

(Laplanche and Pontalis 1973: 456)

What is true of the term 'transference' is, in varying degree, true today of many of the key terms in psychoanalysis. The words may mean vastly different things to different people.

Two notable attempts to solve this problem of multiple, elastic, definitions of terms by creating new psychoanalytic languages were made by Harry Stack Sullivan (1956) and Sandor Rado (1962). Sullivan wanted a language that would help him escape from the lack of an interpersonal perspective in Freud and would make clear his view that one cannot speak of individuals governed by instinct and isolated from social context. Instead, Sullivan believed that one can only speak of interactions and of the individual in relation to his human setting. Rado, sharing some similar views, was also interested in creating an operational language attuned to positivist science that would allow him to escape from the metapsychological language of energies – what Freud referred to as his 'mythology' – that took Freud far from his clinical observations. It was Rado's conviction that Freud's language distracted psychoanalysts, including Freud, from acknowledging the painful and joyful thoughts, affects, attachments and interactions that constituted the substance of the analyst's work with his patient, and that were the substance of Freud's original discoveries. Both Rado and Sullivan, unfortunately, lacked anything resembling literary talent. Sullivan wanted us to talk of 'prototaxic' and 'parataxic' modes, and Rado wanted us to say 'non-reporting cerebral nervous activity' where Freud spoke of unconscious and pre-conscious. It was no contest over whose language would prevail. More recently, Roy Schafer (1976) has suggested that we abandon the old language of psychoanalysis and speak in action language – stating what it is that we actually do either as therapists or as patients in terms of desiring, resisting, defending, attacking, and so on. He, too, wants to lead us toward a vivid sense of the present interaction in analysis and away from the mechanical view of the human being as a set of drives or energies. I believe that his attempt, also, although influential, has failed as a language.

It is as if we cannot bring ourselves to talk a language other than the one that Freud taught us – even in a bad translation – largely because he awakened us to a new sense of what it means to be human, partly because his language was so vivid and has remained so for us, partly because it relates so clearly to the language of classical literature, which is our heritage, and perhaps also because its wonderful vagueness has allowed it to come to mean whatever it is we think it should mean. Freud's terms have taken on such breadth and depth of meaning that they seem to be all-encompassing and the creation of new language seems pointless.

This kind of ambiguity, necessary for great literature, is probably disastrous in the long run for science. Obviously, the situation of psychoanalysis, and probably of the social sciences generally, is vastly different from that of the physical sciences. The physicists gleefully create new words to describe new discoveries and they have a lexicon of quarks, leptons, muons, charm; we get a sense of people playing, rather impishly, with their language. It isn't that the nomenclature of the physicist always signifies objects or ideas that have sharp and agreed-upon definition; the opposite may be the case. More often, however, the physicists' new particle is not just the old particle with a little difference. It is indeed something new and different, not previously observed. Human behavior, however, is not particulate and, in fact, one of our problems is teasing out of the continuity of behavior what might be described as units or structures of behavior suitable for study. The psychoanalyst is rarely in the position of describing a behavior never before observed. Usually, he is either changing the unit of behavior, or causally connecting previously unconnected behaviors, or offering anew explanation of a previous observation. These are not trivial changes, and I shall try to demonstrate that despite the sameness of our language, we have, in fact, not unlike physicists, vastly changed our ideas.

Unlike the physicist, however, psychoanalysts have often been loath to own up to the more radical changes that we have made in our thinking and practice. Psychoanalysts cling to Freud's language as one part of our clinging to our identification with Freud. It takes a courageous and perhaps foolish psychoanalyst to willingly break away from such a magnificent identification. Few professionals have the luxury of attaching their work directly to that of one of the great minds of history. The playwright can admire Shakespeare; he cannot say he is carrying on Shakespeare's work. The physicist can admire Einstein and in a few instances the physicist with a new discovery may feel that he is carrying on Einstein's work. The psychoanalyst however, who makes no discovery at all, sitting in his office with a patient, can claim to be carrying on Freud's work. This powerful identification with Freud has, without a doubt, been a significant part of the history of the development of psychoanalysis, both for better and worse.

For better, it has held people to the highest standard of intellectual, medical, and scientific achievement, and it has provided a model of courage and exploration. For worse, it has created a group of followers guarding the dogma, believing that their primary task is to defend the discipline against detractors and dilution, and this defense has, at times, been ferocious. When, for example, Kardiner (1945) and Horney (1950) were arguing for the significance of the cultural environment of childrearing in determining individual character, they were labeled culturalists, and because they had abandoned aspects of Freud's version of drive theory, some of the leading ego psychological psychoanalysts of that time declared them to be outside of the psychoanalytic circle. More recently, Kohut has been declared outside of psychoanalysis by a leading analyst in a leading journal (Stein 1979). In most sciences, the man with a new idea or a new discovery does all he can to emphasize the uniqueness and newness of his thought. Until recently, at least, the psychoanalyst with a new idea has also had to demonstrate that he remains within the context of Freud's thought.

These different tendencies, then – (1) the power of Freud's language; (2) the difference between the language of human behavior with its inherent ambiguity and the language of more positive science, whether operational or action language; (3) the desire to preserve Freud from potential destroyers; (4) the desire to remain identified with Freud; and (5) the need to prove that one has remained within the orbit of psychoanalysis – all disguise the changing ideas of psychoanalysis. In fact, psychoanalysis today, more than at any time since its earliest years, is in a state of rapid change, with a new attitude of open scientific dispute over data, technique, and theory. New things are being learned and old ideas are being discarded, but you might never know this from listening to the language, since many of our new ideas remain bound and clothed in old words. I will take up a few topics to demonstrate this point.

The newer view of motivation that has gained ascendancy in modern psychoanalysis is a good example of a change in analytic theory of dimensions that would, in most sciences, be called a revolution, but in psychoanalysis the fact is that Freud's concept of 'drive' either has been discarded by many or has been assigned a new meaning that is often left unclear. Freud was explicit in claiming that the mind was driven to work by hypothetical drives or instincts that were rooted in the body. He postulated two drives – libidinal and aggressive – that were the source of all the energies that were available to the mind and that the mind disposed in carrying out all mental activity. The drives, the intermediate conception between mind and body, were conceived as the origin of all behavior and were central in the psychoanalytic scheme, providing the way to conceive of behavior as originating within the individual, who was both the motivator of his needs through his id, and the tamer and gratifier of his needs through his ego. In this view the raw energies of the id, libidinal and aggressive, are partially captured by the ego and superego during development, with the consequence of an endless inner battle among conflicting aims and agencies. The slogan for therapy was, 'Where id was, there shall ego be' (Freud 1933a). A good deal of psychoanalytic literature in America during the 1950s and 1960s was devoted to attempting to understand how these libidinal and aggressive energies were disposed by different parts of the psychic apparatus, and 'fused,' 'neutralized' or 'discharged.'

It became apparent to increasing numbers of analysts after Freud's 'Inhibitions, symptoms and anxiety' (1926a) that individuals were motivated at least as much by their needs, whether for dependency, empathic contact, self-esteem, or safety, as they were by inherent sexual or aggressive drives. The infant is clearly motivated by powerful, often relatively conflict-free, desires for stimulation, satisfaction of curiosity, communication, learning, and object-contact, all resting upon the sense of safety and security that the infant derives from the solid bond to its caretaking object. The anticipation of relatively conflict-free, adaptive pleasures motivates large segments of behavior.

The infant is also powerfully motivated by the need to maintain emotional homeostasis by sustaining desirable internal representations of oneself and one's objects. The infant's and adult's task is to make the best possible adaptation to gratify his or her self-esteem, safe relation to the object, and pleasurable needs, only a few of which derive from anything that can be called an instinctual drive. Affects are not simply the epiphenomena of the drives, but are, in themselves, major motivators of behavior. Today's analyst is far more interested in tracing conscious and unconscious affects than in finding a source for behavior in drives.

Several generations of analysts, including Rado (1962), Horney (1950), Loewald (1970), Winnicott (1965), Kernberg (1984), Kohut (1984) and Sandler (1987), from very different vantages, demonstrated that Freud's meaning for 'instinct' or 'drive' does not fit contemporary clinical and theoretical models and needs. While some psychoanalysts continue to speak of 'the drives,' most no longer mean what Freud meant. Otto Kernberg (1984), for example, speaking of the drives as an amalgam of self and object representations, the relations between them, their affective tone, and the wish attached to the interaction, hardly means the same thing as Freud meant when he spoke of the drive as the demand of the body on the mind for work. Yet Kernberg continues to write of the drives as if his ideas were consonant with the ego psychology and libido economics of the 1950s. It is my view that his work is entirely opposed to that view. Margaret Mahler, whose work has demonstrated the primary role of object attachment and safety as motivators, clearly demonstrated by the infant's 'refueling' behaviors, has stated that her work rests on drive theory, although I can see no evidence for that (Mahler *et al.* 1975). When Sandler speaks of the need for safety as a central motivator or when Winnicott speaks of the role of spontaneous play as central in development, they are far from anything Freud intended. As Stern (1985) has emphasized, one can distinguish multiple, interacting motivational systems, all dependent on a matrix of attachment and developing internal representations. Despite all of these advances, the literature of psychoanalysis continues to refer to 'the drives,' as if this had an agreed-upon meaning.

Our failure as psychoanalysts to communicate the extent of the change in our conception of motivating systems has handicapped our own researches and has hindered cooperation with other disciplines. Clearly, the newer views of motivation are closely attuned to the researches in ethology and infant observation. Such productive interactions will be even more likely if we are less burdened with holdovers of archaic and abandoned meanings that are confusing even to psychoanalysts, but may be daunting and misleading to those who would like to work with us but have no reason to be acquainted with the history of our terminology, and correctly perceive, as Freud did, that the concept of drives was a 'mythology,' useful for its time.

Our changing view of transference is a subtler instance of an important yet partially hidden change in psychoanalytic conception. Freud's idea of transference was a relatively simple, historical one. The patient in the present enacted with the analyst those feelings and thoughts that pertained to a significant figure of the 'real' historical past. In effect, none of us sees the object before us except as filtered through the lens of our individual past. For many years, the analysis of the transference referred to the effort to bring the patient back to, i.e. to reconstruct and reawaken, the original relationship that was being reenacted falsely, as it were, in the analysis.

Over the past several decades, however, there has been a profound shift for many analysts in our view of transference. Influenced by De Saussure's early work in linguistics, changing philosophical currents, new findings in infant observation, and changes in the surrounding culture, psychoanalysts have increasingly adopted a synchronic rather than a diachronic view of the transference. The synchronic view holds that any activity, interaction, or mechanism is best understood by understanding how it functions in all the complexity of the here and now. The diachronic, more traditional, view holds that the deepest understanding of a present event derives from its causal relation to its history. The two views are quite contradictory and represent a very significant change in the view of the transference as it is worked on and experienced with the patient. Freud's view tended to emphasize the connection of present and past, with the assumption that the elucidation of past relationships is explanatory and therapeutic. In the newer view, significance resides in the present experience, the 'here and now,' including the living presence of the past, with the assumption that the reported infantile past may never have existed, but is itself a creation of the actively apperceiving infant, and the later modifications of memory occurring with development.

Freud's earlier view of transference tended to regard the analytic situation as one in which the patient responded out of his past unconscious to a neutral figure, the analyst. Our present view of the transference is of an interpersonal interaction, in which analyst and patient are powerfully influencing and affecting each other's responses, although the degree of influence is not equal. The patient is not writing his script upon the blank screen of the analyst; rather, he is creating a new relationship, in which the analyst, holding one or a few theories into which the patient is more or less subtly inducted, is a co-participant, and during which the analyst as well as the patient will change.

These differences are manifestations of an even more profound change in analytic intent. Where, for Freud, the analytic task of making the unconscious conscious, through the undoing of repression, was an end in itself that had curative consequences, today's psychoanalyst is likely to view the undoing of the repressed past as a portion, and often only a small portion, of the task of bringing to awareness and to affective experience the nature of the patient's ongoing ways of feeling, perceiving and relating; the currently active internal representations that influence those modes; and the nature of the anxieties and dysphorias that are aroused by a prospective alteration of those modes. The lived, affective, changing experience of oneself in the new relationship with the analyst is regarded as crucial to the process, not the undoing of the past. These changes in the view of the transference, and of the nature and purpose of the analytic interaction are not reflected in the standard language of psychoanalysis, and the casual observer might conclude that psychoanalysis has remained static in its continued emphasis on the centrality of the transference and its interpretation.

A brief discussion of the Oedipus complex, that hallmark of psychoanalysis, provides another instance of a deep change in analytic outlook. Freud had no hesitation in stating, in 1923, that it was a shibboleth of psychoanalysis that the Oedipus complex was the nucleus of neurosis. For Freud, the Oedipus complex was the culmination of the development of libidinal drive, with the little boy's desires graduating from his desire for the mother's breast to his desire for the mother genitally. Only the terror of castration from the father deflected him from this aim. This climactic experience of desire and terror form the superego and force the need for acceptance of the full complexity of a multiperson world of ambivalence and ambiguity.

For today's analyst, the story remains true, but is likely to be differently conceptualized. Where Freud had difficulty understanding the central role of the mother in forming the infant's psyche, despite his rapturous description of the mother in *An Outline of Psychoanalysis* (1938), most analysts now would give to the mother a crucial role in forming the child's sense of self, his self-esteem system, even his superego, and his general love affair with the world. The Oedipus complex is today better understood as the culmination of earlier determining events rather than an event *sui generis*, and analysts are in sharp disagreement concerning the centrality of the Oedipus complex. The question of the centrality of Oedipal conflict is an important one because it focuses our therapeutic and research interest. Our hugely expanded knowledge of separation–individuation, of the early affective, cognitive and object-relational capacities of the pre-Oedipal child, of the central role of narcissistic regulation in development, all leads toward an emphasis on pre-Oedipal experience as decisive for most people in determining the flavor of the defenses and capacities that make up character.

The significance of this difference in point of view is clear in a reading of Sophocles' *Oedipus Rex*. Freud, contrary to his usual practice, read the meaning of the play in its surface; Oedipus murdered his father and slept with his mother and, therefore, he must have wished to do so. A closer reading of the play reveals other interesting elements. Oedipus' parents decide, because of the prediction of the gods, to kill Oedipus. Laius puts a thong through his ankles and his mother, Clytemnestra, actually hands him to a shepherd to be killed. Oedipus is an abused, abandoned, adopted child who never, until near the end of the play, knows who his biological parents are. Given this early history it is not surprising to discover that he is dedicated to solving riddles and mysteries – what did the Sphinx mean and who killed Laius? It is also not surprising to realize that he is a severely impulse-ridden character; he almost automatically tries to kill every older man who crosses his path – Laius, Tiresius, the old shepherd, and Creon his uncle; furthermore, he marries an older woman despite knowing the prophecy that he would sleep with his mother. We could go on. The point is that while Oedipus has an Oedipus complex, we might best understand that in terms of his pre-Oedipal history of abandonment and attempted infanticide, and its effects on his development of impulse-control, and capacities for object-relations, self-esteem regulation and self-representation.

This alternate reading of the central significance of the play shows how differently we conduct our investigation, depending on our point of view. The tendency to maintain an old official stance concerning the nuclear role of the Oedipus complex hampers our taking a fresh look at behavior in the light of our newer knowledge of the pre-Oedipal world.

The term 'transference neurosis' and the accompanying concept of the infantile neurosis are excellent examples of how the terminology seriously lags behind the thought. I have written of this elsewhere (Cooper 1987e). Very briefly, at one end of the spectrum, Simons observed that 'the transference neurosis as a new object relation in its own right and as repetition of the infantile neurosis remains a hallmark of psychoanalysis; it is what distinguishes analysis from all other psychotherapeutic endeavors' (Simons 1981: 654–655). In 1984, the 'Standards for Training in Psychoanalysis' promulgated by the Board on Professional Standards of the American Psychoanalytic Association specified as a qualification for an approved training case that 'the supervision should occur over a sufficient length of time so that the development of a transference neu-rosis, or significant transference manifestations can be observed and understood.' Freud and many later followers were explicit in maintaining that a development of a transference neurosis, itself a recapitulation within the analysis of the infantile neurosis, was a necessary event in the psychoanalytic process, during which the patient's conflicts became confined to the analysis while freeing the patient in the outer world. Analytic theory and technique have undergone vast change from the simple task of making the unconscious conscious, or undoing infantile repressions or resolving infantile conflict. Currently we consider an enlarged panorama of early and later faults, failures, deficits, deprivations, and their consequences, as well as conflict resolutions, and the enormous changes wrought during the course of development upon earlier conflicts that may no longer be germane. In this new light it is hard to give a meaning to 'infantile neurosis' or to 'transference neurosis.' Charles Brenner is explicit that 'true transference neurosis is a term, whatever meaning one gives it, that no longer should have a place in the vocabulary of psychoanalysis' (1982). Brenner may be wrong, but it is startling to note how our contemporary literature continues to use a term that is at best under contention, without acknowledgement of the vast changes in meaning if not actual meaninglessness of the concept.

A final example of keeping the words the same but changing the music has to do with the analytic situation. There has been a long debate in psychoanalysis concerning the meaning of the analytic neutrality that Freud recommended and how it translated into the analyst's behavior with his patient. From all our available accounts of Freud's own psychoanalyses, he was clearly quite free and open with his patients, kept an extensive and obviously personal archeological collection in full view and made no effort to hide the force or nature of his personality. He did, however, recommend that the analyst avoid suggestion, and maintain himself as a 'blank screen' against which the patient could project his fantasies. The late Samuel Lipton (1977) suggested that Freud himself, in his mature model of treatment, believed that these recommendations for analytic behavior were separable from the personal behaviors of the analyst, not considering the latter part of the analytic treatment. He, therefore, had no hesitation in inviting the Rat Man into the kitchen to eat a herring when he heard that his patient had not had lunch. Most of us today would consider such a split of analytic roles artificial and impossible, and would assume that all behaviors of the analyst become part of the analytic process, making their way into the transference fantasies of the patient. However, in the 1950s, partly in response to Alexander's suggestion of a flexible analytic model, including a corrective emotional experience, there was a movement to construct the so-called 'classical' model of technique. In this view, the core psychoanalytic activities were interpretation and questions, and any other analytic behavior was considered a departure from appropriate technique that would itself require analysis if the treatment were to maintain its integrity. Out of this arose the caricature description of the silent, unresponsive, unacknowledging psychoanalyst. While no one can know with great certainty what analysts do in the privacy of the treatment situation, it is likely that this caricature version sometimes approached reality, as some analysts substituted remoteness, unresponsiveness, and austerity for benign neutrality.

It was Kohut, with his emphasis on empathic responsiveness and the need for the vivid presence of the analyst for those patients whose childhoods had suffered from the remoteness of a loving parent, who revived the discussion during the past decade concerning appropriate therapeutic behavior. There were two striking features in the debate over Kohut. One was the tremendous outpouring of opposition to Kohut's idea of empathic responsiveness as a key portion of the analytic situation, and the second was the rush by analysts to assure their colleagues that they had, of course, always been empathic and human in their dealings with their patients. Although it cannot be proved, it is my impression from comparing the discussions of analytic technique today with the discussions of a decade or two ago that there has been a profound change in the climate of the analytic consulting room; the weather is warmer, and analysts have been freed to acknowledge their interest in and responsiveness to their patients – still, of course, within the limits of maintaining an analysis, but these limits are now differently perceived. Twenty – or ten – years ago, some analysts would have felt reticent to laugh at a joke told by a patient. Today, most analysts would openly enjoy the joke – and analyze it, if indicated. Again, the difference is important for anyone interested in research on the effective elements of the psychotherapeutic process. Our unchanging language – people still speak of 'classical Freudian analysis' – obscures the changes in what we do.

I hope that I have made the point that psychoanalysis has changed and is changing. Neurobiology has also been changing, and the surge of neurobiological discovery during the past two decades has led sophisticated neurobiologists to an increased interest in models of the mind. This development lends particular urgency to our clarifying our language. After all, the biologists' interest in the brain is primarily as the organ of the mind. The more subtle and interesting indications of the activities of the mind – the changing states of feelings, thoughts, relatedness, defensive capacities, etc. – are the most precise indicators of certain brain activities. It is a psychoanalytic task to provide the biologists with a comprehensive and accurate model of the mind and its functions – conscious and unconscious – and we must assure that this map is available in its up-to-date versions. The tendency for scholars in all fields, who are not themselves psychoanalysts, to read an earlier less accurate map leads to confused and misleading applications of psychoanalysis. The models of psychoanalysis that are in general use today, vastly different from the model of even 20 years ago, and sharply different from the model of Freud's metapsychology, are more amenable to cooperative work with allied disciplines such as neurobiology and ethology. The emphasis on the vicissitudes of the adaptive maneuvers mediating attachment, the emphasis on the primary needs for safety and object attachment and the signal affects that motivate behaviors, the emphasis on separation–individuation, affect development, and the study of memory and the role of learning in all these processes, are just some examples of the convergent interests of the psychoanalyst and the researcher in other fields. The development of hierarchical systems for tension regulation, and the effects of the disruption of attachment, for example, are of central interest to the analyst, ethologist, sociologist, and biologist; although they observe different phenomena by different methods, they can begin to work on concepts of the mediating events, using languages that each understands. As I have said before (1985b) in another context, this newer psychoanalysis, existing in fact and practice, sharply departing from the older model to which our language is still heir and prisoner, is less ambitious in its theory, more particulate, lacking a single overarching theory that covers all eventualities, but potentially more usable by multiple disciplines.

I have tried to show through a brief account of some history and some examples that psychoanalytic theory and practice are in a state of rapid growth and change, more so than at any time since the earliest beginnings of psychoanalysis. The continuing use of the traditional language of psychoanalysis has tended to camouflage the major changes that are occurring within this field of study. While there have been historical and political reasons for our bashfulness about our advances, our failure to announce clearly our changing ideas has hindered our educational activities, has slowed the acceptance of psychoanalysis among the sciences, and has interfered with the most fruitful collaboration with the disciplines at our boundaries. It is my hope, and prediction, that psychoanalysis, now maturing as a science and profession, will increasingly resemble other established disciplines in the eagerness of our academic and research leadership to delineate clearly our latest advances, and to accept the fact that our best ideas have ever shorter half-lives. Freud's writings, certainly one of the great bodies of literature of all time, will remain an endless source of inspiration, but we will not forever be able to preserve his terminology.

5

COMMENTS ON FREUD'S 'ANALYSIS TERMINABLE AND INTERMINABLE'*

'Analysis terminable and interminable' (Freud 1937a) was written in 1937, two years before Freud's death. It is a work that several generations of psychoanalysts have found engrossing, puzzling, rich in ideas as well as disturbing because of its apparent pessimism. This paper was written after Freud had endured decades of suffering with cancer of the jaw and had undergone many operations. He had witnessed the rise of Nazism and was aware of the imminence of world war. He had also experienced the extraordinary success of psychoanalysis as a movement of thought in the Western world and his ideas had triumphed over those of his detractors and competitors. Freud, however, never acknowledged this victory, maintaining that civilization by its nature could not be friendly to him and his ideas. In 1936, as he was being deluged with birthday congratulations and honors on his 80th birthday, he wrote to Marie Bonaparte: 'I am not easily deceived, and I know that the attitude of the world towards me and my work is really no friendlier than twenty years ago. Nor do I any longer wish for any change in it, no "happy end" as in the cinema' (Jones 1957: 202).

Freud, more than anyone, had been responsible for the change that occurred after the early days of analytic triumph in the cure of the symptomatic neuroses with dramatic results in short treatments (although today, as we review the early cases, the results were often less dramatic than they at first seemed). In the later period, there was an increasing demand on analysis to achieve more in the way of 'deep' or 'structural' change, and a tendency for a dismissive attitude toward mere symptom relief as transference cure. Freud himself had always been wary about the possibility that analytic results emanated from suggestion rather than

* A version of this paper was first published in 1987 (Cooper 1987i); reproduced with permission of the International Psychoanalytical Association.

from specific interpretation, and that concern has not yet vanished from psychoanalysis. In trying to understand Freud's thinking in 'Analysis terminable and interminable' it would be interesting to know how much analysis Freud himself was doing in the preceding few years, and what the duration of those analyses was; however, I have not been able to find this information.

Against this background it may be no surprise to find that this work is a restatement of some of Freud's most conservative points of view concerning psychoanalysis. However, at the same time, it is a questioning of the status of psychoanalytic treatment and a daring foray into those aspects of psychoanalysis that some current workers consider the most advanced front of the field. As I shall try to illustrate, the conservatism lies in Freud's tenacity in retaining his metapsychology intact, and in maintaining his focus on the neuroses rather than the character disorders, despite the advances of ego psychology that he initiated. His adventurousness lies in his opening the way to an understanding of the psychoanalytic process as an endless quest. But there is much more in the paper than these two concerns, and I shall discuss some of the other thoughts that a reading of it generates.

This paper seems different, in both tone and intent, from some others written during the same period. 'Constructions in analysis' (Freud 1937b) published in the same year, follows the more typical form of a Freud paper, beginning with a modest disclaimer of having anything new to say, followed by a bold and interesting idea – the understanding of delusions as an attempt at self-curative psychological construction based on an item of historical fact. Delusions were thus parallel to the analyst's use of history in creating constructions with his neurotic patient. 'Moses and monotheism' (Freud 1939), worked on only a little earlier (although it was published later), is, like a late Beethoven quartet, the work of the aged, sick, tormented master fearlessly pushing his genius beyond where anyone has ever trodden before. 'Analysis terminable and interminable' is, in contrast, more of a presentation of the technical and theoretical problems confronting the analytic method at its present limits, a bit of summing up. Part of the fascination of the paper may derive from the slightly forbidding tone it takes toward analytic therapeutic enthusiasm. It is almost as if Freud is telling the numerous followers he has now accumulated to review their fervor for the method he has taught them, and to ponder the limits of their capability. Freud is also, perhaps, informing these followers that he will not permit them easy profit and pleasure from his own hard-won findings, letting them know that they are not yet on solid ground, and that much hard work and new information are needed. At its best psychoanalysis is not a comfortable profession. In fact, it is an 'impossible' one.

Freud begins with a discussion of the social and financial desirability of shortening analysis, a goal even more to be desired today when analyses tend to be so lengthy. He quickly concludes (p. 224) that in the light of more modern demands for what analysis ought to be able to do, analysis will surely not get shorter (p. 219). He discusses the practical aspects of ending analysis. 'This happens when two conditions have been approximately fulfilled: first, that the patient shall no longer be suffering from his symptoms and shall have overcome his anxieties and his inhibitions; and secondly, that the analyst shall judge that so much repressed material has been made conscious, so much of internal resistance conquered, that there is no need to fear repetition of the pathological processes concerned.'

Freud then describes the theoretical meaning of the end of analysis, stating: 'the analyst has had such a far-reaching influence on the patient that no further change could be expected to take place in him if his analysis were continued' (p. 219). These ambitious goals, and this distinctive idea of the ideal termination form the backdrop for the remainder of the discussion.

The question of shortening analysis soon gives way to several others. He briefly refers to how analysis works, assuming that basically we know the answer to that problem and have little to add. 'Instead of an enquiry into how a cure by analysis comes about (a matter which I think has been sufficiently elucidated) the question should be asked of what are the obstacles that stand in the way of such a cure' (p. 221). Freud seems to be closing the book on what analysis is and what its technical capacities are. He goes on, however, to raise questions about how we can tell when the process has been completed, and he reminds us that an analysis is not an event or a structure in itself, such as a work of art, which may be examined in isolation from its context. It is rather a piece of a patient's life, and in that sense can never stand alone but can be examined only as a part of the patient's ongoing experience. He reviews the impediments to a 'complete' analysis, for example conflicts resistant to analysis because the original trauma was too great or because the instinct was too powerful, conflicts unanalyzable because they are not active during the span of the analysis, and insurmountable obstacles arising from derivatives of the death instinct. Finally, there are those hurdles that seem inherent in the elemental castration fear as it manifests itself differently in men and women. He questions how we can know that any successful analysis has produced a 'permanent' cure, in the sense of 'taming' an instinctual demand (p. 225), so that it will not again produce deformations of the ego in its defensive struggle with the instinct. He is explicit that his views on the analytic process have been influenced by his experience of doing training analyses, and by treating severely ill patients in unending, although interrupted, treatment. 'There was no question of shortening the treatment; the purpose was radically to exhaust the possibilities of illness in them and to bring about a deep-going alteration of their personality' (p. 224).

Early in the paper, Freud states the position that dominates the early part of his discussion, revealing the unusually conservative view of analytic work that I mentioned earlier. After defining (p. 225) health as a successful taming of instinct ('That is to say, the instinct is brought completely into the harmony of the ego, becomes accessible to all the influences of the other trends in the ego and no longer seeks to go its independent way to satisfaction'), Freud makes two interesting methodological decisions. First, he decides that, in choosing between ego and instinct, the important variable to be studied is the instinct. Second, he asserts that an understanding of instinct cannot be conducted on clinical grounds but can be approached only through metapsychology. The first decision, to focus on instinct rather than on the ego and its interactions with the environment, is crucial. Despite the great advances of ego psychology and the increasing interest in the superego, Freud returns to his earliest metapsychology, laying the greatest stress on the quantity of instinct and assuming that life can best be understood as the outcome of the struggle of the ego, the representative of civilization, against the instinct that is always inimical toward the ego's aims. The constancy of this view in Freud's theory as well as in his personal philosophy is reflected in the quotation given above from the letter to Marie Bonaparte, in which he refuses to acknowledge the possibility of a friendly cultural attitude towards him and psychoanalysis. We should note that Heinz Hartmann was soon to publish his work on the preadaptedness of the instincts and on the conflict-free sphere of the ego (Hartmann 1937). It seems likely that Freud knew of Hartmann's ideas but this did not influence his work at all. He even seems to be cutting the ground from under Anna Freud and her advocacy of ego analysis and the analysis of defense as being at the core of our analytic work. While Freud is fully cognizant of this position, it interests him less than does a return to his earlier views of instinct. In effect, having described mental health as requiring a balance of id and ego strengths, he chooses to regard the ego's activities as a constant. He examines the consequences of changes in the force of an instinct and also those occasions in life when instinctual force increases, thereby rendering most defensive work impotent. It is almost as if Freud is putting a brake on ego psychology, and on the direction it would take in the future in its emphasis on developmental vicissitudes.

This impression is reinforced by his second methodological decision, when he addresses the question of how instincts are tamed. Rather than pursue this as a clinical issue, perhaps by tracing the affective aspects of the transference, with affects being seen as the mental representation of instincts, Freud decides that the only way to consider the question of taming the instincts is through the 'witch' metapsychology. Using a famous phrase, he says, 'If we are asked by what methods and means this result [taming the instinct] is achieved, it is not easy to find an answer. We can only say: "So muss denn doch die Hexe dran!" – the Witch Metapsychology. Without metapsychological speculation and theorizing – I had almost said "phantasying" – we shall not get another step forward. Unfortunately, here as elsewhere, what our Witch reveals is neither very clear nor very detailed' (p. 225). It is worth noting that despite whatever pessimism, or perhaps even depression, may color this paper, Freud never loses his wit, his pleasure in irony, his literary grace and his total honesty with himself.

Our current attitudes towards the concepts of instinct-taming, one of the central ideas of Freud's early metapsychology, are vastly changed. The work of a generation of infant-observers and child psychoanalysts has cast serious doubt upon the validity of that idea. If we follow Freud in viewing the affects as the mental representatives of the instincts, Robert Emde (1981) and Daniel Stern (1985), in their work on affect development and on the development of the infant's tie to the mother, have independently concluded that the concept of affect taming or instinct taming does not accurately represent what happens in development. The evidence indicates that the infant is at no point confronted with more instinctual charge or affect than he or she is biologically wired to handle. It must also be understood, however, that there is a vast change in point of view reflected in these current studies. The unit under study in the very young infant is the infant–mother pair, not the infant alone. There is increasing agreement among psychoanalysts that an interpersonal and object-relational point of view is essential when conceptualizing the baby's mental life, and one cannot speak of the infant alone, since biology and society both dictate that the infant's affective (instinctual) life is regulated by the mother–infant dyad. In this view it becomes impossible to quantify instinct or affect, since whatever is constitutional always and immediately interacts with behaviors of the caretaker towards the expression of those tendencies. Furthermore, the behaviors of the mother favor the expression of certain aims and the suppression, or perhaps even the deletion, of others. Contrary to Freud's strategy, the contemporary developmentalist is more likely to accept the infant's constitution (instinctual endowment) as relatively constant (although recognizing the importance of temperamental differences) and is consequently more likely to study the variable of mother–infant adaptation.

This brings us to Freud's second decision, i.e. to study instinct-taming metapsychologically rather than clinically. It follows from what we have been describing that contemporary interest is likely to focus on the tension-regulating, soothing and self-controlling capacities that begin to be internalized within the mother–infant dyad. Although theory-guided, the important studies of the workers we have mentioned, as well as those of Sandler (1983), Bowlby (1969) and Mahler (1972), have all been efforts at clinical understanding. Under ordinary circumstances of childrearing, the infant, enjoying the mediating and modulating effects of mothering, is in no greater danger from uncontrolled instinct or affect expression than is the older child or adult, who has largely, but never completely, internalized his regulation processes. The seemingly raw affective expressions of the infant are actually beautifully designed and quite effective for gaining appropriate mothering response. Further, there is reason to consider that the bawling young infant does not yet have fully fledged psychological experiences, so that the question of the ego's being overwhelmed is not apposite. When he has a psychologically significant experience of frustration it seems likely that it is perceived as part of an interaction with a caretaker rather than as a totally internal event. Tension regulation, a developing task for the growing infant, is probably not quite the same as instinct regulation. However, tensions resulting from dysphoric affects are reasonably subject to study. Instincts, as Freud correctly points out, can only be considered metapsychologically.

If we turn to the questions put by Freud concerning the circumstances for the outbreak of psychic illness, it is likely that we would now decide differently in choosing the questions and methods for study. We would be interested in the changes in the environment and in object-relations that could interfere with the ego's regulatory and control functions, and we would choose to study these circumstances clinically rather than metapsychologically. We would be concerned with how affects, object-relatedness and self develop in organizational complexity and subtlety, and in how the infant develops his or her own modulating and self-soothing capacities. Freud, in the language of his time, was also interested in these matters, as he makes abundantly clear in his exposition when, for example, he compares the achievements in analysis with those of the normally developing ego. Why, then, should Freud have relinquished clinical observation in favor of metapsychological considerations? I do not know, but I will suggest two possible reasons. The first is that he lacked our current knowledge of infant development, and the second that he feared the loss of the distinctiveness of psychoanalytic psychology if the theory of instincts was significantly modified. This modification of the dual instinct theory, if not an outright abandonment of it, has occurred in contemporary psychoanalysis – in my opinion to the benefit of psychoanalytic theory and technique. Freud, and Anna Freud after him, were perhaps fearful of the 'widening scope of psychoanalysis' and the resulting tendency towards broadening of psychoanalytic conceptualizations. As I indicated above, it would be interesting to know if Freud was now also some distance from clinical psychoanalysis in his personal work, perhaps not having undertaken a new lengthy analysis for some years, and hence more drawn to theory.

We should also be aware that the challenge to the concept of instinct primacy was already developing during Freud's lifetime. Strachey's (1934) paper on analytic cure was written shortly before the paper we are discussing. In it he emphasizes the analyst's role as an object whose internalization helps in modifying the superego, the real agent of cure. I do not know whether Freud knew of Strachey's paper. It is of interest that, more recently, Loewald (1960, 1970), eager to conserve Freud's metapsychology, including the concept of instinct, has nonetheless felt obliged to alter his metapsychological ideas quite radically. He fully abandons the primordial antagonism of instinct and ego, adopting views much closer to Winnicott and others, and assumes that instinct and ego both develop out of a mother–infant matrix. One cannot even imagine the instincts apart from their developmental matrix. Here, again, ideas of instinct-taming give way to a newer model of mutual adaptation, in which the object of study is the mental structure of object-representations. One's aim can then be to assess the pliancy of the system and its accessibility to psychoanalytic alteration. We come closer here to clinical assessment, rather than to metapsychological speculation. The anti-metapsychology movement begun by George Klein may have gone too far in its effort to bring psychoanalysis back to its clinical roots, but we should surely welcome every opportunity to keep our discussion of a clinical issue such as termination of analysis on a clinical level. Freud was right in saying that he called upon metapsychology as a last resort, but as we would now see it, he had not yet reached the last resort clinically.

Throughout his discussion of clinical issues in this paper, Freud tends to assume that conflicts are relatively isolated from one another, and that the ego has at its disposal specific repressive defenses directed toward each early instinctual conflict. He says, 'the real achievement of analytic therapy would be the subsequent correction of the original process of repression, correction which puts an end to the dominance of the quantitative factor' (p. 227). He goes on to express his doubt that this is ever realized, and thus his belief that the quantitative factor remains paramount. In a brilliant discussion of the treatment of neurosis Freud continues this line of thought, discussing the rigidity of the neurotic ego that results from its being locked in battle against an infantile danger. 'The crux of the matter is that the defensive mechanisms directed against former danger recur in the treatment as *resistances* against recovery itself as a new danger' (p. 238). Many contemporary analysts would add that the prospect of change is viewed as a danger by the neurotic ego not only because it threatens the awakening of forbidden impulses, but also because any change of ego function or attitude threatens the sense of safety and coherence represented by the habitual and familiar. As Freud himself points out (p. 238), 'The adult's ego . . . finds itself compelled to seek out those situations in reality which can serve as an approximate substitute for the original danger, *so as to be able to justify, in relation to them, its maintaining its habitual modes of reaction to them*' (emphasis added). One might interpret this as indicating that the ego is more concerned with its own coherence and consistency than with the original danger. A key question concerning adult pathology is the degree to which the current problem is the continuing need to avoid an original danger, or is the process of miscarried repair itself, rigidified and internally perceived as the essential self. Today there is no agreement on this issue.

All of this brings us to the interesting question Freud raises concerning the ability of analysis to insure the patient against future neurotic illness resulting from the revival of a conflict that is dormant at the time of the analysis. He concludes that such an assurance is not likely, since in analysis we cannot artificially revive a dormant conflict that causes the patient no anxiety at the time. Nor can we strengthen the ego against it since it is inactive, and therefore the defenses involved do not appear in the analytic process. Many analysts today see the psyche as a fully interconnected web – enter at any point, and in principle, one has access to every other point. But Freud, the discoverer of so many different strands of psychic life, tended to think of them as more separated.

One could, adopting the view of widespread internal connection, assume that an ego with a new degree of internal coherence and flexibility could handle the activation of a conflict even without analysis of the specific, previously dormant, conflictual matter. I will return to this interesting question at the end of this discussion, when I examine the narrative view of psychoanalysis in relation to termination. At issue is the question of the primacy of psychic conflict as a determinant of neurosis as opposed to the prominence given to the weakness or abnormality of the structure of the self or ego. Again, although analysts have generally veered from the rather strict isolation of conflicts that Freud implies, there surely is no agreement today concerning how far we should venture from Freud's view. It is conspicuous that in this paper, unlike some earlier ones, Freud gives little attention to what we would now call the world of internal objects. In essence he avoids any aspect of mental representation except for the direct awakening of the original trauma. He also gives relatively little attention to the character disorders, which in modern psychoanalysis have rather fully replaced the neuroses as the objects of therapeutic intent. In fact, a number of the avenues of interest that had been opened up in 'Inhibitions, symptoms and anxiety' (1926a), particularly the opportunity to expand upon the role of affect in mental life and neurosis, are omitted.

Freud goes on to discuss some questions about psychic structure and gives a remarkably advanced view of the inheritance of personality characteristics, concluding that the fact that the ego has inherited (biological) characteristics removes the topographical distinction between ego and id. This leads him to a discussion of those special resistances that cannot be localized in a structure that seem 'to depend on fundamental conditions in the mental apparatus' (p. 241). He describes (1) adhesiveness of libido, (2) excessively mobile libido and (3) excessive rigidity. I find this listing fascinating, because these three groups represent precisely those patients thought of today as suffering from forms of severe character disorder. These are of particular interest because of what we can learn from them about pre-Oedipal development, and because of the presence of excessive separation anxiety, often in personality structures. The first group would be regarded as forms of panic anxiety with potential phobia formation. We would probably agree that there are important genetic elements in such characters, but we would look to pre-Oedipal development for an understanding of the clinging, unadventurous nature of these patients. Many of them prove to be responsive to a variety of anti-depressant and anxiolytic pharmacologic agents. The patients in the second group would probably be considered under the rubric of narcissism, analyzed in terms of a defective structure of the self that either fears attachment or has an incapacity for affective linkage. Again, we would now be interested in the nature of the object-relatedness that had developed in the earliest years and its revival in the transference. The third group is perhaps the most puzzling. One may raise questions about the plasticity of their neuronal structures as well as about their psyches. They are likely to be viewed as having suffered excessive pre-Oedipal damage from failure to establish empathic ties to caretaking persons. While we might share Freud's therapeutic pessimism, we would try to explore the narcissistic wounds that this rigidity may defend against. It is also perfectly clear that we are little, if at all, wiser today than Freud was in understanding this premature hardening of the psychodynamic arteries.

In continuing his exploration of the elements that make for therapeutic success or failure, Freud discusses those characteristics of the analyst that make him effective. He expects 'a considerable degree of mental normality and correctness,' so that his defects will not interfere with his assessment of and his response to the patient. He also 'must possess some kind of superiority, so that in certain analytic situations he can act as a model for his patient and in others as a teacher' (p. 248). Finally, the analyst must have a love of truth. These attributes are interesting in the light of the common joke today that some of the analysts of Freud's generation were so 'crazy' that they would not be accepted for analytic training today. Despite his devotion to his concept of 'psychic reality,' Freud unabashedly maintains that the analyst's view of reality is superior to that of his patient, and that it is necessary for the analyst to be someone who can be idealized. He clearly means that the analyst should have traits that *deserve* to be idealized. He is not referring simply to the patient's transference tendency to idealize. Freud states these personal characteristics with no attempt to relate them to the theory of analytic therapy he has been discussing. But a very different theory of analytic change is implied in the idea of the patient modeling himself on a superior person, or internalizing a good object, than is implied in the idea of undoing repressions via interpretation. These two halves of the theory of cure are not discussed by Freud in this paper, although he often alludes to them elsewhere. The interpersonal context of the treatment process cannot be expressed easily in the language of the intrapsychic conflict – a problem that remains in analytic theory.

It is curious that Freud, while acknowledging the increasing complexity, depth and time that analysis takes, recommends for the analyst in training only a 'short and incomplete' analysis for 'practical reasons' that are not stated. Its purpose is simply to give a 'firm conviction of the existence of the unconscious.' Freud counts on the 'processes of remodeling the ego' continuing spontaneously in the course of the young analyst's education and experience. Why should a short analysis continue spontaneously and satisfactorily for analysts and not for other creatures? Presumably this is because analysts are constantly immersed in psychodynamic processes, and once convinced of the unconscious, will continue to change themselves. One might infer that their model for the superior person of the analyst is Freud himself, and he takes it for granted that anyone committed to psychoanalysis will in a sense unconsciously continue to be his analysand.

At the same time Freud refers to the constant churning up of instinctual demands in the course of doing analytic work, as a source of danger. As a result he suggests that 'Every analyst should periodically – at intervals of five years or so – submit himself to analysis once more, without feeling ashamed of taking this step. This would mean, then, that not only the therapeutic analysis of patients but his own analysis would change from a terminable into an interminable task' (p. 249). It is safe to say that present-day psychoanalysts do not follow Freud's recommendation. Despite the frequency of second analyses, they are usually undertaken out of dissatisfaction with the training analysis or because of a life crisis, and not because of a sense of accumulating instinctual pressure and the weakening of defenses. Should we interpret this as a failure of the seriousness of modern psychoanalysts or as an indication that Freud was incorrect in suggesting that analytic work increased the instinctual danger to the practitioner? I suggest the latter hypothesis. If we abandon the instinctual perspective, then we might consider that being a psychoanalyst is good for one's mental health. The opportunity to review the myriad defense mechanisms displayed by our patients and the almost automatic (and perhaps inevitable) comparison of one's own intrapsychic activity with what one has viewed in a patient, provide innumerable opportunities to bring pre-conscious thoughts and feelings into consciousness. On occasion, even previous unconscious conflicts may be brought to consciousness. I believe that the analyst's position of helping others provides a relatively guilt-free opportunity for acknowledging one's own difficulties, with the disclaimer 'The patient is worse off than I.' While all sorts of instinctual arousals do occur in the course of conducting psychoanalysis, they are carefully bounded by the analytic situation, for the most part posing little threat of action and their detection is condoned – even rewarded – by the code that demands constant self-scrutiny for precisely these currents within ourselves. Our ethic assumes that we bear in ourselves all the flaws in our patients, in different mixtures and quantities. We are also aware that the psychoanalyst in his professional role is not quite the same person as elsewhere in his life. In our protected role as psychoanalysts we are generally able to be far more selfless and empathic than in our life situations in which we may perceive the threats to our feelings of safety far more keenly. It was a part of Freud's genius to design the psychoanalytic situation so that the psychoanalyst is skillfully protected from psychic risk.

In the last section of the paper, Freud returns to one of his recurrent themes, the consequences of the anatomical distinction between the sexes. Here he finds a piece of the bedrock of psychoanalytic possibilities. In one of those statements that aroused feminine ire, he refers to the 'repudiation of femininity,' as it appears in both sexes, as a 'remarkable feature in the psychical life of human beings' (p. 250). He rejects Ferenczi's claim of having successfully analysed female penis envy and the male fear of passivity towards another male. He says:

> At no other point in one's analytic work does one suffer more from an oppressive feeling that all one's repeated efforts have been in vain, and from a suspicion that one has been 'preaching to the winds,' than when one is trying

to persuade a woman to abandon her wish for a penis on the ground of its being unrealizable or when one is seeking to convince a man that a passive attitude to men does not always signify castration and that it is indispensable in many relationships in life. The rebellious overcompensation of the male produces one of the strongest transference-resistances. He refuses to subject himself to a father-substitute, or to feel indebted to him for anything, and consequently he refuses to accept his recovery from the doctor. No analogous transference can arise from the female's wish for a penis, but it is the source of outbreaks of severe depression in her, owing to an internal conviction that the analysis will be of no use and nothing can be done to help her. And we can only agree that she is right, when we learn that her strongest motive in coming for treatment was the hope that, after all, she might still obtain a male organ, the lack of which was so painful to her. But we also learn from this that it is not important in what form the resistance appears, whether as a transference or not. The decisive thing remains that the resistance prevents any change from taking place – that everything stays as it was. We often have the impression that with the wish for a penis and the masculine protest we have penetrated through all the psychological strata and have reached bedrock, and that thus our activities are at an end. This is probably true, since, for the psychical field, the biological field does in fact play the part of the underlying bedrock. The repudiation of femininity can be nothing else than a biological fact, a part of the great riddle of sex. It would be hard to say whether and when we have succeeded in mastering this factor in an analytic treatment. We can only console ourselves with the certainty that we have given the person analysed every possible encouragement to re-examine and alter his attitude to it.

(pp. 252–253)

With these remarks Freud ends his paper, and his conclusion is a curious one, for it calls upon biology to explain a clinical difficulty rather than sticking to analytic tools to try to understand, on purely psychoanalytic grounds, why castration anxiety is so intractable. This parallels Freud's earlier strategy in his paper when he reverts to metapsychology to understand how instincts are tamed. Possibly Freud was loath to return to the pre-Oedipal themes that he almost reluctantly uncovered in his paper on 'Female sexuality' (1931). In an earlier paper (1986), I have suggested that castration anxiety attains its central role in mental life as the representative closest to consciousness of deeper, pre-Oedipal anxieties related to the loss of identity or boundary or body – to some form of annihilation fear related to earliest states of the forming self. Freud's reluctance to see the bedrock of psychic development as prior to the Oedipal phase seems particularly relevant in understanding his conclusions. It is almost as if he set the boundaries to psychoanalysis by claiming that whatever was beyond castration anxiety was pure biology.

We should note several points. Few analysts would agree that for the woman patient her 'strongest motive in coming to treatment was the hope that, after all, she might still obtain a male organ.' Rather, without challenging the existence of penis envy, we believe that a significant portion of penis envy relates not to anatomy but to two aspects of penis symbolization – the penis as representative of male privilege and the penis as a representation of successful separation from the powerful mother of the pre-Oedipal period. There are also important problems of self-esteem and object-relations that are not reducible to penis envy in any form. Freud gave no attention to the social attitudes towards femininity. His lack of interest in these concerns may relate to a hesitation to perturb or interfere with the assumption of unquestioned male authority. This may have impeded his capacity to analyze penis envy to a deeper layer.

The fascinating question of the masculine protest – the inability of a man to accept a passive attitude towards another man – is still quite unresolved. There is an implied demand on Freud's part for submission to him by his male patients – in fact, by all his patients. Treatment requires the patient's acceptance of subjection to the father, or at least acceptance of the idea that he receives his recovery from the doctor. Freud seems to treat this as a fact, rather than as a fantasy to be analyzed. He seems to believe that the resistance to the passivity involved in the treatment situation refers to actual passivity in a real relationship with another person, the analyst, rather than to a frightening fantasy of passivity that is aroused in some fearful males. There is a fine but important line between accepting the recovery from the doctor and accepting with gratitude the doctor's role as *facilitator* of a recovery, for which the patient is responsible. Today, many analysts would understand certain key aspects of passivity as being readily traceable to conflicts with the mother. In this view fear of passivity towards another male would represent a displacement of an earlier fear of a powerful mother. Alternately, we observe homosexuals who are eager to be passive with another man, while unconsciously enacting fantasies of being at the mercy of an all-powerful mother. Freud may have been right in his view of the bedrock, but it is worth querying his conclusion that the masculine protest and penis envy are basic fears, rather than reflecting other underlying wishes and fears that may be analyzed. It would be preferable not to be in the theoretically uncomfortable position of having to assume that nature constructed a masculine world in which all females are doomed to special discomfort because of a biological antagonism to being feminine.

The idea of analytic bedrock (or 'interminability') poses the question of what in the individual personality is inaccessible to analytic exploration, even if it does affect the analytic process. Freud's idea of the repetition compulsion would fit this description, being seen as a force in mental life, perhaps derived from the death instinct and not amenable to verbal exploration. This is implicit in his idea that 'the presence of a power in mental life which we call the instinct of aggression or of destruction according to its aims, and which we trace back to the original death instinct of living matter' (p. 243), a power that is resistant to health or change, accounts for masochism and the negative therapeutic reaction. From a different point of view, a similar idea was put forth by Winnicott (1960) when he wrote of the normal adult as an 'isolate' protecting himself from any intrusion in his true self. Some analysts have long held the view that our patients do not thank us for truly successful analyses that violate the innermost sense of the self. Many of our better analyzed cases remember very little of the analytic process and establish new and firm boundaries against outside intrusions of such depth. Assuming that there is a certain health involved in the protection of the inner self from intrusion, the more ambitious the analysis becomes, not only will it become more difficult, but it may also begin to cross into relatively non-psychological areas of early pre-Oedipal patterning that are only analyzable, at least initially, by their non-verbal manifestations, rather than as free associations. These problems seem much more like a bedrock of analysis than the clinical obstacles described by Freud.

Apart from the particular arguments that Freud put forth in various parts of his paper, we should bear in mind what his overall clinical conclusions are, and whether they ring true to our own analytic experience. Freud reminds us that we have no clear end-points for termination in cases of character neurosis. We would have to agree. He reminds us too of the immanent nature of resistance to change in psychoanalysis. Whether or not one believes in a death instinct, I believe that most analysts are struck by the sluggish pace of analytic change, the seemingly endless repetition required during the analysis of transference and resistance, and the ubiquity of masochistic phenomena. Freud is surely right in his attitude of skepticism toward dramatic analytic success (p. 229). He empha-sizes how small a role is played by knowledge itself and how the importance of the patient's depth of conviction concerning what he has learned about himself in analysis is critical. In fact, depth of conviction concerning the nature of the unconscious is considered by Freud to be the most important achievement of the training analysis. Again, we recognize the old problem of 'knowing' versus 'knowing' in analysis. Indeed, one could go on with a long list of Freud's extra-ordinary insights in this paper.

Finally, I want to discuss one of the ideas implicit in this essay that reaches to the very edge of modern literary and philosophical views about how we construct our universe. An important contemporary view of the psychoanalytic process brings to psychoanalysis ideas that originated in literary criticism, although they are foreshadowed in Freud's paper. Psychoanalysis, according to the hermeneutic view, is a process of narrative construction. Analyst and patient work together to create, during the course of the analysis, increasingly complex, coherent, and complete versions of the patient's life story. Beyond its most primitive core, the self consists of the history or narrative that links together the infinity of thoughts, feelings, and actions that constitute the person. In 'Analysis terminable and interminable' Freud anticipates the most modern trend in contemporary literary criticism in suggesting that the person or life story or narrative never comes to genuine closure; there is no ending. Frank Kermode, a literary critic, suggests in *The Art of Telling* (1972) that there is no closure or genuine ending (termination, if you wish) to any great novel. This lack of ending is explicit in the modern novel, but novels have always been designed to provide for the continuing life of the characters and continuing narrative interpretation. That is why any good novel is pertinent to any age and generates endless new exegesis of its text. Analysis, as Freud describes it in this paper, as well as literary criticism, generates endless endings; another version or interpretation of the story is always possible and every re-reading will generate additional meanings.

Kermode points out that the idea of a clear ending to a story is relatively new and was unknown in medieval literature, in which several different versions of a story existed side by side, with significant alterations of the tale, and with no sense of contradiction. The modern narrative view of psychoanalysis, with its emphasis on large constructions rather than our narrow interpretation of conflict, assumes that there are always multiple possibilities. As with great novels, any human personality will appear different and will be differently understood under different conditions. For the novel, the different circumstance is the different culture that provides a reader who has a different understanding. For analysis a different circumstance is a new set of transference–countertransference relationships, and this difference can be regarded as occurring anew in each session or (more grossly) at different periods of a patient's life or with different analysts.

From this point of view the questions that Freud raises of reawakening dormant conflicts take on a different perspective. As indicated above, analysts are less likely to view conflicts as sequestered, each one having its own set of special defenses devoted to it. Taking a narrative point of view we are likely to view the personality as intertwined, a complex skein in which all the knots are linked. Unraveling may proceed from any point and will lead towards all other points. Conflicts are not isolated but are ongoing aspects of the total personality, and the working through of some conflicts of significance will begin to have effects on those not apparent on the surface. It is a common experience, when doing analysis, that symptoms that have not been addressed during the analytic work disappear as a result of the reorganization of aspects of the character that were germane to other issues. Frequently, for example, mild phobias, sexual symptoms, and eating disorders 'self-cure' in the course of an analysis that may be addressing narcissistic problems. Freud speaks as if the repertoire of conflicts is already encapsulated within the individual, to be uncovered by analysis. Many contemporary analysts are inclined to think of conflicts as unending, creative human acts, and that the overall level of personality organization will determine whether or not any one has pathological consequences. The issue of interminable analysis is not one of reawakening dormant conflicts, but a realization that different perspectives on the person will always arise in the course of adaptation to new life situations. The adaptation of the personality in such different situations will bring different conflicts to the fore, and some of them will not have been capable of being predicted.

Having discussed many different points of view, I wish to emphasize that we end in agreement with Freud. The 'therapeutic' analysis is not one that has analyzed all dormant conflicts but is one that has enabled a sufficient reorganization of ego capacities to take place so that there is a greater coherence of conscious and unconscious elements. There is an acceptance of unconscious trends into consciousness so that new aspects of unconscious conflicts and wishes can be available to an ego that is neither rigidly hostile to the unconscious trend nor passively intimidated before the evidence of an unacceptable wish. Beyond all the technical problems posed by Freud, this is his basic position. Analysis is indeed interminable as the human personality is constantly recreating itself. Our job as analysts is to try to push beyond the bedrock that Freud encountered, to increase this human possibility.

PART II

Challenging the boundaries
of psychoanalysis

6

WILL NEUROBIOLOGY
INFLUENCE PSYCHOANALYSIS?*

Psychoanalysis may be characterized as an attempt to decode, that is, interpret, a patient's communications according to a loosely drawn set of transformational rules concerning underlying meaning, motivations, and unities of thought. The analyst does his best to understand the patient's communications as the patient intends them to be, but both patient and analyst are heavily influenced by a theory, or a group of theories, used by both parties. For example, patients have theories about the nature of responsibility and the causal agents of behavior; these theories may range from extremes of conviction that 'everything is my fault' to 'nothing is my fault' or from 'I intended to do that' to 'something made me do that.' Patients have theories about the nature of their motivation; some are convinced that all their actions are altruistic, while others believe that their most innocent thoughts are evidence of their murderous intent. Patients have theories about the sources of their behavior; some are firmly convinced that all their actions are explained by the nature of their nurturance, and others are convinced that only a bad fate could explain their lives.

We take for granted that these theories, no matter how firmly held, reflect defensive needs and are to be regarded as an entry to different – we usually imply deeper – aspects of the patient's personality. We also assume that all human beings weave their experience and their capacities into a holistic way of understanding themselves and their world and create a theory that provides some degree of comfort. At high levels, these theories may be philosophies, religions, and life attitudes.

Analysts also have a range of available theories with which we are all familiar. While we share many things in common, it makes a difference whether we see

* A version of this paper was first presented at the Babcock Symposium of the Pittsburgh Psychoanalytic Institute in 1984. It was later published as Cooper (1985b) 'Will neurobiology influence psychoanalysis?', *American Journal of Psychiatry*, 142: 1395–1402; reproduced with permission of American Psychiatric Publishing, Inc. www.appi.org

the world through Freud's lens, or Schafer's, Kohut's, Kernberg's, or our own variation of how to view analytic data. The theory will determine how the analyst shapes the patient's material so that he will have the benefit of theory that the patient has; that is, he too will be able to have a holistic, seemingly rational, view that will explain the entirety of his patient's behavior and provide the analyst with a bit of needed comfort and confidence in his professional world. Theories also lead us, no matter how we may try to be merely the recipient of the patient's story, to collaborate with the patient in creating a new personal myth, a life narrative more acceptable to analyst and patient. If we believe that the Oedipus complex is central in neurosis, any patient will provide ample opportunity for demonstrating the existence, vitality, and significance of Oedipal fantasies. If we believe that pre-Oedipal arrests or fixations are determinants, again it is a rare patient who does not provide adequate opportunity to construct the life story so that pre-Oedipal issues will occupy a central place.

I am not nihilistic about the role of theory. I do not think that theories do not matter; rather, I think they matter crucially. But until we have better ways of testing our theories, different theories will coexist, and we will go on, consciously or unconsciously, intentionally or unwittingly, educating our patients to see the world as our theory has already told us the world is. This is inevitable. Because there is a paucity of validating strategies in psychoanalysis, it is important that analytic theories not be out of touch with developing new knowledge in areas adjoining our own area of interest, lest they become idiosyncratic and isolated from the mainstreams of science and the humanities. Information from other disciplines may provide a check on our own findings and theories.

The question posed by my title could be phrased another way: 'What are the possibilities that anything found in neurobiology will change the way an analyst hears his patient talking?' It may be instructive to examine, as an example, the relationship of direct child observation to psychoanalysis. There has always been and still is a significant group of analysts who have maintained that child research is interesting and even worth knowing for its own sake or for some yet unforeseen purpose but has no relevance to the analytic situation in which we are interested solely in the psychic reality verbally conveyed by the patient rather than infantile reality observed by the investigator. That is, psychoanalysis in its working mode accepts as data of infancy only the patient's construction of it or our interpretive understanding of the patient's construction of it and not the so-called objective data.

Despite this claim, however, most of us have seen a quiet revolution in analytic theory and practice secondary to the work of investigators as different as Mahler and Bowlby. Whether or not one subscribes to all their views, the data on the central role in development of attachment behaviors and their consequences in separation–individuation have led most analysts to give far more emphasis to these aspects of development in their reconstruction of patients' lives, to give greater weight to the interpersonal and object-relational portions of the developmental narrative, and to look more closely at pre-Oedipal issues than was the case when libidinal and aggressive drives were seen as more simply derived. Furthermore, the recent and ongoing discoveries of the spectacular range of cognitive and affective capacities of the very young infant, with evidence for very early development of capacities for control and for distinguishing self from other, give rise now to new questions concerning the nature of the infant's early tie to the mother. These findings also are leading to suggestions for new theories of the self and different ideas about the so-called symbiotic phase. We do not yet know how these newer findings and formulations will affect the ways in which we listen to our patients' stories, but it is, I think, unlikely that they will leave us unchanged. Any data or theories on development may fade in significance when we encounter seemingly contradictory evidence from the patient, but we know that the evidence from the patient is always the stuff of our interpretation, not the bedrock, and our interpretations will be, and ought to be, in accord with what is objectively known about development. Our confidence in our interpretations will be strengthened by the knowledge that they are in accord with scientific data. Freud, for example, was significantly handicapped in not eventually knowing the data on infant sexual seduction. While his discovery of his error in believing that all neurosis was caused by seduction led to the development of the core of psychoanalysis, the world of psychic reality, it is possible that better information later would have led him to modify the overemphasis he had given to instinct and to alter his theory to find a role for the environment and for the more interpersonal and object-relational modes that were available to him in his practice but were not included in his metapsychology at that time.

Because it is my thesis that neurobiology ought to, probably already does, and surely will influence psychoanalysis, I want first to emphasize the primacy of our effort to listen, as Freud urged, with freely hovering attention, or, as Bion said, without memory or desire, or, as Kohut said, empathically seeing the world as our patients see it. We should be equally aware, however, of the inherent and inevitable limits to achieving these goals that result from the necessity for an organizing analytic theory. All outside knowledge potentially biases the observer not to hear his patient but to confirm his own a priori knowledge and avoid cognitive dissonance – that great source of anxiety. Knowing that we cannot succeed in achieving 'unbiased' listening does not relieve us of the obligation to attempt it.

Many psychoanalysts believe that psychoanalysis can derive useful data only from its own activities, that the scientific development of psychoanalysis depends solely on findings derived from the psychoanalytic situation. It helps if one realizes that what many accept as the standard psychoanalytic points of view – whether the stages of libidinal development, the nuclear role of the Oedipus complex, or the nature of transference – are not simply derivatives of analytic experience but are amalgams of varieties of analytic experience and other kinds of knowledge. Neurobiologic concepts are built into the core of psychoanalysis. Think for a moment of a few of our core concepts. The pleasure–unpleasure principle is a biologic as well as a psychological concept, whether phrased in Freud's early energic terms (that the individual acts to reduce neural excitation to the lowest level and to maintain homeostasis) or in psychological language (that the individual acts to maximize pleasure and safety and to avoid pain and danger). Those are different ways of phrasing the principle of adaptation, which is at the heart of every consideration of organismic functioning. Much of the modern neurobiology can be seen as an effort at the level of the molecule and the cell receptor to understand the ways in which homeostasis, pleasure, and safety are maintained at levels appropriate to the effective functioning of the organism. Even if one chooses to abandon Freud's concept of drive and to accept the psychological concept of wish, as Holt and others have recommended, I think that most of us would agree that psychoanalysis would benefit from a better understanding of the biologic substrate of wishes, their categories, their mixtures, and the regulators that turn them on or off.

Freud did not hesitate to go outside psychoanalysis for aid in obtaining information useful in forming his concepts. Not only did he model his thinking on the scientific mode of his era, but he also looked for specific data. He used the work of the Hungarian pediatrician, Lindner, to support his libido theory that the sexual drive must be an important part of infantile oral activity even if no overt sexuality, as then conceived, could be demonstrated (Freud 1905b). Lindner's description of the infant's evident sensuality while sucking strengthened Freud's conviction about his new theory. He used the data of Sophocles, as described in drama, to support his view that the Oedipus complex was itself a central drama. Freud used his vivid phenomenologic description of the baby's relationship to the mother to support his view of the core constancy of drive aspects of object-relations and the nature of transference regression. Although Freud gave up his Project, which aimed at making psychoanalysis a branch of, or at least entirely compatible with, neurobiology, he never gave up the desire that psychoanalytic findings accord with and be affirmed by findings in other sciences and the humanities. In a footnote to his paper 'The dynamics of transference' (1912a), Freud said:

> I take this opportunity of defending myself against the mistaken charge of having denied the importance of innate (constitutional) factors because I have stressed that of infantile impressions. A charge such as this arises from the restricted nature of what men look for in the field of causation: in contrast to what ordinarily holds good in the real world, people prefer to be satisfied with a single causative factor. Psychoanalysis has talked a lot about the accidental factors in aetiology and little about the constitutional one; but that is only because it was able to contribute something fresh to the former, while, to begin with, it knew no more than was commonly known about the latter.

We refuse to posit any contrast in principle between the two sets of aetiological factors; on the contrary, we assume that the two sets regularly act jointly in bringing about the observed result. Endowment and Chance determine a man's fate – rarely or never one of these powers alone. The amount of aetiological effectiveness to be attributed to each of them can only be arrived at in every individual case separately. These cases may be arranged in a series according to the varying proportion in which the two factors are present, and this series will no doubt have its extreme cases. We shall estimate the share taken by constitution or experience differently in individual cases according to the stage reached by our knowledge; and we shall retain the right to modify our judgment along with changes in our understanding.

It is in this spirit that we should look at neurobiology today. It may now merit a larger share.

I have suggested a number of ways in which findings of infant observation and ethology already have changed the way we work. Neurobiology, in the broad sense, will almost surely further change some of the ways in which we understand development, affect, learning, sexuality, and the meaning of symptoms. I will mention a few areas of current study in which growing neurobiologic knowledge may require that we reexamine and perhaps alter aspects of the theories with which we listen to our patients and the ways we teach them.

With regard to our understanding of anxiety, we know that Freud had an early theory of anxiety that he did not entirely abandon when he developed his later one. According to his original view, anxiety represented psychologically contentless overflow of neuronal excitation, an overflow of blocked and transformed libidinal energy. In this early view, anxiety was not in itself a psychological phenomenon but signaled homeostatic disturbances elsewhere, either in psychological systems or in neuronal function. Freud's second theory of anxiety treated anxiety as part of evolutionarily evolved biologic warning system, with a signal form of anxiety serving as a mild stimulus for the institution of defense mechanisms in order to ward off more powerful forms of anxiety. Anxiety is part of a biologic fight–flight alerting system, preparing for action to avert dangers either from unconscious impulses or from the environment. It is also assumed that the experience of anxiety is disorganizing and unbearably painful and that it is a major task of the organism to avert that experience.

Psychoanalysis, under the sway of ego psychology and our concern with adaptation, has taken Freud's second theory of anxiety as the basis for our continued thinking on the subject, with various workers constructing lists of the dangers that elicit anxiety. Anxiety in our patients is generally assumed to represent the ego's response to the threatened breakthrough of unacceptable impulses or an anticipated loss of an object necessary for the maintenance of inner stability. In this view, anxiety is always related to psychological content.

Recent neurobiologic findings, however, suggest other interesting possibilities. The discovery of benzodiazepines in 1956 and of benzodiazepine binding sites in the brain in 1977 has led to a series of investigations concerning the biology of anxiety.

On the basis of these 50 years of research, one could postulate that there are several different groups of people that are chronically anxious, often phobic, perhaps with intermittent panic attacks, who have developed their anxious personality structure secondary to a largely contentless biologic dysregulation. Although psychological triggers for anxiety may still be found, the anxiety threshold is so low in these patients that it is no longer useful to view the psychological event as etiologically significant. One group may have a hyperactive alerting system, related to a failure of γ-aminobutyrate (GABA) activity, resulting in excessive anxiety signaling and breakthrough of anxiety states. These individuals are benzodiazepine responsive. The second group may be understood as suffering a lowered threshold for separation anxiety – the postulated trigger for panic. In effect, this is a return to a version of Freud's early anxiety theory: the trigger for anxiety is a biological event, as in 'actual neurosis,' but now the trigger is separation, not dammed-up libido. The newer theory postulates that panic is an evolutionarily constructed response to separation, but the mechanism may miscarry and fire independently of appropriate environmental triggers. That neurons mediating separation responses and the creation of panic both seem responsive to tricyclic antidepressants suggests, of course, the psychologically known links of separation and depression. In these two groups of individuals, the presence of anxiety is not an indication of a primary disorder of conflict or self/object relations; these are secondary to the disorganizing effects of anxiety. Furthermore, the biologic dysregulation is not only a developmental event but also an ongoing one. These persons are currently physiologically maladapted for maintenance of homeostasis in average expectable environments. Klein and Fink (1962) claim that individuals with panic disorder who are treated with imipramine cease to have panic attacks but then require psychotherapy to undo the learned anticipatory anxiety and phobic behaviors that were developed as magical efforts to cope with unpredictable panic.

This theory suggests that the psychoanalyst is now confronted with a diagnostic decision in his anxious patient. What portions of the anxiety are, in their origins, relatively nonpsychological, and what portions are the clues to psychic conflicts that are the originators of the anxiety? The neurobiologic theory does not suggest that all anxiety is a nonmental content but rather that a distinction must be made between psychological coping and adaptive efforts to regulate miscarried brain functions which create anxiety with no or little environmental input and psychological coping and adaptive efforts to regulate disturbances of the intrapsychic world that lead to anxiety and are environment sensitive. Clearly, we have not yet arrived at the point where we can easily make that distinction, but there is good reason to attempt it. In instances in which underlying biologic malfunction is suspected, there is powerful warrant to attempt a biologic intervention that may then facilitate psychological interventions. Let me give an example.

A woman entered treatment describing a history since midadolescence of intermittent depression, timidity in relations with men, and very high rejection sensitivity. Any relationship with a man was colored from the start by her expectation that the man would probably leave her. The prospect of desertion precipitated such anxiety and rage that she was then prone to behave in ways that brought about the rejection she allegedly feared. The patient recalled as a small child always being extremely upset when her parents went out in the evening, requiring hours before she could calm down. She was mildly school phobic. The patient entered analysis and worked through the consequences of a relationship with a profoundly narcissistic mother who, it became clear, was also chronically depressed. A sister of the mother had been hospitalized with an uncertain diagnosis of schizophrenia. In early latency, the patient had turned from the mother toward the father, whose favorite she was, but the father seemed to go through a profound personality change, presumably a depression, when the patient was about ten years old. The patient remembers her father becoming extremely withdrawn, going to work, coming home, and watching television by himself. The patient and father began to have tremendous battles when the patient began to date, as the father regularly disapproved of the patient's boyfriends, most of whom were chosen to elicit that disapproval. The father died when the patient was 16 years old, during a period when they were angry at and not speaking to each other, and the patient felt continuing guilt and rage that she had never had the opportunity to make peace with her father.

From the very beginning of the analysis, the transference was characterized by severe anxiety reactions at every disruption of the tie to me. Weekend breaks were extremely difficult, canceled appointments were a crisis, and vacations seemed a major trauma. As the analysis progressed, the patient became generally calmer, was able to pursue her work successfully, began to develop a much higher level of self-esteem, and had somewhat better relationships with men. Despite these improvements, she episodically reverted to the symptoms with which she had entered treatment: a mixed depressive–anxious state with feelings of shame and worthlessness, terrified that she would be rejected by her boyfriend, a female friend, a work supervisor, me, or anyone else. The termination phase of the treatment was difficult but seemed to be successfully negotiated.

Two years after termination the patient called me, just before the beginning of my summer vacation. She was already on vacation and was in a state of mixed depression and panic, the kind of feeling with which she had entered analysis. There were no apparent external precipitants other than the pre-conscious reminder of my vacation time, and she felt extremely discouraged over this uncontrollable state. While her description of her feelings was extremely familiar, this time it occurred to me that she might be describing a recurrent biologic dysregulation and that a search for further psychological content might not be productive. That thought had also occurred to her. Despite much trepidation, she agreed to a trial medication. She responded well to the medication, despite side-effects, and stated that she felt relieved and reorganized and had the sense that an outside intrusion into her life, the severe anxiety, had been alleviated. On medication, although she was not free of anxiety, she had a feeling that she was in some way more in control of herself than she had ever been.

The case is suggestive. This woman later decided to return for further analysis to deal with aspects of her conflictual life that had not been successfully analyzed while anxiety and mood dysregulation were, perhaps independently, dominating her ongoing psychological life.

Current research indicates, with varying degrees of certainty, multiple levels – cellular, neural network, and experiential – for the organization and regulation of anxiety and for the development and alteration of pathologic anxiety. The elegant research of Kandel (1979) has elucidated the actual neurochemistry of some forms of learning in the snail, including what may be considered aspects of anticipatory and chronic anxiety. The interaction of the environment and the adaptive responses of the organism can now be partially understood in terms of basic cellular neurobiology. The readiness with which an analyst attempts to affect the patient's self or his brain organization through a new relationship or medication has philosophical and ethical connotations, and in the current absence of specific indications for either or both treatments, the treatment choice will reflect individual bias. We are alert to the issues of efficacy. If we can demonstrate that physiologic interventions are more efficient ways to achieve a portion, at least, of the effect we seek – relief of pain and opportunities for new growth – as physicians, we welcome the most effective treatment.

The question may be asked, 'Are psychoanalysts interested in changing the patient's life or changing the symptom?' Analysts used to find it easy to answer this question. We believed that symptoms were surface manifestations of deep disturbance, as in the rest of medicine, and that the symptom was not the target of our ministrations. In fact, we thought that too easy symptom removal would confront the patient with the task of constructing a new symptom to provide defenses against underlying threatening wishes. This idea of symptom substitution has not been borne out by recent work. Experience with behavior therapy, focal psychotherapies, and pharmacotherapies seems to demonstrate that, contrary to expectation, symptom removal, in many although not all instances, may lead to enhanced self-esteem and possibilities for new experiences and renewed characterologic growth. Most analysts have long realized that excesses of dysphoric affect inhibit the effectiveness of psychoanalysis by fixating the patient on the affective state and limiting the patient's cognitive associational capacity. For the patient whom I have described, I believe, retrospectively, that pharmacologic assistance earlier might have permitted a much clearer focus on her content-related psychodynamic problems and would also have made it more difficult for her to use her symptoms masochistically as proof that she was an innocent victim of endless emotional pain.

I would like to draw another implication from the brief clinical vignette I gave. Most analytic treatment carries with it a strong implication that it is a major analytic task of the patient to accept responsibility for his actions. In the psychoanalytic view, this responsibility is nearly total. We are even responsible for incorrectly or exaggeratedly holding ourselves responsible. It is our job to change our harsh superegos, and it is our job to do battle with unacceptable impulses. However, it now seems likely that there are patients with depressive, anxious, and dysphoric states for whom the usual psychodynamic view of responsibility seems inappropriate and who should not be held accountable for their difficulty in accepting separation from dependency objects, or at least they should not be held fully accountable. There is a group of chronically depressed and anxious patients – perhaps they are part of a depression spectrum disorder, as Akiskal (1983) suggests – whose mood regulation is vastly changed by anti-depressant medication. The entry of these new molecules into their metabolism alters, tending to normalize, the way they see the world, the way they do battle with their superegos, the way they respond to object separation. It may be that we have been coconspirators with these patients in their need to construct a rational-seeming world in which they hold themselves unconsciously responsible for events. Narcissistic needs may lead these patients to claim control over uncontrollable behaviors rather than to admit to the utter helplessness of being at the mercy of moods that sweep over them without apparent rhyme or reason. An attempt at dynamic understanding in these situations may not only be genuinely explanatory, it may be a cruel misunderstanding of the patient's effort to rationalize his life experience and may result in strengthening masochistic defenses.

Turning now to our understanding of sexuality, psychoanalysts have long been torn by arguments over the appropriate attitude toward homosexuality and other 'gender-deviant' behaviors. Neurobiology will not settle the argument, but advances in neurobiologic understanding of gender role add intriguing new insights to our outlook on homosexuality. There is evidence from research with mice that there are two independent brain systems for sexual behavior – one for male behaviors and one for female behaviors, the activity of each depending on genetic, prenatal, environmental, and hormonal influences. It seems that females may be masculinized, defeminized, or both, and, conversely, males may be desmasculinized, feminized, or both. Hofer reported that:

Females whose uterine position was between two males show slight modi-fication of their genitals in the male direction, are more aggressive, do more urinary marking of their cages (a male trait), and are less attractive to males than their litter mates with uterine positions between two females. The implication is that the proximity to males *in utero* and some sharing of their placental circulation resulted in their being exposed to somewhat more testosterone during the prenatal period. However, it was found that these masculinized females were not defeminized. They were no different in their response to estrogen and they were as capable of all female reproductive functions, including maternal behavior and the raising of young, as their female littermates who had been together in the uterus. Thus, with different amounts and timing of exposure to testosterone in male animals, behavior may be feminized without being demasculinized.

(Hofer 1981: 273)

Hofer concluded that 'a number of sex related behaviors may depend to a certain extent on the presence of testosterone in early development, that both genetic males and genetic females possess the potential for both masculine and feminine behavior traits, and that traits for the opposite sex may be increased or decreased without necessarily impairing the behaviors related to the genetic sex' (1981: 273). In other words, depending on the amount of testosterone present in the environment, we can produce effeminate males, fully capable of male sexual function but with female behavioral traits, or we can produce demasculinized males, incapable of male sexual behavior later on even in the presence of testosterone; the converse can be done to females. The fetal mouse brain is exquisitely sensitive to the organizing effect of hormones.

Psychoanalysts tend to assume that the presence of effeminate characteristics indicates the presence of a feminine identification and is a result of that identification. The data of neurobiology indicate that there may be more than one source for effeminate behaviors and that effeminate behaviors may not connect with identifications except in complex secondary ways and may be totally distinct from homosexual tendencies. Moreover, a recent, unconfirmed study by Zuger (1984) suggested that early effeminate behavior in male children is congenital and is the best single indicator of later homosexuality.

Another study, in a human population, was done of a group of genetic males with an enzyme defect that did not permit them to convert available testosterone *in utero* into an effective genital-masculinizing substance (Imperato-McGinley *et al*. 1979). Although their brains were exposed to normal intrauterine androgen, they were born with female-appearing genitalia, were given female sex assignment, and were brought up as girls. As these phenotypic females entered puberty, they began to produce their own testosterone and at that time developed normal male genitalia. What makes this group especially interesting is that these individuals seemed to have little difficulty in changing their gender identity and gender role at puberty; of the 18 studied, 15 married and showed no evidence of undue stress or distortion of their male role. This result is contrary to both the studies of Money and our current wisdom, which conclude that core gender identity is firmly fixed by 18 months and very little affected by later changes of external genitalia (Money and Ehrhardt 1972). In this group of patients, it is as if the fetally hormonally masculinized brain maintained masculine neuronal networks that made later masculine role behavior easily available, overriding the usual psychological influences. Very early intrauterine patterning of the CNS seems powerfully determining for later sexual behaviors. In yet another experiment:

> male rats born to mothers stressed during their last trimester of pregnancy by periodic restraint and bright light failed to develop normal male sexual behavior in the presence of receptive females and assumed female sexual positions when approached by normal experienced males. They were thus demasculinized and feminized as a result of their mother's experience during pregnancy. Treatment of the affected animals with testosterone did not fully correct the deficiencies in male sexual behavior and only served to exaggerate the inappropriate female-type behavior. This means that the alteration was in the *neural systems mediating the behavior*, not in the amount of male sex hormones produced in childhood. Individual animals showed different patterns that were consistent for them. Some were asexual, responding neither to normal females nor normal males. Some were bisexual, some only responded with female behavior to males, and some were indistinguishable from normal heterosexual males.
>
> (Hofer 1981: 180; emphasis added)

These experiments indicate rather conclusively that prenatal experience patterns the brain, at least in mice, and may do so to such a degree that later experience does not significantly alter the early neural patterning. It is a large leap from animal studies to humans, even though there are suggestive data in humans supporting similar conclusions. It seems reasonable, in the light of the studies I have cited combined with earlier psychoanalytic studies, to suggest that there are several pathways to the same end behavior – for example, effeminate behavior in males or perhaps even obligatory homosexuality. The influence either of specific molecules on the brain *in utero* or of special forms of learning through identification may lead to altered, that is, effeminate, behavior. At this time we have no way of determining the preponderance of biochemical or interactional etiology (both considered biologic) in any individual, nor do we yet know whether it matters in terms of later plasticity. Is the chemically determined effeminate male any more or less likely to give up his effeminacy, if that were desired, than the psychologically determined one? What are the limits of the plasticity of the adult brain? We do not know. Without an answer, it at least behooves the psychoanalyst to be aware that he should proceed with caution. A conviction that all homosexuality is part of a normal range of variability or a conviction that all homosexuality is psychopathologic is unwarranted at this time.

There are now many experiments in human and animal infants that demonstrate the lasting effects of very early life experiences and the powerful shaping of later behaviors by even single early traumas or particular behaviors of the mother. In some instances, a fair amount is known about the chemical regulators of these brain changes. At this borderline of neurobiology and psychoanalysis, we are quite in the dark concerning the question of later plasticity of both neural networks and behaviors. Are some treatment failures and endless analyses a result of the too rigidly prewired brain? It is a potentially convenient excuse, but it is possible that some of these cases represent such neural prepatterning. Again, we need more knowledge before we can usefully address the question; in the meantime, it might be wise to keep the possibility in the back of our minds. One other example illustrates an experience that is becoming increasingly common in the psychoanalytic community.

I recently saw in consultation a 36-year-old male scientist who came to see me for referral to a new analyst because for external reasons he had to interrupt his previous treatment. He gave a classic description of himself as someone with a narcissistic personality disorder: grandiose, self-inflated, full of unfulfilled promise although innately well endowed and perhaps even potentially brilliant – a brilliance that showed in flashes but never in steady achievement. He was married and had three children; he had married a passive, frightened woman and was himself emotionally detached, remote, and distant. He had entered treatment because he recognized his pattern of making a superb first impression and then disappointing his admirers and himself. He had passed the stage of boy wonder in his early thirties and had begun to worry that he would burn out.

He had been in analysis for a few months when he experienced his first clear manic episode, which lasted several months. During the next year he had his first major depression and clearly began a bipolar course. His analyst refused to consider medication, so the patient medicated himself with lithium obtained from a friend, with his analyst's knowledge. His own description of the result was, 'The lithium stopped the crazy swings during which I couldn't do any analytic work and I was in great danger of either wrecking my life with my financial schemes during my manic periods or killing myself during my depressions. On lithium, I knew I had a severe character problem and needed analysis.' The treatment had been enormously helpful, and he was eager to resume.

Possibly, the stress of analysis and the specific address to this patient's characterologic defenses played a role in the appearance of his bipolar disorder. It also seems possible that he would have been untreatable, and would perhaps not have survived, if medication had not been available for the disorder of affect. I cannot think of a significant analytic advantage gained by withholding the medication, and although many transference issues were not resolved at the time he came to me for consultation, there seemed to be no great impediment to his continuing a genuine analysis while taking medication. It was my view that the medication should be properly supervised by a physician, thus probably assuring him better care and interfering with a bit of the narcissistic grandiosity of his conviction that he could do everything himself. This combination of neurobiologic advance and psychoanalytic effort seems at least additive and perhaps even synergistic. Analysts will have to learn how to do this better than we have in the past, developing appropriate criteria for combined treatments.

We should not be surprised if advances in neurobiology continue a centuries-old process of whittling away at the realm of psychiatry. It was not very long ago that diseases such as tuberculosis, Parkinson's, tertiary syphilis, and neurodermatitis were considered psychiatric diseases. More recently, syndromes such as Gilles de la Tourette, rheumatoid arthritis, ulcerative colitis, essential hypertension, dysmenorrhea, premenstrual syndrome, and temporal lobe and petit mal epilepsy were considered by some to be psychological in origin and suitable subjects for psychoanalysis, at least in part because the disease course seemed at one time to be event-responsive. Current work in personality disorders indicates that some of the behaviors of obsessive–compulsive, explosive, depressive–masochistic, or borderline patients may reflect genetically determined biologic abnormalities that are in part pharmacologically modifiable. Psychoanalysts should welcome any scientific knowledge that removes from our primary care illnesses that we cannot successfully treat by the methods of our profession because the etiology lies elsewhere or that facilitates our analytic treatment by assisting us with intractable symptoms. We should also not be excessively modest about the contributions we can make to the care of these patients. Psychoanalysis is a powerful instrument for research and treatment, but not if it is applied to the wrong patient population.

It is most unlikely that there will be any direct bridges from neurobiology to the unconscious or to consciousness. Neurobiology explains at a different level than psychology, and knowledge of the brain will not fundamentally alter our mode of inquiry about the mind. What modern neurobiology does is to make it increasingly apparent that knowledge of the brain can help us to refine our knowledge of the mind and, in some instances, by its effects on our theory at its boundaries, it will set different limits to what we consider to be the mind. As Kohut (1980) pointed out, the realms of material observation and experimentation and intrapsychic observation and experimentation are discontinuous. Introspection and extrospection are different processes. Again, what is to be sought is congruence and limit setting on both sides. Psychoanalytic knowledge of unconscious operations poses interesting problems for the biologists and provides important hints for experimental work. The flow goes both ways.

Psychoanalysis requires a theory of development that will help explain the phenomena important to us: the world of internal representations and meanings, the world of attachment and object relations, the world of sexual differentiation, the world of fantasy and wish, the world of intrapsychic conflict, and the modes of learning and the biologic substrate that make these worlds possible. We also

93

need far better data, experiments, and theories for understanding the effective agents in the complex undertaking of analysis; neurobiology can help us to understand which of our concepts are unlikely and which are congruent with biologic experimentation. We should be extremely uncomfortable with any theory that is incongruent with neurobiologic discovery. Eric Kandel put the matter succinctly. He said:

> The emergence of an empirical neuropsychology of cognition based on cellular neurobiology can produce a renaissance of scientific psychoanalysis. This form of psychoanalysis may be founded on theoretical hypotheses that are more modest than those applied previously but that are more testable because they will be closer to experimental inquiry.
>
> (Kandel 1983: 1282)

I think Freud would have been pleased by this prospect.

7

INFANT RESEARCH AND ADULT
PSYCHOANALYSIS*

Analysts generally agree that the primary psychoanalytic task is the understanding of the patient's psychic reality, rather than his material reality, and that,
ultimately, we are interested in the genetic point of view, not the developmental
one. Analytically, the past that the patient has internalized, rather than some
'realistic' past, is the past that is relevant to his present. For example, a toddler
who has just been spoken to sharply by his mother runs to his father and says
'Mommy pushed me down and bit me.' The discrepancy of fact and report is
clear, but the child may internalize his fantasied version rather than the realistic
one, since at the moment a feeling of overwhelming injustice done to him is
more satisfying to his injured narcissism than an admission of being a bad boy
who is too small and helpless to ward off punishment. It is that genetic past –
the past as experienced, including the distorting defenses that make experience
tolerable even at the expense of some observable truth – that his future analyst
will attempt to unravel.

The question of the role of infant research in adult analysis can be approached
by asking how the analyst brings himself to the task of understanding psychic
reality, including the genetic past. We know that none of us is naively open-
minded. Thousands of years of naive open-mindedness did not lead to the
discovery of psychoanalysis. Rather, each of us approaches the patient with a
limited array of mental templates that predetermine the shape that we give to
the communications we receive from the patient. While being psychoanalysts
will impose some uniformity upon our approaches to listening and understanding, there are broad areas of differences among analysts that are relevant to
our question.

* A version of this paper was first presented at The American Psychoanalytic Association
Workshop for Mental Health Professionals in Seattle, WA, 1988. It was published as Cooper
(1989f); reproduced with permission of International Universities Press, Inc. © 1989 by IUP.

Even though it may be obvious, I want to emphasize that we have never derived our data solely from our patients. Freud, while creating the genetic and developmental points of view for understanding the patterns and details of adult life, patterned the patient's associations according to his own inner vision of the infant's early life, as have all analysts since Freud. We now know those visions vary enormously, but all of them are limited. Freud, discovering the Oedipus complex within himself, looked for corroboration from developmental observation of children (Freud 1905b). The two pioneers of child analysis, Melanie Klein and Anna Freud, 'observed' very different children; neither was able to make a theory-free observation. The Freudian baby, driven and frightened, is quite different from the Kleinian baby, rageful, paranoid, and depressed, who is, in turn, very distinct from the Kohutian baby, ambitious and relatively content. Significantly, the intent of the early child analysts was quite dissimilar from the aims of the developmentalists during the past few decades. The earlier analysts were interested in extending and expanding an existing theory of the meanings and origins of adult psychological function; the newer baby-watchers, on the other hand, have been doing their best to find out what babies actually do, unencumbered by immediate therapeutic aims, and trying hard to put aside accepted theory. This scientific effort has now accumulated a vast amount of data, some of it well known to analysts, and some of it still quite obscure. I believe that the science of infant observation has done three things for psychoanalysts of adult patients: (1) it has challenged and changed some of our core theories in important ways that influence our therapeutic endeavors; (2) it has opened the way for us to hold a far richer and more varied vision of baby life, thus changing the way we listen to our patients' associations and providing more interpretive possibilities than were previously available; and (3) it has placed relative limits and regularities on possibilities, so that we know that certain adult psychic constellations probably do not appear without accompanying childhood circumstances. Buckley, in his recent volume on object relations, says:

> Direct observations of young children and their mothers by Margaret Mahler and her colleagues has [*sic*] resulted in a body of 'objective' behavioral data upon which a developmental model of the infant's psychological separation from the mother has been built, a model which has major implications for object relations theory and for therapy, since some clinicians now emphasize pre-Oedipal mother–child dyadic issues in their work with patients and trace transference back to early mother–child interactions.
>
> (Buckley 1986: xii)

Buckley is, I believe, correct in deriving these changes in our practice from Mahler's observations on children. I would add only that Mahler is one of a number of researchers who have brought this newer perspective to analytic work. David Levy, Bowlby, Stern, Emde, Sanders, Ainsworth, Greenspan, and others have enriched our vision of the baby and his activities, while demonstrating the profound effects of the vicissitudes of the early dyadic relationship on later life. I think the case can be made that the growth of object-relations theory in this country and our increased focus on pre-Oedipal constellations have been enormously reinforced by what we have learned from infant and child development. Not only has that work led many people away from instinctual motivational theories toward object-relational ones but, more importantly, that work has altered the narrative possibilities, the plot paradigms of growth and development, that the analyst is inevitably creating with his patient as he hears his or her story.

As much as we try to keep our focus on the patient's experience with us, that experience will always be, to some significant degree, more complex than we can comfortably contain. Therefore, in our inevitable attempt to impose some intellectual and affective order on the unfolding life story, we call upon the familiar pictures in our minds of the circumstances of pain and suffering that we imagine might engender our patients' neurotic patterns, and that make our empathic responses possible. The modern analyst has a number of experiences that, I believe, indelibly imprint his intellectual and affective psychoanalytic world. For example, seeing Harry Harlow's movies of maternally deprived infant monkeys (Harlow 1960), or George Engel's movies of his patient Monica (Engel 1953), or James Robertson's movies of children going to the hospital (Robertson and Robertson 1952) conveys a sense of the child's experience of loss that will inevitably color the way the analyst hears his patient speak of experiences of helplessness, loss and disappointment in love. Similarly, our newer knowledge of the infant's extraordinary communicative and attachment repertoire and range of affective and cognitive capacities has changed our sense of the 'personhood' of the baby. It is inevitable that our listening and interpreting will be somewhat reductionistic, but we want it to be as minimally reductionistic as we can manage, a goal that requires our openness to many versions of both the current narrative that the patient unfolds with us and its possible precursors in the past. As a result of child developmental research, the newer versions of patient life stories that we weave have a much greater role for mother, and a much more active infant, eagerly seeking experience, responding not only to his instinctual needs, but developing his needs in accord with the interaction he experiences with his mother.

Freud was explicit (Freud 1920b) in claiming that no prediction could be made from the past. The direct prospective study of development, however, shows us not only how difficult it is to understand the detailed present out of the past, but also how much can, in fact, be predicted from a knowledge of the past. Prospective work in temperament (Thomas *et al.* 1968) and Engel's work with Monica and her children (Engel *et al.* 1985) show that some predictions can be made, and that some patterns laid down very early are extraordinarily enduring, Monica, a child with an esophageal fistula, was fed lying flat on her back with a feeding tube inserted into a gastrostomy. Later, as an adult, she fed her own infant child in the same position, and that child was observed feeding her dolls in the same fashion (Engel *et al.* 1985). I think we would probably agree that something so basic as the feeding pattern between mother and child will have powerful and lasting effects on later developmental stages. Bowlby's recent review (Bowlby 1988) stresses that we must assess personality structure and its attendant personal vulnerability and resilience, rather than current functioning alone. He states that while there are important discontinuities in development, there is a solid basis for predicting that:

> Given affectionate and responsive parents who throughout infancy, childhood and adolescence provide a boy or girl with a secure base from which to explore the world and to which to return when in difficulty, it is more than likely that a child will grow up to be a cheerful, socially cooperative, and effective citizen and to be unlikely to break down in adversity. Furthermore, such persons are far more likely than those who come from less stable and supportive homes to make stable marriages and to provide their children with the same favorable conditions for healthy development that they enjoyed themselves. These, of course, are age-old truths, but they are now underpinned by far more solid evidence than ever before.
>
> (Bowlby 1988: 9)

While it remains true that individual outcome is an unpredictable resultant of genes and environment, we know the actual effects of developmental vicissitudes on later function far better than we once did. It is likely to matter in the course of analytic work whether we are dealing with an individual whose temperament or genetic makeup is such that only the most skillful and sensitive handling could avoid traumatizing him during childhood, or whether we are dealing with someone whose temperament or genetic makeup allows him to respond healthily to a broad range of environments, and for whom only gross failure of parenting will cause damage. Analytic outcome may be heavily dependent on this variable, which may be assessable in the course of treatment. Our knowledge of the infant, derived from infant research and from direct observation, has contributed to a major intellectual shift in psychoanalysis. Infant research now provides the biological underpinning for modern analytic work, replacing the theory of instincts which served this role in the earlier period of psychoanalysis. This research provides new insights into the interpersonal world of the infant as well as a more detailed and precise set of inferences concerning the infant's experiential world; together these will provide the boundaries for the narrative of hermeneutic reconstructions which many today believe are the core of analytic clinical effort.

Direct empathic child observation also permits us a sense of the kinds of child–environment interactions and maturational events that may directly contribute to certain affective and object-relational constellations. With knowledge of these we are in a better position to recognize the ways in which our patients' stories may be defensive, disguising other constructions. The Sandlers' concept of past unconscious and present unconscious is useful in this regard (Sandler and Sandler 1987), pointing to the layering of the narrative. Developmental knowledge helps us to help the patient sort out differences between experience as he now perceives it, influenced by all the defensive aspects of development, and experience as it may once have been. The better our knowledge of actual plots of early interpersonal life, the more likely we will be to enable our patients to relive those plots within the transference. It is equally true that child observation may set limits to the genetic narratives that can be reasonably entertained; if a patient's story contradicts our knowledge from direct observation, it will be listened to very differently from one consonant with the data of observation. Sometimes a patient will tell us an unfamiliar story that will open up a developmental possibility that can now be sought in direct observation. More likely, the patient's story alerts us to a new inventiveness of defenses and screens, and directs us to look beyond the tale as told. We know that there are some reports of developmental patterns that cannot be developmentally true. The patient who reports that he was never held or touched by his mother and yet has grown up to be a functioning human being, is, in all likelihood, reporting a fantasy. This is important in itself, but the importance is tempered in the analyst's mind by the conviction that the fantasy is serving defensive needs. As analysts, we question the source of the discrepancy between the developmental and genetic histories. In this sense, one may view infant observation as refining and redefining our ideas of infantile trauma. The newer views not only will alert us to a different order of traumatizing conditions, but will emphasize developmental pathways rather than fixations.

All of us looking back at our own analytic material, or reviewing reports of others, have little difficulty detecting instances in which the analyst, believing that he was helping the patient to understand his own experience, was, in fact, forcing the patient to a view of the experience that was determined by the analyst's view of what that experience must have been. The analyst's limitation in envisioning possible plots stems not only from countertransferential blind spots but also from the analyst's failure to recognize important story lines other than the ones that he has already learned. When Freud discovered the Oedipal plot it was not self-evident that it must be true or universal, as indeed it seems to be. Our task is to be on the alert for all of the variants of that plot, since it is those variations that are important for our interpretive purposes. But, even more, our task is to look for other basic plots. Empathic observation of infant maturation and development is helping us achieve that task; our vision has been extended by knowledge of the early infant.

I shall present some clinical material indicating how the knowledge of infant observation influences my clinical work. I am powerfully influenced by the work of Stern and Emde on the early interactive nature of a child's relationship to its mother; by the work of Greenspan showing the profound effects on child behavior of alterations of the mother's psychic state, and her attitude toward the child; by the work of Bowlby on the effects on the infant of separation from its mother; and by Harlow's work with baby monkeys. I take away from each of these workers a conviction of the profound effects of early mothering on the developing self and on the defensive attitudes and activities that are set in motion in the effort to maintain well-being under less than optimal circumstances. It also seems to me that many of these characterologic attitudes, strongly entrenched before the Oedipal phase, are readily expressed in the transference, often in nonverbal aspects of the relationship, and can be worked with.

A 35-year-old professional woman explains that all her life she has been fearful of new activities; she has never learned to swim or ride a bike. Anorexic during early adolescence, she has felt unattractive and sexually uninhibited. She has been successful in her scholarly pursuits, but is lonely, with few friends. She is polite, reserved, precise in her speech, plainly dressed, as if hiding her sexuality, and looks sad. In fact, at times during our initial interviews, her facial expression was that of a sad child as we have come to know it from child researchers; the anxious look, the down-turned eyebrows, the pinched facies. She describes her father as an artistic genius, who was attentive to her and very interested in her development. Her mother was a 'nice person' who was content to serve and idolize the father. For reasons she cannot imagine, since she believes she had good parents who loved her, she recalls being a terribly unhappy child, school phobic, and only moderately comfortable at the side of one of her parents. During our first interview, she also described a previous therapy during which the therapist made affectionate advances toward her, and she was concerned that I, too, would find her sexually attractive and make an advance.

In the analysis she was also unhappy, convinced that any activity on my part, whether an effort to probe a bit of her past, or to understand her current feelings toward me or toward herself, could only succeed in making her more unhappy by forcing her to see things that were even more unpleasant than the things she knew. Any attempt to understand this conviction brought the same response. How does one listen to this story?

Although some believe that we should listen without memory or desire, presumably theory-free, I believe, for the reasons I have already indicated, that such a mode of listening is inherently impossible and, therefore, I think it desirable to be aware of all that we bring to the story that is told. As I hear her tale, I have several reactions. I think it most unlikely that her parents could have been as supportive as she describes. I base this belief partly on her conviction of my pernicious intent, which I take to be a manifestation of her expectations of caretakers. But I think it also, and perhaps primarily, because the data of child development do not support the idea of the development of such a glaring lack of self-esteem and such fearfulness in a loving and sympathetic atmosphere. One can, of course, construct numerous Oedipal dynamic constellations that could help to explain the phenomena, but as I read the data of child observation, it is extremely unlikely that such an extensive sabotage of self-esteem could occur without important early precursors. Again I emphasize that I am not imposing a foreign theory on the patient, but I am doing what every analyst inevitably does, both consciously and unconsciously, when ordering the story in accord with an analytic worldview. As the analysis proceeds, it becomes apparent that the father was a severely narcissistic character, interested in the daughter only to the extent that she admired and imitated him; the one positive aspect of her identification with him was her capacity for scholarly work. On the other hand, he was devoid of affection, and spoiled all her attempts at independent play or pleasure by demanding her attention for himself.

Another aspect of her behavior has become increasingly apparent as the treatment proceeds. She often speaks in the tremulous, fearful, sad voice of a three-year-old, a voice one might expect of a child who has been left alone by its parents and is fighting not to show her tears. When asked about this she begins to describe her mother in more detail. Her mother had only one aim in her life – not to anger the father. This meant that no one in the family was allowed to display any anger, or make a fuss of any kind; everyone's needs were secondary to those of the father. The children were dressed as the father wanted, and the food on the table was what suited the father. At about age five, the patient recalls, she was often left at home to 'look after' her demented grandmother while her mother accompanied her father to an art event. No matter what was happening, the mother insisted that everything was fine, and under no circumstances was the child allowed to be angry, nor did she ever receive sympathy for her unhappiness; her mother simply denied the possibility of unhappiness. The picture of the mother that emerged over time was of a severely emotionally limited woman who had been brought up in a foster home, and who was determined to avoid all affective display, and do nothing that would jeopardize her role as the person who allowed nothing to interfere with the father's serenity, the source of her own safety. The patient, eager to avoid any semblance of criticism or conflict with her parents, needed great encouragement, and persistent focus in the transference upon her negative expectations, for this material to emerge. The issue, while conflictual, is more importantly one of understanding the background of affectivity, the capacity for tension regulation, and the experience of safety. Unless this is addressed, all later conflictual issues can be resolved only within the limits set by these convictions or anticipations.

I think that several decades ago, without the impact of object-relations theory and the data of the interactiveness of early childhood, one might have seen this patient differently, focusing on her obvious Oedipal attachment to the father, and her guilty self-denigration and avoidance of self-assertion as penance for her Oedipal desires. That is not a false story; rather it is a later story, easier for her to cope with. In fact, she thrusts it forward at the first session, but it fails to

101

deal with the recoverable earlier origins of her difficulties. I do not want to be misunderstood; what we see in the adult is not a simple reproduction of child-hood. Development has occurred, and the persistence of early patterns has undergone numerous epigenetic alterations of form and meaning in different developmental stages. For example, the sadness seen in this adult patient is not just a continuation of her childhood feelings; rather, that sadness now reflects her masochistic attachment to those feelings, a desire to expose her bad parents by demonstrating her suffering, a demand for reparations for her suffering before she will relinquish it. However, the knowledge from child observation of the responses of the child to the parent during the early years, and the emphasis on affective interaction rather than on instinctual satisfaction, were important in helping to sort out her current defenses.

In summary, the increasingly precise and emotionally compelling data of infant observational research must exert an influence, both conscious and unconscious, on the form and content of the plots that we construct with our patients in our continuing struggle to make sense of our patients' life stories. Child observation has alerted us to a variety of infant behaviors, interactions, and potentialities that are part of the background of psychological development; their derivatives may appear in adult mental life. The closer our reconstructions within the transference are to the patient's developmental experience, the more likely it is that our interventions will be genuinely empathic and effective, eliciting more associations and loosening rigid defenses.

8

PSYCHOTHERAPY AND PSYCHOANALYSIS

The same or different?*

My answers to the question of whether psychotherapy and psychoanalysis are the same or different are inconsistent, depending on who is asking and why. To those who already believe that they are different, I usually go to great lengths to describe the difficulty in proving that difference, and assert all the advantages of blurring that difference. To those who are sure that they are the same, I happily drag out all the answers that prove the reverse. I think I am not just being contrary or Talmudic. Rather, the question does not have a simple answer at this time, and so it is better to recognize the advantages and disadvantages of each point of view. Certainly, the question has generated important discussion, along with lots of poorly founded certainty and defensiveness. I do, however, hold to a firm belief in all of these discussions; whether or not psychoanalysis is more like psychotherapy or more different from it, there is such a thing as psychoanalysis, and its practice, if not its ideas, is relatively fragile and needs protection both from its excessively zealous supporters who might strangle it in their loving grasp, and from its vehement detractors who would prefer that it disappear. Furthermore, the external cultural influences are not always friendly to psychoanalysis – whether in the form of insurance companies, governmental regulations, competing therapies, or popular culture – and so some of us have to be ready to support psychoanalysis unless we come to the conclusion that it doesn't merit our blessing. The topic, therefore, in addition to being clinically and theoretically important, is at least in part political and it always was. The question of whether psychoanalysis and psychotherapy are the same or different involves issues of money, status, social class and elitism, in the perception of both

---

* A version of this paper was presented at a symposium on 'Interpersonal Frontiers in Psychoanalytic Practice' sponsored by the William Alanson White Institute, New York, in 1990.

our patients and ourselves. This inescapable political dimension to the topic colors the discussion.

The need to assert the uniqueness of psychoanalysis as a form of treatment different from all other mentalist treatments began almost at the moment that psychoanalysis began. One of Freud's earliest concerns was to assure his scientific audience that the spectacular results he was obtaining in the cure of the hysterias were entirely unrelated to suggestion (Freud 1923b). It was critical for the validity of Freud's theory that suggestion be removed from consideration because otherwise there was little reason to consider that free association and interpretation were the curative factors, and if they were not the curative factors, there was nothing really new about psychoanalysis. How did Freud rule out suggestion? He did not. He informs us that suggestion was in no way a part of the technique. Of course, as we read through his cases it is very clear that Freud was capable of enormous imaginative leaps, probably some of them incorrect, which he imparted to his patients in the form of interpretations to their associations long before there could be any assurance that alternate interpretations would not have fit as well. The power of Freud's personality, the intensity of his desire that the patient should get well, and the ferocity of his defense of his ideas, of course, all left suggestion as a strong contender for many of his patients' responses to him. Freud, however, ever alert to this possibility, in one of his brilliant discoveries, urged the analysis of transference, the vehicle of suggestion, as an assurance that suggestion was not at work. While Freud wasn't always sure that the positive transference should be analyzed, or at least not quickly, Stein (1979) has emphasized the importance of analyzing the unremarkable positive transference, and Gill (1982) has emphasized the importance of analyzing all transference, especially inadvertent analyst-induced transference effects. Most analysts, following Freud's lead, would today share the view that an attempt at thorough analysis of transference rather than manipulation of transference is a hallmark of analysis, distinguishing it from psychotherapy.

I am bringing up this bit of history because Freud's concern over the uniqueness of the psychoanalytic method has never left us. While analysts today are not defending a new discovery, we have many other uncertainties. We have still not validated the effectiveness of our treatment and even more, we are unable to specify which elements of the treatment situation are the curative or ameliorative ones. We have no convincing evidence that our hugely labor-intensive method really produces better or more lasting results than more economical techniques and we are frequently accused of not even being a scientific field of exploration. This situation is anxiety-provoking for psychoanalysts. The problem is complicated by the fact that analysis has never had and probably never will have a clear definition that is convincing both to analysts and to others interested in psychological therapies. Available data indicate (Erle and Goldberg 1984) that patients selected for analysis often do not have what analyst reviewers think was an analysis (Huxster *et al.* 1975), even though the patient attended four or five times a week, used the couch, and the analyst thought he was doing analysis. Similarly, all of us have had the experience of psychotherapy patients, who are in what we thought would be psychotherapy, but in fact seemed to be engaged in an analytic process. In other words, neither by selection of the patients, nor by the analyst's conscious selection of the desired modality, nor by the patient's conscious intent to participate with one or another mode of therapy, are we able to assure that the therapeutic dyad will conduct the prescribed treatment, according to some predetermined versions of what the treatments are. It is against this background that analysts are particularly concerned to distinguish psychoanalysis from psychotherapy. Because our enterprise lacks definition, and because this arouses so much anxiety among its practitioners who cannot escape the dread that psychoanalysis is not more effective than are simpler, proven, shorter treatments, an enormous amount of energy has misguidedly been directed toward finding a categorical distinction between analysis and psychotherapy. Many conferences on the topic have, in my opinion, been equally unsuccessful in placing psychoanalysis and psychotherapy in different categories. Unfortunately, the parochial, often zealous, effort to demonstrate that psychoanalysis exists in a pure form and is subject to precise definition has significantly hindered our efforts to participate as psychoanalysts in modern psychotherapy research. Most recently Gill (1984), who gave a seemingly crisp and clear definition of the distinction between psychoanalysis and psychotherapy in 1954, gave an equally crisp and clear but quite different definition in 1984. His newer, more fluid definition would allow many forms of what some would insist had been psychotherapy to be relabeled psychoanalysis.

While the topic is an old one, several new theoretical and practical considerations have catalyzed our renewed interest in the 'psychotherapy or psychoanalysis' question. On the theoretical side, our acceptance of multiple points of view within psychoanalysis, including our acknowledgment of the interpersonal aspects of psychoanalysis and our renewed interest in the patient—analyst interaction as an aspect of transference, has required a renewed and deeper consideration of the relationship of psychoanalysis to psychotherapy. Practically, the financial constraints of analytic practice, the changes in the patient population, the scarcity of the ideal analytic patient, and the desire for quicker treatments have led many practitioners to reexamine the alleged difference. Wallerstein's recent exhaustive review (Wallerstein 1986) demonstrates once again what many of us have long maintained – that psychoanalysis and psychotherapy exist along a spectrum, and that there is a large blur in the middle. The distinction can be made, although not always. In the easy cases it is like telling a robin from a bluejay, in the difficult cases it is like trying to distinguish one yellowish warbler from another. Certainly a part of our difficulty in distinguishing psychoanalysis and psychotherapy derives from a misguided attempt to find radically, that is categorically, different theoretical formulations for the two processes. If, however, we regard them as variants of a single process of exploratory psychotherapy we may have less difficulty in distinguishing them and arrive more easily at an understanding of the worth of each.

If we accept that psychoanalysis and psychotherapy exist on a continuum with sharp differences apparent only at the ends, then we are freer to ask a more interesting set of questions concerning what are the many elements that are always present in both therapies, and which appear more frequently in one version or the other, or is there no difference? To what extent are they independent or dependent variables of each other, and how may we study these variables in relative isolation? Which is the more fundamental or basic discipline: psychoanalysis or psychotherapy? We must also be aware that there are practitioners and theorists of psychotherapy who would claim any or all of the processes we label 'psychoanalysis' for psychotherapy, even brief psychotherapy. Davanloo (1980), for example, further blurs matters by claiming that the early Freud, who used interpretation as a direct measure for symptom relief, had it right, and that the later method of long-term reconstruction and working through was an abandonment of the desirable analytic technique. Where once one could define analysis in terms of the development of a transference neurosis and the subsequent exposition of the infantile neurosis, I have elsewhere (Cooper 1987e) tried to show that those terms no longer have meaning in analytic discourse, and are therefore entirely unsuitable bases for founding a definition.

Similarly the attempt to define a process by a technique trivializes our field. The heart of analysis cannot be a matter of how many times a week we see the patient and the patient's posture. We mean something deeper than that. I think that analysis refers to a process in which the patient has an ongoing, compelling interest in progressive self-exploration, of which the transference is both the engine and the occasion. The attachment to the analyst propels the patient's continuing exploration and provides the ever-changing text and context for his self-exploration. Implicit is a degree of neutrality to foster the curiosity that propels progress, as well as the gratifications that are inherent in the analytic situation. Within this broad definition, all of the relational, technical and topical issues that have at one time or another been labeled the core of analysis, or have been forbidden to true analysis, come to bear in the specific needs of particular patients at particular times. Analysis is an intention guided by our psychoanalytic theories, initially sometimes an intention of only one of the dyad, later of both. I personally believe that the odds of an analytic process taking place, in our present state of knowledge, are greatly enhanced by the traditional techniques of very frequent sessions, at least four per week, and the use of the couch. The traditional analytic situation and setting are designed to facilitate the intention to analyze for most patients, but for some analytic patients at some times this may not be the optimal setting. The past decade of openness has made it possible to begin to explore the full potential of psychoanalytic insights and techniques.

In general, patients are placed in psychotherapy rather than analysis, leaving out extraneous factors of time and money, for three reasons: (1) The patient is regarded as lacking psychological capacities for deeper self-exploration. This may be regarded as a specific developmental deficit. (2) Their areas of difficulty are limited, exist in a surround of reasonably adaptive psychological functioning, and one may expect that a treatment of limited goals and ambitions may achieve symptom remission and the limited characterological alteration that may be indicated. (3) The patients are too sick for analysis – they lack adequate psychic structure to tolerate either the frustrations of the analytic situation or the special limited form of intimacy that analysis fosters, or the deconstruction of existing adaptive functions that can occur in analysis.

By far the most comprehensive study of the difference between psychoanalysis and psychotherapy has been the Menninger psychotherapy research project (Wallerstein 1986). While the methodological flaws in that project were significant, the groups were not adequately matched, and the opportunities for doing psychotherapy or psychoanalysis were not equal in the two groups. Nonetheless, Wallerstein's overall impression is that psychoanalysis did not show a treatment advantage nor were there clear process differences that enabled one to make sharp distinctions. Wallerstein has given a description to me of how trained analysts are not able to distinguish, at least in single sessions, a psychotherapy session from an analytic session with any confidence. More recently, Blatt (1992) has suggested that if one matches the treatment modality to the character type based on whether it is more 'analytic' or 'introjective,' then in fact psychoanalysis and psychotherapy as conducted in the Menninger project did show differential results.

But again, that begs the question of whether psychoanalysis and psychotherapy are qualitatively different processes or whether psychotherapy is a diluted version of psychoanalysis, with the same elements of transference, holding environment, insight, etc. I think we might agree that psychoanalysis in contrast to psychotherapy has larger goals. We hope in analysis to understand the transference experience in detail and in depth, to achieve a more thoroughgoing reconstruction, to focus on characterologic structure rather than symptom formation, and to insist upon creating a treatment situation that will probably, in most instances, lead to the patient's intense focus on the analytic experience as a major ongoing life experience. The analyst is willing to give up short-term gains for the sake of long-range goals. Some analysts have said that psychotherapy has specified goals but psychoanalysis does not. A few have adopted an above-the-battle view, essentially saying 'It does not matter to me whether or how my patient changes. My intention is to try to understand the patient and have the patient understand himself. If that has beneficial effects, well and good, and if not, equally well and good, since our purpose is to do analysis and beneficial results are a secondary matter.' This rather lofty, perhaps airy, view does away with the anxiety of whether I am doing good for my patient, who is devoting enormous personal and financial resources to this enterprise, and leaves one with the contentment that certainly my patient and I have understood a great many things, and that is undoubtedly true. Most analysts, however, continue to believe that patients come for help, not philosophical enlightenment, and it remains important that the help obtained should in some way be commensurate with the effort and expense. Some of us would be very unhappy if psychoanalysis and psychotherapy were distinguished by the greater improvement shown by the latter group.

I shall give a brief example to illustrated some of the ambiguities between psychotherapy and psychoanalysis. A 25-year-old woman came for treatment after breaking up with her boyfriend. She had been depressed partly over the loss of the boyfriend but also because his loss pointed up the extent of her inhibition in every aspect of her life. She had not finished college, and had drifted through a number of jobs that she had enjoyed, but she felt that none of them had challenged her or had provided a sense of direction. She was deeply suspicious of men, a feeling that she attributed to her experience of her father. The patient reported that her father was never able to tolerate her independent activity, particularly as she became pubescent, and that he was furious at any evidences of her budding sexuality. He had an unpredictable rage that frightened her throughout her childhood and she believed he favored her brother and her less rebellious older sister. Her parents were recently divorced. The boyfriend with whom she had just broken up was in the mold of several previous boyfriends, rather remote, ungiving, self-involved and passive. She was very concerned with issues of control and preoccupied with which partner had 'the power.'

It seemed to me that my patient had the kinds of inhibitions and characterologic distortions that would be best treated by analysis. She, however, could not consider the possibility of coming more than twice a week or lying down. She was terrified of the idea of becoming so involved with me that, as she perceived it, she would be at my mercy, presumably to be exploited sexually and abused by the rage that she would not be able to escape. We agreed, reluctantly on my part, to begin a psychotherapy; I was explicit in saying that it was not the treatment of choice. I will not try to summarize the entire treatment, but will just mention that issues of control were a dominant theme and the transference experience revolved around her paranoid suspicions of me, and her conviction that I was manipulating her into her growing acknowledgement of her strong ties to me, both positive and negative, while I myself was emotionally uninvolved with her. The depth of positive feeling as well as the full extent of her rage seemed clear in the sessions but they were never fully probed. Penis envy was a major theme, with numerous dreams of being cut by knives, or having palms slit open, but she was never able to work with any consistency or at any depth with these themes, although social aspects of her competitive and envious feelings were explored. After a year of twice-a-week therapy, I again raised the question of analysis and she again declared it to be out of the question for her. We compromised at her coming three times a week. At the end of the second year of treatment she was in many respects a different person. The androgynous, even masculine self-presentation she displayed when I first met her had given way to an open femininity. She had finished school, had entered graduate school, and was pursuing an independent project with great success as well as considerable anxiety. She had been through another failed romance, with a clearer sense of what it was about, and her relationship to me was more trusting, permitting her to express some greater although still limited range of positive and negative feelings. When at this time I again suggested the possibility of analysis, she was able to talk about the alarm she experienced at the prospect of that degree of passivity with regard to me, the terror of not being able to look at me and of her potential loss of control, which she vaguely realized had sexual connotations. While aware that she might be limiting her progress, she felt unable to do it. We agreed to terminate and we set a termination for four months ahead. During this time the patient went through a period of work paralysis, feeling dependent on me and rebuffed by me. We were able to reconstruct more clearly than before many aspects of her relationship with her emotionally unavailable father, her secret demand on him and her defensive inability either to be dependent or to assert herself. She was hyper-aware of a new level of positive feeling toward me and tempered the full experience of termination with the thought that she might one day return for analysis. She came to see me for one visit a year and a half later. She became deeply involved in a creative project, did not have a boyfriend and was optimistic about her future.

It is my impression that one of the features distinguishing some psychotherapies from some analyses is the difference in internalization of the therapist and of the therapeutic process as revealed at termination. After the psychotherapy the patient often remembers it vividly, long after the treatment is over. It is an experience of power and importance, but an experience that retains an objective quality; it is an event rather than an experience. In contrast, after an analysis, the patient often remembers it poorly. This reflects not only the difference in specificity of goals, but in successful analyses, it reflects the greater degree of internalization. The experience is no longer one that is 'out there,' but is so much a part of one's self that the analysis does not have a clear separate existence to be remembered as an event or sequence of events. I believe that in the termination of successful psychotherapies, the patient often takes the therapist with him as an available introject. Patients often can ask themselves, 'What would my doctor have said on such-and-such an occasion, or what did I learn about myself that I can successfully use now?' In contrast, the analytic patient is more likely, though by no means entirely so, to find that he does not try to recreate his analyst's voice, but rather that he has internalized from the analyst an available part of himself and his behaviors are more automatic. Presumably this is part of what we mean by structural change, a change of self-representation.

Even if psychotherapy and psychoanalysis belong under the same general heading of exploratory psychotherapy, the attempt at the present time to maintain a distinction between them is important for a number of reasons. The primary reason is educational. I think Freud was right in warning about the continuing cultural and individual pressure to relieve ourselves of awareness of unconscious conflicts. The educational experience of being analyzed and of analyzing with four or five sessions per week is, in my view, the best way to assure that the analyst-to-be will have had the best chance to experience the full depth and range of analytic process. While some gifted analysts and some gifted patients can do as well with less, we owe our students the chance to have the best – not the economy version. The high frequency of the sessions and the special character of the setting in which the patient is lying down and the analyst is sitting up provides the optimal opportunity at our present state of knowledge for the most detailed analysis of transference and patient–analyst interaction; it is this expertise that characterizes the psychoanalyst.

It is essential for the analyst-to-be to experience and understand the processes of working through, regression, and reconstruction. For most of us, we require the intense analytic experience to develop fully our analytic skills and our confidence to experiment with technique. The therapist's conviction concerning what he does may be critically dependent upon his own analytic experience. To the extent that we are aware of unanalyzed conflicts that we manage to keep away from analytic scrutiny, we are prone to corrupting the analyses we conduct either by steering them away from conflictual matter that is too hot, or by attempting to correct our own deficient experience by demanding that our patients immerse themselves in painful conflict beyond their capacity to bear. Even if one never does another analysis using this traditional description, the experience of having done it will inform one's psychotherapeutic work. Here, I think, we have a vast experience subject to the error of all vast experience. Unfortunately, we have no data. If there is no difference between psychoanalysis and psychotherapy, the intensive psychoanalytic educational experience I recommend will make no difference, but it will do no harm. If there is a difference, it is crucial for the maintenance of this valuable exploratory technique both in the individual and in the profession that the education of the analyst include this analytic experience.

9

DISCUSSION ON EMPIRICAL RESEARCH*

Psychoanalysts have for some time comfortably debated the question of whether psychoanalysis is science or hermeneutics. The arguments on both sides have been stated clearly and frequently, and the controversy has been a useful one in helping us to understand the dimensions of psychoanalysis. However, to the extent that psychoanalysis lays claim to being a method of treatment, we are, for better or worse, drawn into the orbit of science, and we cannot then escape the obligations of empirical research. As long as we develop practitioners who are members of a profession and charge for their services, it is incumbent upon us to study what we do and how we affect our patients. As most of psychiatry has embarked on brain studies, psychoanalysts and our collaborators in the psychotherapies retain responsibility for the continuing study of mental processes.

Furthermore, while some psychoanalysts still believe that our activity is separate from, and unrelated to, advances in psychiatry, most analysts have come to appreciate that there are significant interactions between psychiatric empirical research and psychoanalysis that profoundly affect how we think about and practice our profession. It was not so long ago that psychoanalysts undertook to provide complete explanations of tics, phobias, depression, obsessive–compulsive behavior, etc. Today we are quite aware that some of our explanations were simply wrong, while others were not wrong, but incomplete. We have learned that, contrary to our earlier views, some analyses can be conducted better, or only, if the analysis is combined with appropriate medication. Some disorders for which there was no treatment available other than analysis will, we now know, respond as well or better to varieties of treatments in addition to, or instead of, psychoanalysis or psychoanalytically derived psychotherapies. Like it or not, we are being powerfully influenced by empirical research.

* A version of this paper was first published as Cooper (1993d) in *Journal of the American Psychoanalytic Association*. Reproduced with permission.

The history of empirical research in psychoanalysis has not been a happy one. Beginning with Freud's contempt for American-style empirical research, many analysts have eschewed the methodology of empirical research, and few analytic institutes equip their candidates with the basic skills required either to conduct such research or to evaluate it intelligently. Ironically, it would seem that although, by the end of his life, Freud was far more interested in psychoanalysis as an investigative method than as a therapy, he did little to bring psychoanalysis into the orbit of empirical research. Over the past several decades a small group of determined and inspired psychoanalysts have sought to redress the paucity of empirical research in our field, and the five papers published in a recent supplement of *The Journal of the American Psychoanalytic Association* (1993, 41S) are an exemplary sample of what has been achieved and an illustration of the problems involved.[†] Empirical studies are being conducted in psychoanalysis with a degree of encouragement from the profession that would not have occurred just a few years ago. When Karush and his group began, in the 1960s, to do empirical research on prediction of outcome using the Adaptive Balance Scale for patient ratings, none of the existing analytic journals would publish the paper, which was published in the *Journal of Nervous and Mental Diseases* (Karush *et al.* 1964). Although biases against empirical methods are still strong in our field, the publication of the *JAPA* supplement illustrates how far we have come. In 1990, The International Psychoanalytical Association, under Joseph Sandler's leadership, began a section on research, a significant portion of which is devoted to empirical research, and the American Psychoanalytic Association is now sponsoring an empirical research project on outcome.

What do we mean by empirical research? We can briefly define empirical research as the systematic study of any phenomena by a methodology that allows for some form of statistical analysis, simple or sophisticated, that gives a measure of confidence concerning the truth or falsity of the hypothesis under study, and that reports the phenomena and the tests applied to them in a way that allows others to attempt to replicate the experience. All portions of this proposition have presented special difficulties for psychoanalysts. We have found many

[†] This paper was written as a commentary for 'Section Three: Outcome Studies,' published in *The Journal of the American Psychoanalytic Association*, 1993, 41, Supplement. That volume has since been republished as a monograph 'Research in Psychoanalysis Process, Development, Outcome,' Edited by Theodore Shapiro, Robert N. Emde. IUP, 1995. Section Three of that volume is on outcome studies and included five papers – four of which I allude to in my commentary: 'The Columbia Records Project and the Evolution of Psychoanalytic Outcome Research.' Henry M. Bachrach; 'The Effectiveness of Psychotherapy in Psychoanalysis: Conceptual Issues and Empirical Work.' Robert S. Wallerstein; 'Outcome Research in Psychoanalysis: Review and Reconsiderations.' Judy L. Kantrowitz; 'The Era of Measures of Transference: The CCRT and other Measures.' Lester Luborsky and Ellen Luborksky. A fifth paper in that section, integrating experientially based concepts and behavioral observations in developmental and intervention research by Christopher Heinicke, was omitted in my commentary.

of our hypotheses difficult to cast in the form of a research question that would allow a test of the validity of the hypothesis, and we have found it difficult to describe our concepts so that we can be sure that someone else discussing the phenomenon is referring to the same thing. Empirical research may vary from the simplest tests of the reliability of an observation to complex experimental arrangements. It is clear that psychoanalysis is not intrinsically unavailable for empirical research; rather, the culture of psychoanalysis and the failures of our educational system have inhibited the appropriate development of an appreciation of the importance of empirical research for the continued advance of the field. Without empirical studies we have no way ever to discard a hypothesis. Whether a particular presentation of the self, for example, is a result of deficit or conflict cannot be decided by argument alone, but will finally require some form of evidence. Many of the controversies in psychoanalysis endure not because the questions are philosophically unamenable to research scrutiny, but because we have not yet attempted to frame the research questions. Psychoanalysts have leaned heavily on clinical experience to give us confidence in our activities, although the history of medicine is replete with tenaciously held false beliefs based on clinical experience. We can be quite certain that eighteenth-century doctors using leeches had great confidence in their method, based on their clinical experience. They happened to be wrong.

It may be unfortunate that the greatest spur for empirical research in psychoanalysis is the perceived need for efficacy (outcome) studies, not only to support our confidence in our treatment, but also to participate as a beneficiary of mental health funding. Clearly any rational healthcare system will increasingly, often incorrectly, demand efficacy data. While it seems entirely reasonable to demand evidence of effectiveness and safety, we are also aware that a large portion of every physician's time is devoted to activities that are untested and, in fact, are not clearly related to a diagnosable illness. Reassurance, encouragement, and all the aspects of transference that enter into a desirable doctor–patient relationship are largely untested. Furthermore, the majority of clinical treatments have never been subjected to rigorous clinical trial.

Although we urgently desire the information, psychoanalytic outcome data are probably the most difficult measure for which to achieve scientific reliability and validity; for psychoanalysis, therefore, to use its resources to demonstrate its effectiveness may be a serious misdirection of research capacities. (Since this paper was published the Committee on Psychoanalytic Research of the International Psychoanalytic Association has released *An Open Door Review of Outcome Studies in Psychoanalysis* (Fonagy 1999).) The cost of a serious clinical trial seems overwhelming. Wallerstein's masterly review of the Menninger project reminds us how difficult outcome studies are. Three major students of analytic outcome contributing to the supplement, Wallerstein (1993), Kantrowitz (1993), and Bachrach (1993), have each deviated from their original intent. Wallerstein is now more interested in studying how specific psychological capacities can be

113

measured and how they change with a variety of psychotherapies, Kantrowitz is studying the effect on outcome of the match of therapist and patient, and Bachrach suggests that in place of large-scale multivariate outcome designs we return to scientific individual case examination and the pursuit of specific questions that are amenable to empirical research design. Each of them has given up broad outcome studies in favor of a different order of question. In addition, the odds that mental health policy makers are interested in funding psycho-analysis seem so long that we may be better advised to pursue the empirical researches that are most promising rather than most expedient. Intellectually, the most interesting aspect of psychoanalysis is not its outcome but its process ideas. It may well be that from a public health vantage psychoanalysis is most valuable as the clinical and research field that has spawned the ideas and techniques of dozens of other therapies that, while less ambitious, are more easily studied and administered. Like most analysts, I have no doubt that psychoanalysis is efficacious and is the treatment of choice for an important group of patients. I am dubious that proving this is possible with the resources that can be brought to bear.

It is useful to compare three of the studies described in the *JAPA* supplement. Although each of the outcome studies reported here has significant problems, we must be struck by the consistency of the findings among the authors, using quite different methodologies. Our capacity to select cases for analysis is poor, with less than half of carefully selected patients ever experiencing an analytic process, however that is defined. Patients show improvement, but it cannot be demonstrated that the improvement is the result of the specific psychoanalytic components of the therapy, and there is excellent evidence that the reverse is true. Patients who see therapists more often and for longer periods do better, but this may only reflect that the patients whom the therapist likes and feels gratified by and are getting better are the ones he keeps in treatment, or perhaps that there are no clear endpoints to treatment, that we can all get better than we are, and therapeutic relationships are helpful. Wallerstein, who has dedicated his life to empirical research in psychoanalysis, is the most radical in accepting these findings (Wallerstein 1986, 1993). Wallerstein is explicit in stating that within the limits of his study, the Psychotherapy Research Project, psychotherapy and psychoanalysis did not have clearly distinctive outcomes. Most important is his finding that within their use of the concept of structure, structural change was as likely with more supportive techniques as through interpretive insight-oriented techniques, and that conflict resolution was not necessary for deep and enduring psychic change. He concludes that we cannot tie the type of change to the mode of intervention, that the tie of theory to practice is poor, and that we are best advised in our studies of patient outcome to study capacities that can be behaviorally defined rather than structures that are not really subject to measurement. That structural change can be produced by noninterpretive means ought not to be surprising in the light of our changing views of the analytic process. For example, for many it has for some time seemed clear that the new experience with the new object is critical in the analytic process, and the relation of this new experience to interpretation and insight is not well understood (Cooper 1989b).

Wallerstein concludes that our differences of frame of reference preclude the possibility of consensus on broad concepts such as structure. His group has, therefore, abandoned the psychoanalytic conceptual perspective and has adopted a psychological perspective of capacities, describing 17 of them. (In passing, I note that this conceptualization is remarkably close to Karush's effort, but at a far more sophisticated level.) Wallerstein suggests that the capacities being measured – such items as hope, zest for life, flexibility, commitment to relationships, trust – are so clearly core aspects of character that one would accept that a change in these capacities reflects a change in underlying structures, no matter how defined. It may not be such a radical step to substitute capacities for structures for the purpose of research methodology, but it does raise the question of the value of our structural concepts. Unless one can show a clear derivation of these capacities from structural concepts, structure may become superfluous in analytic conception, and analysts might be advised to move closer to psychological schemas that better describe what it is we are interested in. Analysts are, I am sure, reluctant to speak a language of capacities and give up yet another piece of metapsychology. Wallerstein's research may be leading us in that direction. Psychologists such as Benjamin (1974) and others who have devised circumplex personality descriptions may yet contribute greatly to our analytic thinking. It is always a pleasure to watch a brave thinker who follows his findings where they go, ready to abandon an idea when the weight of data against it becomes unbearably burdensome.

Kantrowitz (1993), faced with the same problem of difficulty of broad outcome studies, has raised a different question about outcome. Outcome may be a variable dependent on the patient–analyst mix rather than on patient characteristics. She has evidence that certain characteristics of certain psychoanalysts foster some processes and inhibit others. In fact, the same characteristics may be desirable at one point in an analysis and undesirable at another. This brings up the topic of analytic style, the analyst's character (Cooper 1982d), and the analytic attitude. What is empathic at one stage of the treatment may not be at another. This is an important and interesting field of study attuned to our current recognition that psychoanalysis is a two- (at least) person system, rather than the observation of processes in a single individual. Kantrowitz, like Wallerstein, found that all patients in all treatments get better, and less than half of the patients ever engaged in an analytic process; that they were unable to relate outcome to any of the preassessment factors; and that researchers and psychological testing found less improvement than doctors and patients claimed. Kantrowitz has shown that selecting by narrow rather than wider scope does not lead to better prediction of analyzability. Her evidence seems to contradict another analytic shibboleth, that the self-analytic function is an essential part of a successful analysis. In her data the self-analytic function seemed unrelated to therapeutic gains. Our inability to predict who will engage in and benefit from psychoanalysis must disturb us. Bachrach's (1993) work, with the large data set of the Columbia Psychoanalytic Center, is concordant with Wallerstein and Kantrowitz in demonstrating that less than 50 per cent of cases carefully chosen for psychoanalysis ever develop an analytic process. Bachrach is discouraged about whether outcome studies will tell us much, and considers the possibility that each treatment is unique and cannot be grouped with others, and that we will learn most from systematic individual case study.

Luborsky, another pioneer of empirical research in psychoanalysis, has shown that psychoanalytic propositions can be put in the form of researchable questions and elicit reliable and valid data relevant to the therapeutic process (Luborsky and Crits-Cristoph 1990; Luborsky and Luborsky 1993). Luborsky has done this with transference. Whether or not he has captured all the aspects of transference that are of interest psychoanalytically, he certainly has described aspects of the transference that all analysts would agree are central to the concept, and he has described how they can be specified in ways that allow for reliable and replicable empirical research about the phenomenon of transference. It is worth asking why so little use is made of the Core Conflictual Relationship Themes (CCRT) methodology for the elucidation of transference. Luborsky has shown that therapists can learn to identify the elements of the CCRT, and that if they do so, they are likely to conduct their therapies with greater efficacy. The data are good enough so that in most other healthcare fields, practitioners would feel an obligation to master and use the technique. While all therapeutic fields are slow to make use of research findings, there can be no doubt that psychoanalysis is by far the slowest. Analysts, to my knowledge, rarely consciously use the CCRT techniques as part of their ongoing analytic work. One part of the answer is in the intellectual climate of psychoanalysis. There is almost no formal encouragement from the analytic establishment to utilize instruments or objective criteria to check our formulations. Until recently, analysts were not encouraged to regard their technique as an objectifiable activity to be scrutinized by empirical methods. We are usually content to assure ourselves that our formulations are in accord with the theories we currently hold, whether explicit or obscure.

Many psychoanalysts have the uneasy sense that while Luborsky may be able to objectify core aspects of transference, this is not entirely relevant to what we do when we are doing analysis. It is felt as a constriction of our capacity to think imaginatively and a constraint on our capacity to make further discoveries, continually deepening the transference. It is also likely that most analysts prefer to see themselves as closer to being artists than artisans. The idea of carrying out a manualizable, prescribable treatment is anathema to the majority of analysts. Furthermore, asking analysts to specify and bring full cognitive awareness to the analytic process may, for many analysts, seem to conflict with their desire to engage in freely hovering attention. While freely hovering attention is, of course, only a data-gathering method, the data of which should then be subjected to rigorous scrutiny, many analysts prefer to retain a vague openendedness in their thinking.

One of the consequences of empirical research is that we are required to give up favorite ideas, ideas we cherish and consider parts of ourselves. Empirical research now clearly shows that some old analytic shibboleths are untrue. For example, transference cures may be lasting; so-called structural change can occur without insight; conflict resolution is not necessary for change; and real treatments are not pure, and supportive measures are an integral part of analysis. The boundary between psychoanalysis and psychotherapy is fluid.

It is now abundantly clear that, whether we like it or nor, empirical research methodology is developing rapidly. It will be applied to psychoanalytic propositions, and many of our favorite ideas will be shown to be wrong or, what amounts to the same thing, not useful. Psychoanalysts should learn to entertain this prospect as good news rather than bad news. Psychoanalysis is still the treatment of choice in selected cases, as well as a superb training experience. New information will make us even more effective. Of even greater importance is that psychoanalysis provides a unique opportunity for studying unconscious and conscious mental processes, and continues to be an extraordinarily fruitful source of new ideas, able to incorporate within it the findings not only of its own studies, but of those of its neighboring fields – psychology and neuropsychology. Psychoanalysis is invigorated by the increase of our empirical research and by shedding concepts that no longer yield new knowledge. We are learning new things about our field and we are contributing enormously to our psychotherapeutic offspring, the variety of brief and supportive psychotherapies we have spawned. We are coming closer to achieving a passing grade in a critical test for any healthy therapeutic field – we change as we gain new knowledge and experience. That change is likely to be increasingly rapid, and analysts dedicated to the preservation of a theory or a technique are likely to be left only with ideology.

PART III

Vicissitudes of narcissism

THE NARCISSISTIC–MASOCHISTIC CHARACTER*

There is an old Chinese curse: 'May you live in interesting times.' These are analytically interesting times, in which, more than ever before in the history of psychoanalysis, accepted paradigms have been called into question, and a congeries of new and old ideas competes for attention and allegiance. In intellectual history, such periods of enthusiastic creative ferment have led to the development of new ideas. Sciences make their great advances when new techniques lead to new experiments, when new data contradict old theories, and when new ideas lead to new theories. Since the early 1970s, much of the interesting creative tension in psychoanalysis has focused on the crucial role of pre-Oedipal experiences and the centrality of issues of self or narcissism in character development. I propose that masochistic defenses are ubiquitous in pre-Oedipal narcissistic development and that a deeper understanding of the development of masochism may help to clarify a number of clinical problems. I suggest that a full appreciation of the roles of narcissism and masochism in development and in pathology requires that we relinquish whatever remains of what Freud referred to as the 'shibboleth' of the centrality of the Oedipus complex in neurosogenesis. I further suggest that masochism and narcissism are so entwined, both in development and in clinical presentation, that we clarify our clinical work by considering that there is a narcissistic–masochistic character and that neither appears alone.

The problem of reformulating our ideas was foreshadowed over half a century ago, when Freud (1931), in speaking of the intensity and duration of the little girl's attachment to her mother, wrote:

* A very early version of this paper was presented first as 'The masochistic character' at the Association for Psychoanalytic Medicine in New York City in 1963. A later, more complete version was presented as 'The narcissistic–masochistic character' at the Joint Meetings of the Psychoanalytic Societies of the Metropolitan Area in Mohonk, New York in 1973. It was first published as Cooper (1988a); reproduced with permission of The Analytic Press.

The pre-Oedipus phase in women gains an importance which we have not attributed to it hitherto. Since this phase allows room for all the fixations and repressions from which we must trace the origin of the neuroses, it would seem as though we must retract the universality of the thesis that the Oedipus complex is the nucleus of neurosis. But if anyone feels reluctant about making this correction, there is no need for him to do so.

(Freud 1931: 225)

Freud then went on to reveal some of his own difficulties in accepting his new findings by stating that those who are reluctant to make this clearly necessary revision need not do so, if they are willing to accept a redefinition of the Oedipus complex to include earlier events. He said:

Our insights into this early pre-Oedipus phase in girls comes to us as a surprise like the discovery, in another field, of the Minoan–Mycenean civilization behind the civilization of Greece. Everything in the sphere of the first attachment to the mother seems to be so difficult to grasp in analysis – so gray with age and shadowy, and almost impossible to revivify, that it was as if it has succumbed to an especially inexorable repression.

(Freud 1931: 226)

Perhaps this is an indication of Freud's and our own difficulty in accepting the breadth of theoretical revision that our data may require. The fact is that in his posthumous work, 'An outline of psychoanalysis' (1940), he again stated without reservation that the Oedipus complex is the nucleus of neurosis.

It is questionable whether it was ever the case that most analytic patients presented with primary Oedipal pathology. Edward Glover in his *Technique of Psychoanalysis*, published in 1955, was already lamenting the scarcity of cases of classical transference neurosis. He referred to 'those mild and mostly favorable cases which incidentally *appear all too infrequently* in the average analyst's case list' (Glover 1955: 205; emphasis added). I suspect that few of us have ever seen many cases of 'classical transference neurosis' and yet it has been difficult for us to give up the accompanying clinical idea, so dear to Freud, that the nucleus of neurosis is the Oedipus complex. I in no way depreciate the immensity of the discovery of the Oedipus complex and its vital role in human affairs. But we need not share Freud's reluctance to place the Oedipus complex in perspective as one of a number of crucial developmental epochs, and not necessarily the one most significant for our understanding of narcissistic and masochistic pathology, and perhaps not even for understanding neurosis generally.

Kohut's (1971) self psychology represented the most radical attempt to date to address, and resolve, the various dissonant elements in psychoanalytic developmental research, clinical experience and general theory. As I have written elsewhere (Cooper 1983b), I believe it is this exposure of some of the major

122

unresolved problems of psychoanalytic work that accounts for much of the passion – positive and negative – that was generated by self psychology. For more than a decade, psychoanalysis has been productively preoccupied with developing a new understanding of narcissism in the light of our newer emphasis on pre-Oedipal events. The scientific and clinical yield of this investigation has been high, and it should prompt us to apply these methods to other of our metapsychological and clinical formulations that are a bit fuzzy. Prominent among these are the concepts of masochism and the masochistic character.

Our major ideas concerning masochism date to an earlier period of psychoanalytic thinking, when the focus was on the Oedipus complex. The cultural climate of psychoanalysis was different then. A reexamination of masochism at this time, using our newer ideas of separation–individuation, self-esteem regulation, the nature of early object relations, and so on, might help clarify our understanding of masochistic phenomena.

Review of theories and definitions

The literature is vast, and I will mention only a few salient points. The term *masochism* was coined by Krafft-Ebing in 1895 with reference to Leopold von Sacher-Masoch's (1870) novel, *Venus in Furs*. The novel described, and Krafft-Ebing referred to, a situation of seeking physical and mental torture at the hands of another person through willing submission to experiences of enslavement, passivity and humiliation. Freud (1920a) used Krafft-Ebing's terminology, although in his early writings on masochism he was concerned with perversion masochism with clear sexual pleasure attached to pain, and only later was he concerned with the problems of moral masochism in which humiliation and suffering are sought as part of the character formation and without evident sexual satisfactions. Freud postulated several explanations for these puzzling phenomena.

1   It is the nature of physiology that an excess of stimulation in the nervous system automatically leads to experiences of both pain and pleasure.
2   Masochism is a vicissitude of instinct; sadism or aggression, a primary instinct, turns against the self as masochism, a secondary instinctual phenomenon.
3   Masochism is defined as 'beyond the pleasure principle,' a primary instinct, a component of the death instinct, a consequence of the repetition compulsion, and thus an independent, automatically operating regulatory principle. Masochism as a primary instinct is, in the course of development, directed outward, and as a tertiary phenomenon, is redirected inward, as clinical masochism.
4   Moral masochism is the need for punishment, consequent to the excessive harshness of the superego. Persons feeling guilty for sexual, generally Oedipal, forbidden wishes seek punishment as a means of expiation.

5 Masochistic suffering is a condition for pleasure, not a source of pleasure. That is, masochists do not enjoy the suffering *per se*; rather they willingly endure the pain as an unavoidable guilty ransom for access to forbidden or undeserved pleasures.
6 Masochism is related to feminine characteristics and passivity.

I think it is fair to say that Freud struggled throughout his lifetime for a satisfactory explanation of the paradox of pleasure-in-unpleasure. In 'Analysis terminable and interminable,' (1937a) he wrote:

> No stronger impression arises from resistances during the work of analysis than of there being a force which is defending itself by every possible means against recovery and which is absolutely resolved to hold on to illness and suffering. One portion of this force has been recognized by us, undoubtedly with justice, as a sense of guilt and need for punishment, and has been localized by us in the ego's relation to the super-ego. But this is only the portion of it which is, as it were, psychically bound by the super-ego and thus becomes recognizable; other quotas of the same force, whether bound or free, may be at work in other, unspecified places. If we take into consideration the total picture made up by the phenomena of masochism immanent in so many people, the negative therapeutic reaction and sense of guilt found in so many neurotics, we shall no longer be able to adhere to the belief that mental events are exclusively governed by the desire for pleasure. These phenomena are unmistakable indications of the presence of a power in mental life which we call the instinct of aggression or of destruction according to its aims, and which we trace back to the original death instinct of living matter. It is not a question of an antithesis between an optimistic and pessimistic theory of life. Only by the concurrent or mutually opposing action of the two primal instincts – Eros and the death-instinct – never by one or the other alone, can we explain the rich multiplicity of the phenomena of life
>
> (Freud 1937a: 242).

The death instinct, as we all know, is an idea that never caught on; it serves in lieu of an explanation.

The vast subsequent literature on masochism was well summarized by Brenner (1959), Stolorow (1975), Maleson (1984), and Grossman (1986), and a Panel of the American Psychoanalytic Association, in which I participated (Cooper and Fischer 1981). I will not repeat these summaries, which succinctly convey the large array of functions and etiologies ascribed to masochism. Stolorow's paper deserves special note because he also concerned himself with the narcissistic functions of masochism, pointing out that sadomasochistic development can aid in maintaining a satisfactory self-image. I will, through the remainder of this paper, confine my discussion to so-called moral masochism,

124

or, as some have referred to it, 'psychic' masochism. I will not discuss perversion masochism, which I believe to be a developmentally different phenomenon. (See Maleson (1984: 350) for a brief discussion of this issue.) Perverse fantasies, however, are common in persons of very varied personalities.

While many definitions of masochism have been attempted, Brenner's (1959) definition has remained authoritative. He defined masochism as 'the seeking of unpleasure, by which is meant physical or mental pain, discomfort or wretchedness, for the sake of *sexual* pleasure, with the qualification that either the seeking or the pleasure or both may often be unconscious rather than conscious' (Brenner 1959: 197; emphasis added). Brenner emphasized that masochism represented an acceptance of a painful penalty for forbidden sexual pleasures associated with the Oedipus complex. He agreed that masochistic phenomena are ubiquitous in both normality and pathology, serving multiple psychic functions including such aims as seduction of the aggressor, maintenance of object-control, and the like. Brenner believed that the genesis of the masochistic character seemed related to excessively frustrating or rejecting parents.

A somewhat different, highly organized view of masochism was put forth in the voluminous writings of the late Edmund Bergler. Because his theories seem to me relevant to topics that are currently of great interest, because they have influenced my own thinking, and because they are so little referred to in the literature, having been premature in their emphasis on the pre-Oedipal period and narcissism, I will present a brief summary of his work. As long ago as 1949, Bergler stated that masochism was a fundamental aspect of all neurotic behavior, and he linked masochistic phenomena with issues of narcissistic development, or development of self-esteem systems. Bergler described in detail a proposed genetic schema out of which psychic masochism develops as an unavoidable aspect of human development. I will mention only a few elements that are particularly germane to the thesis of this paper.

1 Bergler assumed that the preservation of infantile megalomania or infantile omnipotence (today we would say narcissism) is of prime importance for the reduction of anxiety and as a source of satisfaction on a par with the maintenance of libidinal satisfactions. This formulation is not dissimilar to Kohut's many years later.
2 Every infant is, by its own standards, excessively frustrated, disappointed, refused. These disappointments always have the effect of a narcissistic humiliation because they are an offense to the infant's omnipotent fantasy.
3 The infant responds with fury to this offense to his omnipotent self, but in his helplessness to vent fury on an outer object, the fury is deflected against the self (what Rado (1969) termed retroflexed rage) and eventually contributes to the harshness of the superego.
4 Faced with unavoidable frustration, the danger of aggression against parents, who are also needed and loved, and the pain of self-directed aggression, the

125

infant nonetheless attempts to maintain essential feelings of omnipotence and self-esteem, and in Bergler's terms, he 'libidinizes' or 'sugarcoats' his disappointments. He learns to extract pleasure from displeasure for the sake of the illusion of continuing, total, omnipotent control, both of himself and of the differentiating object. 'No one frustrated me against my wishes; I frustrated myself because I like it.'

It was Bergler's belief that some inborn tendency made it easy and inevitable that a pleasure-in-displeasure pattern would develop. He insisted that this develops at the very earliest stages of object differentiation and perhaps, I would add, becomes consolidated during the disappointing realization of helplessness that occurs during the rapprochement phase of the separation–individuation process as described by Mahler (1972).

According to Bergler, these hypothesized early events of psychic development resulted in the 'clinical picture' of psychic masochism, which was characterized by the 'oral triad.' The oral triad, a phrase he used many years before Lewin (1950) used the term for a different purpose, consists of a three-step behavioral sequence that is paradigmatic for masochistic behavior.

Step 1. Through his own behavior or through the misuse of an available external situation, the masochist unconsciously provokes disappointment, refusal, and humiliation. He identifies the outer world with a disappointing, refusing, pre-Oedipal mother. *Unconsciously*, the rejection provides satisfaction.

Step 2. Consciously, the masochist has repressed his knowledge of his own provocation and reacts with righteous indignation and *seeming* self-defense to the rejection, which he consciously perceives as externally delivered. He responds, thus, with 'pseudoaggression,' that is, defensive aggression designed to disclaim his responsibility for, and unconscious pleasure in, the defeat he has experienced. Step 2 represents an attempt to appease inner guilt for forbidden unconscious masochistic pleasure.

Step 3. After the subsidence of pseudoaggression, which, because often ill-dosed or ill-timed, and not intended for genuine self-defense, may provoke additional unconsciously wished-for defeats, the masochist indulges in conscious self-pity, feelings of 'this only happens to me.' Unconsciously he enjoys the masochistic rebuff.

This clinical oral triad, or, as Bergler calls it, the mechanism of 'injustice collecting,' is, I think, an excellent description of a repetitive sequence of events observable in almost all neurotic behavior. The term 'injustice collector' was coined by Bergler, and later used by Louis Auchincloss (1950) as the title of a collection of stories. In Bergler's view, all human beings have more or less masochistic propensities. The issue of pathology is one of quantity.

Theoretical issues

I would like now to explore some of the theoretical issues that have been raised in previous discussions of masochism.

Today there is little disagreement that we can explain masochism in terms of its defensive and adaptive functions without recourse to a primary drive. The extraordinary ease with which pleasure-in-displeasure phenomena develop, and their stickiness, suggest a psychic apparatus that is well prepared for the use of such defensive structures, but there is no theoretical need to call on a primary instinctive masochism.

What is the nature of the pleasure in masochism? The generally accepted formulation that the pleasure is the same as any other pleasure and that the pain the necessary guilty price has the great merit of preserving the pleasure principle intact. There has always been a group of analysts, however, including Loewenstein (1957) and Bergler, who insisted, to quote Lowenstein, that 'in the masochistic behavior we observe an unconscious libidinization of suffering caused by aggression from without and within' (p. 230). The operating principle seems to be, 'If you can't lick 'em, join 'em.' Perhaps, more simply, one may speculate that the infant claims as his own, and endows with as much pleasure as possible, whatever is familiar, whether painful experiences or unempathic mothers. The defensive capacity to alter the meaning of painful experience so that it is experienced as ego-syntonic has also been described in certain circumstances in infancy by Greenacre (1960) and Jacobson (1964). Greenacre reported that babies under conditions of extreme distress will have genital, orgastic-like responses, as early as the second half of the first year, and that these early events may result in ego distortions creating sexual excitation arising from self-directed aggression. This is similar to Freud's original formulation, and I think we must leave open the possibility that there is a dialectic here of excessive quantity changing quality.

From a different point of view, we may ask, what are the gratifying and constructive aspects of pain? We do not dispute every mother's observation that painful frustration, disappointment, and injury are inevitable concomitants of infancy. It is rare that any infant goes through a 24-hour period without exhibiting what we adults interpret to be cries of discomfort, frustration, and need. Even the most loving and competent mother cannot spare the infant these experiences, and, indeed, there is good reason to believe that no infant should be spared these experiences in proper dosage. It seems likely that painful bodily, particularly skin, experiences are important proprioceptive mechanisms that serve not only to avoid damage, but also, developmentally, to provide important components of the forming body image and self-image. There are many cases in the literature, summarized by Stolorow (1975), of persons who experience a relief from identity diffusion by inflicting pain upon their skin.

A typical pattern for borderline self-mutilators is to cut or otherwise injure themselves in privacy, experiencing little pain in the process. They later exhibit the injury to the usually surprised caretaking person, be it parent or physician, with evident satisfaction in the demonstration that they are suffering, in danger, and beyond the control of the caretaking person. A prominent motivation for this behavior is the need to demonstrate autonomy via the capacity for self-mutilation.

Head-banging in infants, a far more common phenomenon than is usually acknowledged and quite compatible with normal development, is also, I suggest, one of the normal, painful ways of achieving necessary and gratifying self-definition. Skin sensations of all kinds, and perhaps moderately painful sensations particularly, are a regular mode of establishing self-boundaries. Hermann stated:

> In order to understand masochistic pleasure, one has to recognize that it is quite closely interwoven with the castration complex but behind this link is the reaction-formation to the urge to cling – namely the drive to separate oneself. At this point, we have to go far back to early development. Our guess is that the emergence of the process of separation of the mother and child dual unit constitutes a pre-stage of narcissism and painful masochism; normal separation goes along with 'healthy' narcissism.
>
> (Hermann 1976: 30)

Hermann then went on to describe the manner in which pain is a necessary concomitant of separation but is a lesser evil than the damage and decay of the self, which would result from failure of separation in infancy. He referred to a healing tendency within the psyche and the erotization of pain, which facilitates healing of a damaged psychic area. Hermann viewed all later self-mutilations, such as self-biting, tearing one's cuticles, pulling hair, tearing scabs, and the like as attempts to reinforce a sense of freedom from the need to cling: 'pain arises in connection with the *separation that is striven for*, while its *successful accomplishment* brings pleasure' (p. 30; emphasis added). Hermann viewed masochistic character traits as a consequence of failure of successful separation with reactive repetition of separation traumas.

Pain, it is suggested, serves the person's need for self-definition and separation–individuation and is part of a gratifying accomplishment. Mastery – not avoidance – of pain is a major achievement in the course of self-development; mastery may imply the capacity to derive satisfaction and accomplishment from self-induced, self-dosed pain. The tendency for such an achievement to miscarry is self-evident. The pleasurable fatigue after a day's work, the ecstasy of an athlete's exhaustion, the dogged pursuit of distant goals, the willingness to cling to a seemingly absurd ideal – all of these represent constructive uses of pleasure in pain and a source of creative energies.

All cultures at all times have idealized heroes whose achievement involves painful and dangerous feats, if not actual martyrdom. The achievement is not valued unless it is fired in pain. No culture chooses to live without inflicting pain on itself; even cultures seemingly devoted to nirvana-type ideals have painful rituals. Rites of passage and experiences of mortification, 'baptism by fire,' are means of assuring essential aspects of cultural and individual identity, and their effectiveness may be proportional to their painfulness and sharpness of definition. A circumcision ceremony at puberty is obviously a clearer marker of a stage in self-development and onset of manhood than is a Bar Mitzvah ceremony.

The question of aggression in the induction of masochism is interesting but, I think, not satisfactorily answerable at this time. Regularly in the course of development, aggression is distributed in at least five directions: (1) in legitimate self-assertion; (2) in projection; (3) turned against the self; (4) toward the formation of the superego; and (5) used defensively as 'pseudoaggression.' The proportions vary, but in the narcissistic–masochistic character legitimate self-assertion is in short supply. I will not discuss here the many issues of the relationship of sadism to masochism, double identifications with both aggressor and victim, and so forth. It seems clear that experiences of frustration and the absence of loving care, whether in infant children or infant monkeys, induce self-directed aggression and mutilation. The usual explanations involve ideas of retroflexed rage or failure of instinct fusion. These concepts are convenient, but not entirely adequate. Stoller (1975) states that hostility, in retaliation for and in disavowal of early experiences of passivity and humiliation at the hands of a woman, is the crucial motivation in *all* perversions, not only masochistic perversion. (Hostility, in his view, is an important aspect of all sexuality.) Referring to the risks that perverts take, he says, 'But the true danger that perversion is to protect him from – that he is insignificant, unruly – is not out there on the street but within him and therefore inescapable. It is so fundamental a threat that he is willing to run the lesser risk, that of being caught.' Dizmang and Cheatham (1970), discussing the Lesch-Nyhan syndrome, have suggested a psychobiological basis for masochistic behavior in the postulate of a low thresh old for activation of a mechanism that ordinarily controls tendencies toward repetitive compulsive behaviors and self-inflicted aggression.

At what stage of development do the decisive events leading to masochistic character disorder occur? It is clear from what I have been describing that I feel it is now evident that the masochistic conflicts of the Oedipus complex are reworkings of much earlier established masochistic functions. In the later character development, these defenses, by means of the mechanism of secondary autonomy (Hartmann and Loewenstein, 1962), function as if they were wishes.

An attempt at clarification

If even part of what I have been suggesting is correct, then masochistic tendencies are a necessary and ubiquitous aspect of narcissistic development. I think there is convincing evidence that Freud was right – the pleasure principle alone is inadequate to explain masochism, nor does the dual instinct theory add sufficient heuristic power. If we add an instinct or tendency toward aggression, we still lack heuristic power. Our knowledge of early development and our knowledge derived from the studies of borderline and psychotic disorders make it abundantly clear that a newer theoretical perspective requires that issues of self-development and object-relations be accorded their proper weight as crucial factors in early psychological development. Libidinal pleasures and aggressive satisfactions will be sacrificed or distorted if necessary to help prevent the shattering disorganizing anxieties that arise when the self-system is disturbed or the ties to the object disrupted. Whether one refers to Kohut's (1972) narcissistic libido, or Erikson's (1963) basic trust, or Sullivan's (1953) sense of security, or Rado's (1969) basic pride and dependency needs, or Sandler and Joffe's (1969) feelings of safety, or Bergler's (1949) omnipotent fantasy, or Winnicott's (1971) true self – all are ways of addressing the crucial issues of the organism's primary needs for self-definition out of an original symbiotic bond. In fact, Freud, under the unfortunately termed 'death instinct,' was making the same point. The organism will give up libidinal pleasure for the safety, satisfaction, or pleasure of maintaining a coherent self.

Let me summarize my view of the relevant issues.

1 Pain is a necessary and unavoidable concomitant of separation–individuation and the achievement of selfhood. Perhaps *Doleo ergo sum* (I suffer, therefore I am) is a precursor of *Sentio ergo sum* (I feel, therefore I am), and *Cogito ergo sum* (I think, therefore I am).

2 The frustrations and discomforts of separation–individuation, necessary events in turning us toward the world, are perceived as narcissistic injuries – that is, they damage the sense of magical omnipotent control and threaten intolerable passivity and helplessness in the face of a perceived external danger. This is the prototype of narcissistic humiliation.

3 The infant attempts defensively to restore threatened self-esteem by distorting the nature of his experience. Rather than accept the fact of helplessness, the infant reasserts control by making suffering ego-syntonic. 'I am frustrated because I want to be. I force my mother to be cruel.' Freud (1937a), of course, often discussed the general human intolerance of passivity and the tendency to assert mastery by converting passively endured experiences into actively sought ones. The mastery of pain is part of normal development, and this always implies a capacity to derive satisfaction from pain.

4 Alternately, one may consider that the infant, out of the need to maintain some vestiges of self-esteem in situations of more than ordinary pain, displeasure, failure of reward, and diminished self-esteem, will still attempt to salvage pleasure by equating the familiar with the pleasurable. Survival in infancy undoubtedly depends on retaining some capacity for receiving pleasurable impressions from the self and object. We may theorize that the infant makes the best adaptation he can and familiar pains may be the best available pleasure.

5 What I am terming narcissistic–masochistic tendencies are compatible with normal development and with loving, although never unambivalent, ties to objects.

6 Where the experience of early narcissistic humiliation is excessive for external or internal reasons, these mechanisms of repair miscarry. The object is perceived as excessively cruel and refusing; the self is perceived as incapable of genuine self-assertion in the pursuit of gratification; the gratifications obtained from disappointment take precedence over genuine but unavailable and unfamiliar libidinal, assertive, or ego-functional satisfactions. Being disappointed, or refused, becomes the *preferred* mode of narcissistic assertion to the extent that narcissistic and masochistic distortions dominate the character. Nietzsche, quoted by Hartmann and Loewenstein (1962), said, 'He who despises himself, nevertheless esteems himself thereby as despisor' (p. 59). One can always omnipotently guarantee rejection – love is much chancier. If one can securely enjoy disappointment, it is no longer possible to be disappointed. To the extent that narcissistic–masochistic defenses are used, the aim is not a fantasied reunion with a loving and caring mother; rather it is fantasied control over a cruel and damaging mother. Original sources of gratification have been degraded, and gratification is secondarily derived from the special sense of suffering.

7 It seems clear that the pleasure sought is not genital-sexual in origin, is pre-Oedipal, and is the satisfaction and pride of a more satisfying self-representation, a pleasure in an ego function, the regulation of self-esteem. Psychic masochism is not a derivative of perversion masochism, although the two are often related. Exhibitionistic drives, pleasures of self-pity, and many other gratifications play a role secondarily.

8 Inevitably, when narcissistic–masochistic pathology predominates, superego distortions also occur. The excessive harshness of the superego is, in my view, a feature of all narcissistic and masochistic pathology and often dominates the clinical picture.

9 In any particular instance, the presenting clinical picture may seem more narcissistic or more masochistic. The surface may be full of charm, preening, dazzling accomplishment, or ambition. Or the surface may present obvious depression, invitations to humiliation, and feelings of failure. However, only a short period of analysis will reveal that both types share the sense of

deadened capacity to feel, muted pleasure, a hypersensitive self-esteem alternating between grandiosity and humiliation, an inability to sustain or derive satisfaction from their relationships or their work, a constant sense of envy, an unshakable conviction of being wronged and deprived by those who are supposed to care for them, and an infinite capacity for provocation.

Trilling (1963), in his brilliant essay 'The fate of pleasure,' based on Freud's 'Beyond the pleasure principle,' spoke of the change in cultural attitude from the time of Wordsworth, who wrote of 'the grand elementary principle of pleasure,' which he said constituted 'the named and native dignity of man,' and which was 'the principle by which man knows and feels, and lives, and moves.' Trilling referred to a:

> change in quantity. It has always been true of some men that to pleasure they have preferred unpleasure. They imposed upon themselves difficult and painful tasks, they committed themselves to strange 'unnatural' modes of life, they sought after stressing emotions, in order to know psychic energies which are not to be summoned up in felicity. These psychic energies, even when they are experienced in self-destruction, are a means of self-definition and self-affirmation. As such, they have a social reference – the election of unpleasure, however isolated and private the act may be, must refer to society if only because the choice denies the valuation which society in general puts upon pleasure; of course it often receives social approbation of the highest degree, even if at a remove of time: it is the choice of the hero, the saint and martyr, and, in some cultures, the artist. The quantitative change which we have to take account of is: what was once a mode of experience of a few has now become an ideal of experience of many. For reasons which, at least here, must defy speculation, the ideal of pleasure has exhausted itself, almost as if it had been actually realized and had issued in satiety and ennui. In its place or, at least, beside it, there is developing – conceivably at the behest of literature – an ideal of the experience of those psychic energies which are linked with unpleasure and which are directed towards self-definition and self-affirmation.
>
> (Trilling 1963: 85)

The model for Trilling here is Dostoevsky's 'Underground Man,' the provocateur without peer. One could add Melville's 'Bartleby' as the other pole of the masochistic–narcissistic character who dominates through his seeming passivity. I believe that Trilling was, with his usual extraordinary perspicacity, describing at the level of culture the same shift we have experienced in psychoanalysis at the level of clinical practice. This new type that he described was the same new type with which psychoanalysis has been struggling now for years, the so-called narcissistic–masochistic character. Trilling clearly perceived that this character type struggles to achieve self-definition through the experience of unpleasure. When this occurs within socially acceptable limits we have 'normal' narcissistic–masochistic character development. The narcissistic–masochistic character as a pathological type, of varying severity, is marked by the preferential pursuit of suffering and rejection with little positive achievement. Every quantitative gradation occurs between normal and severely pathological or borderline. The mildly neurotic 'plays' with self-torture, while the borderline or psychotic may cause irreparable self-damage.

Clinical examples

I would like now to illustrate this thesis with a clinical vignette and a condensed account of an analysis. Once again, I emphasize that I will not in this brief presentation elaborate a great many significant elements but will focus on a few of these relevant to the view I am suggesting.

Clinical vignette 1

Miss A, a 26-year-old student, entered treatment with complaints of chronic anxiety and depression, feelings of social isolation, and a series of unfortunate relationships with men. She was the younger by three years of two sisters, who were the children of an aloof, taciturn, successful businessman father and a mother who was widely admired for her beauty and who devoted herself almost full-time to its preservation. Miss A recalled having had severe temper tantrums in childhood that would intimidate the family, but between tantrums she was an obedient child and an excellent student. Although she always felt cold and distant in her relationships, she recalled that almost up to puberty she had continued to make a huge fuss whenever the parents were going out for an evening. She couldn't bear their leaving her alone. When she began to date at age 14, this middle-class Jewish girl chose lower-class black boys for her companions and insisted on bringing them home to meet her parents. As a consequence, she and the father fought and literally did not speak to each other from that time until the father died when she was 16. By the time that she entered treatment, she had repeated several times the following pattern with men: she would become intensely involved with a man who she knew from the start was unsuitable. He might be married, or someone who was intellectually her inferior, or someone she really didn't like. From the beginning of the relationship, she would be aware that this could not last. She would project this feeling and become intensely angry at the man because he, in her view, was unreliable and threatened to leave her. She would in her fury become increasingly provocative, finally bringing about the separation she both desired and feared. She would then become depressed and feel abandoned.

The repetition of this pattern was a major element in the transference. She was never late for an appointment, paid her bills on time, tried hard to be a 'good patient,' although she found it difficult to talk. She was convinced that I eagerly awaited the end of every session, the break for the weekend, or the start of a holiday because I was delighted to be rid of her, and she felt that she could not survive without me. (She had dreams of floating in space, isolated, and dreams of accidents.) On the surface, her idealization of me was complete, but dreams and other data revealed the anger and devaluation that permeated that seeming idealization. Idealization in the adult transference is, in fact, never pure idealization but is always merged with the hidden rage that the child experienced in the course of separation–individuation. She would never allow herself to take a holiday or miss an appointment, obviously to maintain the clear record that I was the one who did all the abandoning. This was analyzed at length. Midway in the analysis, in the spring of the year, she planned her summer holiday before knowing precisely what my holiday dates would be. We discussed her plan at length, and for the first time she felt confident and pleased about being able to go away on a self-initiated separation. Several weeks later, I mentioned in the course of a session that the vacation dates had worked out well because, in fact, my holiday would coincide with hers. She immediately was enraged and self-pitying that I would go away and leave her, and it became utterly unimportant that she had previously made her own arrangements to go away. Several things became apparent in the analysis of this episode.

1 A major portion of her self-esteem and self-knowledge consisted of her representation to herself of herself as an innocent abandoned martyr.
2 She felt a comfortable familiarity and control of her intimate objects only in the context of her ability to create a feeling of abandonment or to provoke an actual abandonment by the object. This was at its basic level pre-Oedipal in nature and clearly reflected her sense of being uncared for by her narcissistic mother.
3 Additionally, this constellation represented the repetition of oedipal issues, and in the transference she was also reliving aspects of her Oedipal relationship to her father. All pre-Oedipal constellations have another reworking during the Oedipal phase, but the latter does not constitute all the recoverable content of the genetic constellation.
4 The intolerable frustration of the original infantile demands for love and union had led to narcissistic–masochistic defenses. What she *now* sought in her relationships, disguised as an insatiable demand for attention, was the repetition of the painful abandonment, but with the hidden gratification of narcissistic control and masochistic satisfaction. The demand for love had been given up in favor of the pleasure of rejection.

This is the paradigmatic sequence for narcissistic–masochistic pathology.

Clinical vignette 2

A 40-year-old, successful corporate executive entered analysis because he had plunged into a deep depression following an accusation of minor wrong-doing in some financial maneuvers. In fact he was innocent of the charge, which had arisen out of an equally innocent error of one of his assistants, whom he had inadequately supervised. He had been officially cleared of any taint, and the whole matter was minor to begin with. However, this was one in a lifelong series of actually, or potentially, self-damaging provocations in important situations, which were further characterized by his inappropriate failure to defend him-self with sufficient vigor in the face of the attack that followed his provocation. These incidents had regularly been followed by feelings of depression and self-pity, but this time the feelings were severe. He could not rid himself of the feelings that he had shamefully exposed himself to his colleagues, that his entire career would collapse, and that he would turn out to be a laughing-stock with fraudulent pretensions to greatness. The presenting symptom thus combined masochistic, provocative self-damage and self-pity with a sense of narcissistic collapse. I will present only a few relevant aspects of the history and treatment course. I will deliberately neglect much of the Oedipal material that arose during the course of the four-sessions-a-week analysis and that was interpreted; instead I will concentrate on earlier aspects of development. This will be a sketch, and many significant issues will not be elaborated.

He was the youngest of three children, the only boy and, as he acknowledged only later, the favorite child. He viewed his own childhood with great bitterness. He felt he had received nothing of value from his parents and that they had played no positive role in his life. He regarded himself as a phoenix – born out of himself, his own father and mother. These feelings of bitter deprivation – nobody ever gave me anything – had formed a masochistic current throughout his life. His mother had been a powerfully narcissistic woman, who saw in her son the opportunity for realizing her ambitions for wealth and status, cravings she unceasingly berated the father for not satisfying. The patient recalled little affection from his mother and felt she had used him only for her own satisfaction and as an ally against his weak, passive father. His father had been a modest success until the Depression hit, when the patient was four, and both the father and his business collapsed, never to recover. This probably provided a serious blow to whatever attempts at idealization may have been underway. The parents fought constantly, mother reminding father daily of his failure, and the boy remembered great anxiety that they would separate and he would be abandoned.

The sharp edge of his depression lifted shortly after analysis began, revealing a level of chronic depression and a character of endless injustice-collecting and self-pity, covered by a socially successful façade of charm and joviality. He felt that although many people regarded him as a friend and sought him out, he had no friends and felt no warmth toward anyone. Perhaps he loved his wife and children, but he arranged his work schedule so that he would never have to be near them for any length of time. He felt isolated and lived with a constant dread that some disaster would befall him. The incident that precipitated his depression bothered him partly because he felt he was being hauled down by something trivial rather than by an episode fittingly grandiose. He battled endlessly with his associates in business, making wildly unreasonable demands and feeling unjustly treated when they were not yielded to. At the same time, he maintained a killing work pace and never asked for the readily available help that might have reduced his workload. He had a mechanically adequate sex life with his wife and fantasied endlessly about the beautiful women he wanted to sleep with. In fact, he was convinced that he would be impotent with anyone except his wife, and he never dared to attempt an affair.

Early in the treatment, he expressed two major concerns with regard to me. First, that it was my goal to make him 'like everyone else.' 'I couldn't bear to live if I thought I was like everyone else. I'd rather be bad or dead than not be a somebody. Before I give up the feeling of awful things happening to me, I want to be sure I won't be giving up my sense of being special.' Second, he was convinced that I had no interest in him, that I saw him only because I wanted the fee. That suited him fine because he had no interest in me, but it worried him that I might not need the fee badly enough so that he could count on my availability for as long as he might want me. Interestingly, convinced that I only saw him for the money, he was regularly late in paying his bills and would worry about the consequences, but not mention it himself. When I would bring up his tardiness, he would feel a combination of terror that I was now going to be angry with him and throw him out and fury that I had the nerve to dun him for money, when everyone knew he was an honest man. Quickly, then, the transference, like his life, developed a variety of narcissistic and masochistic themes.

The early transference combined both idealizing and mirror forms. These narcissistic transferences are, in my view, always equally masochistic, since they are regularly suffused with rage and the expectation of disappointment. The idealization often is the façade for constructing larger, later disappointments. As adults, narcissistic–masochistic characters no longer have genuine expecta- tions of their grandiose fantasies being met. Rather, grandiose fantasies are the occasion for re-enactment of unconsciously gratifying disappointments. The seeming insatiability of so many of these patients is not due to excessive need; instead, it represents their raising the demand for love, time, attention, or whatever to the level necessary to be sure it cannot be met. This man, for example, seemed to look forward to sessions, was friendly, felt that my most obvious remarks were brilliant, seemed happy to attribute to me all of the intelligent ideas that he had in the analysis. The other side of this coin, however, was his angry conviction that I used my intelligence totally in my own behalf and had no interest in helping him. He felt that all the work in analysis was being done by himself. A typical dream was of him and a guide scaling a high mountain, making remarkable progress but never speaking, and with him in the lead. In discussing this dream, he said, 'All you do here is nudge me along. Why don't you help me more? The work is all mine. I can't bear the thought that anyone else has a part in anything I do.' Fantasies of this sort have the double purpose of maintaining a grandiose, omnipotent image of himself and of maintaining an image of the totally refusing mother. The narcissistic portion of the fantasy requires the masochistic portion. 'I give myself everything; my mother gives me nothing.' A sense of grandiosity and a sense of self-pitying deprivation paradoxically are sides of the same coin, and neither can exist without the other. The narcissistic grandiose self as seen in the adult can never be the original germ of narcissism but is always tempered by the experiences of frustration, which then become part and parcel of the narcissistic fantasy. 'I am a great person because I overcome the malice of my refusing mother.'

At a later stage of treatment, when I insistently brought up the issue of his feelings about me, he reacted fiercely, saying, 'This is a process, not a human relationship. You are not here. You are not. There is just a disembodied voice sitting behind me.' As I persisted and discussed how difficult it was for him to acknowledge that he received something from me and felt something for me, he reported, 'I feel creepy. I have a physical reaction to this discussion.' He was experiencing mild depersonalization, related to the disturbance of self and narcissistic stability, which resulted from the revival of remnants of the repressed affectionate bond toward his mother. The acknowledgment of this bond immediately induced feelings of terrifying weakness, of being passively at the mercy of a malicious giant. On the other hand, this masochistic, passive, victimized relationship to a maliciously perceived mother was an unconscious source of narcissistic gratification (I never yield to her) and masochistic gratification (I enjoy suffering at the hands of a monster). One could see much of this man's life as an attempt at narcissistic denial of underlying, passive masochistic wishes.

As further memories of affectionate interactions with his mother were recovered, he began to weep, was depressed, and dreamed that I was pulling a big black thing out of the middle of him, a cancer that wouldn't come out but that would kill him if it did come out. The analysis, which had been pleasant for him before, now became extremely painful, and he insisted that I was deliberately humiliating him by forcing him to reveal his stupidity, because I knew the answers to all the questions that I was raising with him and he did not. I enjoyed making a helpless fool out of him. He dreamed he was in a psychiatrist's office in Brooklyn, which for him was a term of derogation, and receiving a special form of treatment. 'I was hypnotized and totally helpless. People are ridiculing me, screaming guffaws like a fun house. Then I run down a hill through a big garage antique shop.' In another dream at this time he was driving a huge shiny antique 1928 Cadillac in perfect condition. 'As I am driving, the steering wheel comes apart, the right half of it comes off in my hand, then the big black shiny hood is gone, then the radiator cap is gone.' He was born in 1928. At this time he also developed a transitory symptom of retarded ejaculation, which was a form of actively withholding the milk he insisted was being withheld from him.

The revival of repressed positive ties to his mother threatened his major masochistic and narcissistic characterological defenses. His entire sense of being exceptional depended on his pride in having suffered unusual deprivation at the hands of his mother, and his entire experience of being loved and favored by his mother had been perceived by him as a threat of passive submission to a superior malicious force. He perceived this turn in the treatment as endangering his life of narcissistic and masochistic satisfactions and exposing him to the hazards of intimacy, mutual dependence, and a genuine recognition of the extent of his unconsciously sought-for bittersweet pleasure in self-damage and self-deprivation. The increasing recognition of a bond to me was accompanied by an exacerbation of the fantasy that I was the all-powerful, withholding mother and he was the victimized child. Loewenstein (1957) has remarked, 'Masochism is the weapon of the weak – of every child – faced with the danger of human aggression.' I would only emphasize that, indeed, every child, in his own perception, faces the danger of human aggression.

At this stage in treatment his injustice-collecting surged to new refinements. Frequent requests for appointment changes, complicated dreams to which I did not have magical, brilliant interpretations, the fact that he was not already cured, my insistence that sessions had to be paid for, all of these were proof of my malicious withholding and of his innocent victimization. The injustice-collecting, partly a result of fragile and fragmented self-representation and object representation, is also a guilt relieving, rage empowering, reinforcement of masochistic and narcissistic defenses. These patients are indeed singled out for mistreatment by especially powerful figures to whom they have a special painful attachment.

After a great deal of working through, two incidents occurred that signaled a change in the transference. The first was that I had made an error in noting the date of an appointment he had cancelled. Instead of his usual reaction of outrage and indignation, he sat bolt upright on the couch, looking at me as if this were the first mistake I had ever made and said, 'You mean, you make mistakes too?' The second incident occurred a few weeks later. After a particularly resistant session, I said, 'I wish we could better understand your relationship to your mother.' He was again startled and said, 'You mean you really don't know the answer?' I assured him that I did not and that we would have to work it out together. He now began to acknowledge my reality as a human being, fallible and yet concerned for his welfare. Increasingly from this point the case tended to resemble that of a classical neurosis, although with many, many detours to deep masochistic and narcissistic issues.

138

One could further discuss the nature of the Oedipus complex in this type of patient, from this point of view, but that is beyond the scope of this paper.

Summary

I have attempted to suggest, on the basis of genetic hypotheses and clinical data, that the themes of narcissism and masochism, crucial in all human psychic development, achieve their particular individual character at pre-Oedipal stages of development. Furthermore, narcissistic tendencies and masochistic defenses are intimately and inevitably interwoven in the course of development; so interwoven, in fact, that I further suggest that the narcissistic character and the masochistic character are one and the same. I think the vast literature on these entities may become more coherent when considered from the point of view of a single nosological entity – the narcissistic–masochistic character.

In any particular person either the narcissistic or masochistic qualities may be more apparent in the lifestyle, as a result of internal and external contingencies that may be traced and clarified in the course of an analysis. A closer examination, however, will reveal the structural unity and mutual support of the two characterologic modes, despite the surface distinctions. Neither can exist without the other. Interpreting masochistic behavior produces narcissistic mortification, and interpreting narcissistic defenses produces feelings of masochistic victimization, self-pity, and humiliation.

The analysis of the narcissistic–masochistic character is always a difficult task. I hope that our changing frame of reference and the beginning elucidation of the genetic and clinical unity of the seemingly disparate pathologies may help to make our efforts more consistent, coherent, and successful.

THE UNUSUALLY PAINFUL
ANALYSIS

A group of narcissistic–masochistic characters*

I have, for some years, maintained that what we label as the narcissistic character should more accurately be called the narcissistic–masochistic character, since masochistic defenses are inextricably interwoven with narcissistic pathology. Futhermore, it is my view that narcissistic and masochistic personalities are not clearly distinguishable nosological entities, and there is great theoretical and technical advantage in conceptualizing a single narcissistic–masochistic character with different clinical presentations at different points in life and therapy. I will try to illustrate this thesis by focusing upon a subset of narcissistic–masochistic patients who present an unusual transference manifestation; they experience the treatment itself as terribly painful and dysphoric, and they place a great burden on the analyst's capacity to maintain the analytic setting.

I have in an earlier paper (see Chapter 10) described a proposed psychodynamic and behavioral profile of the narcissistic–masochistic character. The genetic and clinical description with its emphasis on narcissistic development as the major thrust of infantile psychic development, with libidinal and aggressive satisfactions secondary to narcissistic intactness, is, in some respects, similar to the formulations of Kohut. The emphasis, however, on the pattern of pleasure in displeasure as a regular and inevitable pattern of repair to narcissistic injury deserves more attention than it has heretofore received. It focuses our interest on the role of painful events in mental life – that psychic area beyond

* An early version of this paper was presented as 'The painful analysis' at the Chicago Psychoanalytic Society and Institute 50th Anniversary Celebration symposium on 'Transference in Unusual Personality Organization' in 1981. A later version, 'The unusually painful analysis: a group of masochistic–narcissistic characters,' was presented for the first time at the Michigan Psychoanalytic Society in 1984. It was first published as Cooper (1984b); reproduced with permission of International Universities Press, Inc. © 1984 by IUP.

the pleasure principle. I have in an earlier paper (see Chapter 10) reviewed the historical and theoretical issues that enter into a discussion of masochism, concluding that masochism — that is, making pleasure out of pain — is a ubiquitous phenomenon and is often key to understanding certain forms of psychopathology. I will in this paper present two clinical vignettes, illustrating a particular manifestation of masochistic psychopathology.

Case 1

Miss Z, a patient whom I treated many years ago and in whom I first observed the constellation I am discussing, was a thirty-year-old female teacher who entered analysis because she was not yet married, despite several long-lasting romances, and felt that she would soon lose her opportunity to have children. She felt a general undefined unhappiness, an absence of joy. Furthermore, she said that her enjoyment of her work had begun to decline and she mentioned almost casually that she was unable to achieve orgasm except through masturbation. During our first meeting she told me that she had been in treatment twice before. She first saw a therapist shortly after beginning college, when she felt depressed, frightened, and lonely, away from home for the first time. She felt that the therapist was harsh and unsupportive, and after several months of treatment, during which she felt considerably better, she discontinued. Her second treatment occurred in graduate school and was a dynamic psychotherapy that lasted several years, twice a week, with a young psychiatrist who was friendly and clearly appreciated the patient. Toward the end of the first year the therapist began to embrace the patient, and soon each session ended with their engaging in some mild sexual petting. The patient found these advances pleasurable and felt, at the time of starting treatment with me, that this sexual contact had at worst been harmless and even, perhaps, had benefited her.

During her first session she said she was worried about beginning treatment with me for fear that her seductiveness was so powerful that I, too, would not be able to resist her. She seemed pleasant, rather formal, spoke with great precision, and showed some eagerness to begin analysis. Initial history described an admirable, intellectually successful father, a devoted, energetic, relentlessly cheerful mother, and a happy childhood devoted to her infinite pleasure in being taught by her devoted father and being a superb student at everything she undertook. An older sister was a poor student. It was apparent, even while the patient was describing her family, that her actual childhood experience had been rather different from her description. The father was revealed as a severely self-centered, unaffectionate man, totally unable to praise his children, who expected them to serve as an admiring claque of students while his professional ambitions dwindled and he became more embittered. The mother, who later remarked to the patient that she could remember hugging her only twice in her life, emerged as a frightened woman, hoping to escape the father's scorn and refusing to acknowledge the child's experience of injury and neglect. The mother always insisted that everything was fine and everyone in the family should smile around the father.

Within the first weeks of treatment, the patient began to recall her childhood feelings of being the most unhappy of children. As I began to suggest that she was beginning to give a description of the family setting which might relate to her present unhappiness, she began to express the view that she could see no benefit in recalling those old unpleasant matters. In fact, she saw no purpose to treatment if all it did was to make her feel bad because it gave her bad thoughts.

It became clear that as the patient unraveled her pre-conscious and conscious, thinly disguised feelings of hatred and disappointment toward her parents, this knowledge was defensively experienced as imposed by me and an attempt on my part to make her feel bad. The cheerful, good-little-girl demeanor with which she entered treatment quickly gave way to a sad, pouting, fragile quality, and her voice sounded like that of a child about six, a kind of heartbreaking whimper conveying sadness and helplessness. Episodically, however, she would make the harshest, most damning reproaches against me without any change of tone of voice or expression of anger. She felt it was a self-evident fact, requiring no discussion, that I was cruel, unsympathetic, and uninterested. She did not protest this, but merely registered it. She wept in almost every session and expressed intense anger at the treatment, although not directly at me, restating that she saw no point to a treatment that brought her only bad news.

She claimed to be totally without curiosity and didn't understand why anyone in the world would be curious to learn bad news. She experienced no relief from the more coherent, though certainly unfortunate, tale of childhood that began to emerge. While she cognitively understood that her bitterness toward me and the experience of the analysis were aspects of her life pattern, emotionally that knowledge was of no interest, and the paranoid sense of my desire to injure her and cause her pain reached magnitudes where I feared for the intactness of her reality testing.

While much of what I am describing can be understood as routine transference in a severe narcissistic character, or as a negative therapeutic reaction, I want to emphasize the unremitting painfulness for this patient of the process of analysis itself, which I felt was proceeding rather unaffected by any interventions of mine, no matter how empathic I thought them to be, or by any events in the outside world. Four months after the treatment began, her father died, an event that was announced in a matter-of-fact way and not brought up again. References by me to her feelings about it over many ensuing months elicited only the unemotional statement that she hated him and was sorry he died before she had a chance to tell him so. Professional successes during the second year of the analysis were reported similarly flatly and had no effect upon her treatment behavior, which was unremittingly sad, tearful, and distant.

Although she frequently spoke of wanting to leave therapy, I never seriously feared that she would, nor did she ever attempt to do so. She never missed an appointment. On the other hand, she never gave the slightest indication that she felt there was any point in coming or that she expected anything good from me. She kept the appointments the way obedient children go to a bad school every day. The content of the sessions was taken up with the daily injustices dealt out to her by both past and present, the hopelessness of her life, the uselessness of the analysis, and the utter triviality of any issue that seemed of interest to me.

I have, in this sketch, tried to describe a woman whose only rewarding experience in childhood was that she would be allowed to admire her father if she learned well. She was never admired herself. She was apparently significantly sad throughout childhood and saw the treatment situation, especially when it would not yield to her escape into seductiveness, as an unrelieved repetition of the worst aspects of childhood. When she discovered, a year after analysis began, that her mother, shortly after the father's death, had taken up with a young, fun-loving boyfriend in clear repudiation of the father's intellectual pretensions, the patient was enraged that her mother had fooled her into obedience to a father whom the mother knew to be fraudulent, and hated. Further, the mother had backed the father in his insistence on the patient's adolescent sexual abstinence – she was carefully watched over – while the mother took the first chance she could to steal her own sexual satisfactions. Although one might think this discovery, although depressing and enraging, might also be liberating, her response in treatment was only to deepen her sense of hopelessness and her conviction that I, too, was carrying out the analysis purely because of the satisfaction I derived from the analytic routine, rather than out of any regard for her needs. The only tie to me that was ever acknowledged was the sense of being forced into humiliating and depressing self-revelations. This characterized the first two years of her analysis.

Needless to say, this unremitting state of affairs created severe pressures upon me. I wondered in what way I had failed her empathically; I worried over whether she was in danger of psychotic decompensation; I felt guilty over my periodic anger and disappointment at her consistent inability to provide me any acknowledgement of our work together, and I thought a lot about whether someone else would be better for her. At the same time, of course, I realized that nothing would serve her less well than abandoning her. She felt that everyone had abandoned her and, despite her complaints, she was sticking it out, and it was clear that I would, too. This state of affairs continued for two years during which there was a gradual improvement in her external life circumstances which presaged a gradual change in her treatment behavior.

Case 2

Mrs B, a woman in her late thirties, entered treatment – four-times-weekly psychoanalysis – because she was depressed shortly after discovering that her husband was having an affair with a neighbor. This revelation precipitated a total sense of failure in her own eyes, feeling that she had given up whatever talents and skills she once had in order to be a mother, now in an emptying nest, and she contrasted herself to her husband's girlfriend, who was a successful career woman. The patient was plainly dressed, attractive in a nonsexy way, and it was not surprising to learn that she had been the good girl of her family, which contained an older sibling who had been a behavior problem all through childhood. Her parents were described as steady, drab, depressed without distinguishing individual qualities, overwhelmed by the sister's problems. She felt somewhat closer to her intellectual, detached father than to her harassed, overburdened mother. Shortly after graduating from college, she married a brilliant and erratic young man whom she regarded as her intellectual superior and whom she admired for his emotional storminess, which she contrasted with her own levelheadedness. They had several children, and the marriage had seemed adequate to her until she discovered her husband's affair.

It was clear that she looked forward to treatment and an opportunity to release herself from what she perceived to be lifelong inhibitions. She never missed a session, and entered the office with a bright, cheerful expression. However, within seconds she would be in tears. She wept uncontrollably throughout each session. The tears seemed unrelated to the content of the session, since the content was not uniformly sad by any means, but the weeping never stopped. It became clear that the treatment itself was, for her, a reminder of painful events of her past, and it became equally clear that she, like Miss Z, was one of those exquisitely masochistic characters for whom no past injury had ever lost any of its poignancy. Time never healed. Recalling an insult from her mother, or a mistreatment at the hands of a teacher, would release even more copious tears of self-pity and fury, as fresh as on the day decades ago when the event occurred.

What seemed at first like a somewhat unusual, but understandable, opening phase of the treatment established itself as the treatment mode, unresponsive to what appeared to be some progression in her psychic organization. Outside the treatment, she conducted her life fairly well, as she always had, with some increasing capacity for self-assertion, but with a chronic tentativeness and almost an air of confusion. Her facial expression during treatment was often that of an innocent lost child, not knowing how she got where she was and unable to understand her complex surroundings. This childlike quality was, on several occasions, startlingly interrupted by reports of her outbursts of impulsive aggression: once striking her husband, once throwing her shopping bag down in a crowded supermarket, and once striking a policeman who was ticketing her for a traffic violation. These events, which seemed to her utterly out of character, but justified and not worth discussion, had occurred intermittently throughout her adult life.

After many months of treatment, she mentioned that she had almost nightly nightmares throughout childhood, had never told anyone about them, and never went into the parents' bedroom or discussed them the next day. She recalled struggling awake from her nightmares, calming herself down, pulling the covers over her head, and forcing herself to remake the dream into something less frightening. Even as a child, she insisted she did not require and could not receive help from anyone and even attempted to control her own dreams. She never recalled being soothed by her parents at any time. It was after several years of analysis that she told me that she had continued to have nightmares throughout her adult life. She was surprised that I was surprised to learn this, and it emerged that she felt if I were genuinely interested in her, I would have figured that out, although she withheld the information from me. She suffered, she wanted me to know she did, but not in ways that might enable me to help her.

The treatment situation created for me the most severe doubts concerning whether she ought to be in analysis, whether I was unattuned to her needs, whether I was missing some obvious content related to her endless bitter sadness, and in what way I was not responding to the bewildered, beseeching look that she wore during each session. In short, I felt de-skilled, impotent, and bad.

Discussion

I believe we have all seen patients of this type. I can add several more vignettes to the ones I have given. I have not attempted to give complete case histories, but rather I have tried to describe a phenomenon and a few of the surrounding circumstances. What characterizes these patients, in my view, is their special relationship to the analytic situation, which is in important ways separated from their relationship to the analyst. The analytic situation, with its inward focus and its invitation to adhere to the fundamental rule, precipitates a reaction that these patients both welcome and cannot control. They perceive an opportunity for the indulgence of their sense of masochistic injury and narcissistic entitlement which, for one or another reason, has never been so openly indulged before. Tears of bitterness, self-pity, and self-righteousness seem without end.

In the case of Miss Z, the maintenance of any tie whatever to her parents required joining the mother in a hypocritical admiration of the father's narcissistic mediocrity and a total denial of her dissatisfactions or unhappiness. Any of her childhood complaints were greeted both with threat and with the mother's moral reproach that this was unseemly behavior. The second patient realized her sense of total neglect within her family, and the husband's affair revived the bitter feeling that all of her good behavior went unrewarded; in fact, only bad behavior was rewarded. This fury episodically emerged in her relatively harmless acting out. Both patients perceived their behavior in analysis as ego-syntonic, and while the first patient complained bitterly, it was also clear that she had no thoughts about how she might change, or about the desirability of changing her dysphoria. For both of them, no amount of sadness or tears would ever adequately match their own sense of having unjustly suffered at the hands of cruel parents who did not reward their special qualities. It was also apparent that the treatment setting, and the basic rule, were viewed by these patients as an enforced return to humiliating dependency, primal-scene curiosity, and trauma.

I have given only the barest sketch of their circumstances, but let me suggest a formulation that I believe applies to patients of this type. They are all women, and their backgrounds include severe narcissistic injury, from earliest develop-ment on, at the hands of mothers who seriously lacked the capacity for warmth, joy, and responsiveness. They then moved on to an attempt to identify with fathers who were narcissistically withdrawn, but who, one way or another, held out, at least temporarily, the possibility of the child's maintenance of a satisfactory idealization of a rewarding parent. This possibility shattered as the child was increasingly confronted with the father's narcissistic pathology and basic passivity, and his incapacity to reward the child in her own right.

This second blow is decisive and is crucial in the construction of masochistic defenses that focus on hidden satisfactions in the feelings of self-pity, injury, and vengeance – hidden because neither parent had the slightest interest in hearing about the child's suffering. This unconscious, bitter sense of disappoint-ment of grandiose and idealizing wishes was strengthened by the child's growing awareness of the hypocrisy dominating the household, in which the mother was sacrificing the daughter for the sake of keeping peace with a frightening and ungratifying father. Aware of the mother's failure to support her, the child further strengthened her masochistic defenses with the sense that no one was reliable, and 'I will gratify myself in the only way available to me. I will cling to my frustrating parents and enjoy, endlessly, the completely private mastery of their cruelty to me. No one else pities me and so I will pity myself.' Self-pity becomes the only form of coddling and anger available. This constellation is heightened by consequences of early narcissistic humiliation through lack of response to exhibitionistic and voyeuristic needs. Primal-scene fantasies, leading to feelings of exclusion and a stifling of curiosity and dependency, are an important part of the dynamic picture.

When these children enter the Oedipal phase, penis envy becomes the final element in the structure, confirming their sense that they have been cheated and fooled and lied to and deprived of everything they wanted. These are the patients for whom Freud's statement is true: that what they want out of an analysis is to be given the missing penis, and it cannot be provided. Contrary to Freud's view, however, I see this not as the bedrock of their deprivation, but rather as a later constructed symbol of their crucial earlier deprivation.

For these patients, then, the analysis itself provides the opportunity, for the first time in their lives, for exhibiting to themselves and to the analyst the full extent of their suffering, their specialness, their exclusion, and their pseudo-independent defenses. Since they have sustained themselves through their lifetimes through their pride in being able to endure their special misfortune, their aim in the analytic situation is to have it observed and admired, rather than altered. Furthermore, the analyst is present only as an audience for their suffering – a neutral screen without characteristics. The analyst is made to feel as the patients themselves felt throughout their childhood – inept, ineffectual, unnoticed, without individual qualities, unrewarded. Even the expressions of anger that came more frequently from the first patient lacked individual quality and were directed towards me as part of the process, quite unnoticing of my actual behaviors. More usually, in the treatment of narcissistic patients, one can readily relate the patient's anger to some cue provided by the interaction of patient and analyst. With these patients, however, although there may well have been such interactions, they were surely more subtle and difficult to detect; at least they were for me.

None of us regards the psychoanalytic process as simply fun and games. We are prepared for our patients' distress and for our own difficult times in our relationship with severely regressed narcissistic patients. These patients, however, are a subgroup for whom the ordinary ups and downs of the analytic process are irrelevant, and the process itself sets in motion the release of reservoirs of injustice-collecting and self-pity that have been underneath the surface during the patient's lifetime. They are convinced that their suffering has been so severe that nothing can now compensate, and all they ask is to be appreciated as sufferers for whom nothing can be done. Penis envy is an important secondary psychic construction, confirming the feelings of being cheated.

These patients function at relatively high social levels, partly because remaining a 'good girl' provides even more poignancy to their plight and feeds the endless dream of unconscious masochistic feelings of rejection, narcissistic self-righteousness, and deprivation. Their superego structures are superficially intact, but within analysis it becomes apparent that a certain amount of lying or cheating in one or another area of their lives, and certainly with regard to the basic rule in analysis, is taken for granted as their due because of their background of having suffered more than was their share.

What is the prognosis for such cases? Excellent, in most instances. Let me give an example from late in the analysis of the second patient, Mrs B. She had at this time undertaken a creative enterprise of her own, and her marriage had been restored with a new balance, in which she began to see herself as having talents that were worthy of both her and her husband's attention. She had the following dream: 'I was in a huge, huge airplane sitting or lying in the belly of the plane. It was huge, it was about to crash against a forest of dark trees. It was night time. Suddenly the plane lifted itself. I could see how it cleared the line of trees. There was a beach below. I was impressed by the size of the plane. It was huge – gigantic.' Her associations then included the feeling that she was able, with me, to lift herself off the ground. She recalled an earlier dream in which the plane had crashed due to pilot error, and then, following her usual technique of denying the analytic experience, she said, 'This is nothing but coincidence.'

Having made her now-expected statement denying any connection with the analysis, she went on to say how strange she felt in the dream. 'I was both frightened and surprised. I guess this is related to my rushing on to new experiences at my time of life. It is odd that I should be doing that. I am so unlike my mother. I feel like a little girl. I think how small things are when going back to the scene of childhood. The plane was so big.' I commented that the image seemed to be a baby in the mother's belly. She said, 'More like a baby in the father,' and she laughed. 'I am fixed on my father these days. It was a baby in the belly, a baby attached to a huge penis. The baby is being saved; it just occurs to me I was tiny in the dream.' And then, again, her disavowal breaks through and she says, 'Maybe I am just making all this up.' She goes on to say, 'I envy people who have a strong father who could teach them things and make a child feel secure. I made a hero out of my father, but I knew it wasn't true. He never taught me anything. My father frightened me. When you were out ill, it gave me fears like my father gave me fears. Somehow, maybe you are the plane, but I no longer feel I have to go where the plane takes me. I always used to think I had to go where I was taken. Now I feel I want to try things my own way even if I am crushed. It is very irrational.' I think this conveys some idea of the flavor of her concerns with attachment and autonomy, and her concern with penis envy.

Summary

Certain severely regressed narcissistic–masochistic characters find, in the psychoanalytic situation itself, an opportunity for the exhibition of severe, previously hidden, feelings of injury, self-pity, and deprivation. These painful affects dominate the analysis and are resistant, for long periods of time, to progressive changes in other aspects of the analytic work and unresponsive to events within the analytic situation. All these patients seem to be women, and penis envy, as a secondary phenomenon confirming their childhood deprivation, is an important factor. A specific family constellation and fixation on exhibitionistic–voyeuristic struggles are suggested as relevant for these patients. The enactment of their masochistic and narcissistic propensities creates severe countertransference responses, with the analyst experiencing the treatment situation as the patient experienced her childhood: shut out, irrelevant, ignored. The severe sustained regression cannot be short-circuited, but the analyst's interest, combined with his persistent curiosity and insistence on clarificatory and interpretive efforts, is likely to be productive. Psychoanalytic treatment is the treatment of choice, and an analysis informed by a knowledge of the dynamics of the narcissistic–masochistic character may enable such patients to achieve new psychological and life capacities.

WHAT MEN FEAR

The façade of castration anxiety*

George Stade (1984) has discussed the American fantasy that the achievement of manhood requires liberation from apron strings, a process that is never finally completed. As a result, 'all men will remain boys trying to become men' (p. 22), and real men are those who are immune to the control of women even in the form of love. At least a major portion of this feeling is innately consequential to the fact that all men have spent a significant formative part of their lives totally in the care of women who wiped their bottoms, fed their mouths and their egos, and held their hands whenever there was danger or difficulty. The prevalence of forms of macho behavior can be generally understood as counteracting the inner fear of reversion to this earlier state.

Rather than attempting to sort out fears that are culturally induced from fears that are inevitable, as a consequence either of the anatomical distinction between the sexes or of the fantasies of infancy, I will discuss, briefly, male fears as they appear in the psychoanalytic setting.

Brief review of literature

Depending on how it is defined, with few exceptions, psychoanalysts are agreed that castration anxiety is ubiquitous, although there are sharp differences of opinion about whether it is central. In discussing Little Hans, Freud said:

> Anyone who, in analyzing adults, has become convinced of the invariable presence of the castration complex, will of course find difficulty in ascribing

* A version of this paper was presented as 'What do men fear: some origins of castration anxiety' at a symposium on 'The Psychology of Men' sponsored by the Association for Psychoanalytic Medicine, New York, 1985. It was published as Cooper (1986c); reproduced with permission of Basic Books.

its origin to a chance threat – of a kind which is not, after all, of such universal occurrence; he will be driven to assume that children construct this danger for themselves out of the slightest hints, which will never be wanting.

(Freud 1923a: 8)

Rado (1956) and Kardiner (1939) seemed to be among the exceptions, adopting the view that significant amounts of castration anxiety arose only in those cultures where there was specific threat of castration or severe prohibition on infantile genital play.

It is generally accepted today that although castration anxiety may appear ubiquitously, the underlying meanings and origins of the phenomenon vary greatly. When we examine castration anxiety closely in the clinical situation, we find that sometimes it is just that, but that often it is a less fearful disguise for other kinds of fear. What are these other fears? A significant portion of the history of psychoanalysis may be viewed as a reordering of the sources of fear, and I will review some of these dismal lists. Freud, in his earliest version of psychoanalysis in *Studies in Hysteria* referred to a broad range of unacceptable thoughts and feelings that aroused anxiety or shame. As he developed his system he suggested that inhibited or unacceptable specifically sexual wishes aroused anxiety. In 1926 he reformulated his theory of the nature of anxiety, and described a developmental sequence of fears: fear of the loss of the mother or the mother's breast, fear of the loss of the mother's love, fear of the loss of the penis, fear of the loss of the superego's love. These were the universal fears. Castration anxiety, although only one in this sequence, and not the ultimate fear, nonetheless was given special place as the heir to the boy's Oedipal strivings and the motive for the consolidation of the superego.

Starke (1973) elaborated this sequence into the idea that each individual learns to fear the loss of what he loves. The experience of weaning, the experiencing of the loss of exclusive possession of the mother, the loss of feces, the loss of baby teeth, are the templates for the imagined loss of the penis.

Melanie Klein (1957), using her object-relational model of infant development, wrote of the very early paranoid fear of the mother's hostile destructiveness, followed by the depressive fears of the loss of the mother. These were the elementary affective states out of which all other fears, as well as other affects, differentiated in the course of development. Other authors have given special emphasis to the fears of the anal phase as determining for development.

Using a somewhat different early object-relational model and interested primarily in the 'basic neurosis' of psychic masochism, Edmund Bergler (1952) described a septet of baby fears ranging from earliest oral fears to later anal and phallic fears. It was his view that these fears represented the combination of misinterpreted ordinary experiences of infancy and the need for esteem-saving explanations to help avoid the full recognition of infantile helplessness. His septet included the fear of starvation, of being poisoned, of being choked, of being chopped to pieces, of being drained, of being trampled, and finally of castration. It was his view that everyone experiences each of these fears more or less sequentially, in varying degrees. These fears arise out of the narcissistic need to attribute to the fantasied malevolence of the mother the narcissistic injuries inevitably sustained as a result of the discrepancy between infantile omnipotent fantasy and relatively passive reality. While the genetic explanations of Klein and Bergler are, of course, speculative, there is little difficulty identifying adult versions of these fears, and one can view them as derivatives of these early universal experiences.

Psychoanalysts, all impressed by the primitive nature of fears that can be uncovered in adult patients, have continued the attempt to adduce the early experiences that would account for these unconscious contents. Recently Joyce McDougall (1984), a French psychoanalyst speaking from the point of view of object-relations theory, described the three great critical and frightening events of infantile life as the discovery of otherness, the discovery of the sexual difference, and the discovery of mortality, each of these an occasion for terror and trauma. Chasseguet-Smirgel (1984), also of the French school, added to these the discovery of the frightening difference between the generations with their attendant differences in size and power. In her view, the little boy's conviction that his penis is too small to service his mother is a severe trauma to his developing self-esteem.

Heinz Kohut (1984) has described the core fear of annihilation anxiety – the fear of the dissolution of the sense of self or the experience of self-fragmentation. He stated that all later fears, including castration anxiety, are disintegration products arising secondary to the indescribable core annihilation fear. The need to maintain a cohesive and developing self is the organism's essential innate program, and interference with this inherent push toward self-realization sets in motion all fears and rages. Kohut, who saw development in terms of optimal, empathic experiences, nonetheless was explicit in stating that structure building through transmuting internalizations occurs only in the presence of optimal frustration, and that frustration carries with it the threat – that is, the fear – of the loss of a necessary self-object.

Roiphe and Galenson (1981) have suggested that there is an early pregenital stage at about a year and a half when the anatomical sexual difference is noted and when castration anxiety becomes manifest in both sexes. For example, male children at this time, in their view, normally engage in denials of the frightening sexual difference as shown by hyperactivity, increased holding and play with the penis, and a slowed development of fantasy play and body-image integration. Roiphe and Galenson note that some children are significantly traumatized during this period, and pathological castration anxiety may begin pregenitally, showing later pathological manifestations appropriate to later developmental stages.

One could continue to add to this list of fears. Incidentally, I find it an interesting footnote that Kinsey and his associates' study (1948) of male sexual behavior contains no reference to castration anxiety. I chalk that up to midwestern optimism. The variety of pregenital terrors that have been described by different authors, each claiming primacy for the fear described, is, I believe, testimony to the pervasiveness of primitive, fantastic terror that is present in the unconscious life of adults and, therefore, by implication in the developmental life of the child. Clearly, no existing data will support one theory over another, nor are these theories necessarily contradictory rather than complementary. They reflect the theoretical predilections of the theorists and the psychoanalytic need to postulate an early version of unconscious phenomena.

With the possible exception of Bowlby's point of view (1969), every significant psychoanalytic theory has assumed that disappointment, frustration, fear, and rage are inevitable and necessary, at least in some degree, if the baby is to separate, individuate, and develop psychic structure. Fear and rage, the inevitable accompaniments of frustration, are significant motivators for all growth processes, and the infant's frustration is an inevitable consequence of being alive. The central role of anxiety as the guide for adaptation was, of course, the theme of Freud's 'Inhibitions, symptoms and anxiety' (1926a) and is built into the core of analytic theory.

A newer view of castration anxiety

While psychoanalytic researchers have differed in their view of what is the basic fear or the sequence of fears, there has been almost no disagreement concerning the special significance of castration fear and the castration complex in shaping male behavior. It is now a very long time since Freud (1905b: 226) proclaimed as a shibboleth of psychoanalysis that the Oedipus complex was the nucleus of neurosis, and today the focus of much of our analytic literature is on pre-Oedipal phases and their fateful outcome in later life. There has been a profound shift by many psychoanalysts in their clinical work, from listening primarily for the cues to Oedipal conflicts to picking up the nuances of earlier events and their reverberations in the analytic situation. Under the circumstances of our current knowledge and interest, what is the appropriate place to assign to castration anxiety as an organizing fear for the formation of psychic structure, a central fear of the male? Freud (1937a), in 'Analysis terminable and interminable,' concluded that the basic fear for men is the fear of passivity toward another male, a form of castration anxiety. At this late point in Freud's work, it was, I think, no longer clear whether he regarded castration anxiety as primarily an Oedipal event or the final form of expression of the earlier losses and fears.

That castration anxiety occupies a special place, at least in conscious thinking, is as evident to any clinician as it is to the man in the street and is illustrated by endless clinical and anecdotal data. Bomber crews in World War II reported that when antiaircraft flak became particularly terrifying, some crew members would remove their flak vests, obviously intended to protect the vital organs, and place the vests over their genitals – what the crew members perceived to be their vital organ. Many men report that frightening stories, or looking at a gory wound, lead to sensations in the groin, sometimes accompanied by tightening of the scrotum and shriveling of the penis. The vernacular is replete with expressions of castration.

It is my suggestion that castration anxiety so close to consciousness is so because it is, in some respects, the *least* feared of the baby fears, representing the compromise formations arising out of earlier fears and hiding within it the earlier fears, which are far more threatening. As our knowledge of the signifi- cance of earlier object-relational and interpersonal events in early development has increased during the past two decades, it is desirable to try to specify the manifestations of castration anxiety in terms of the developmental events to which they refer. Earlier literature already refers to anal and oral castration. We may wish to refer to castration anxieties secondary to failures of body-image integration or secondary to empathic failures of one or the other parent, or secondary to faulty identifications with one or the other parent, or secondary to difficulties in separation–individuation. In this light, we might look upon castration anxiety as a manifestation of the defensive compromises achieved in the effort to resolve past crises and as a significant indicator of the nature of those crises for the particular patient.

Referring to the phallic phase, Fenichel said:

> The boy at the phallic phase has identified himself with his penis. The high narcissistic evaluation of the organ can be explained by the fact that just at this period it becomes so rich in sensations, and distinct tendencies actively to pierce with it come in the foreground . . . The fear that something might happen to this sensitive and prized organ is called castration anxiety. This fear, to which such a significant role for the total development of the boy is ascribed, represents a *result* and not a cause of this high narcissistic evaluation. Only the high narcissistic cathexis of the penis at this period explains the efficacy of castration anxiety; its forerunners in oral and anal anxieties over loss of breast or feces lack the dynamic force characteristic of phallic castration anxiety.
>
> (Fenichel 1945: 77)

Our current views of narcissism are far more object-relational than libidinal, and we might well consider that it is precisely the anxieties over the loss of the breast or of the love of the mother that can provide quite sufficient dynamic force to propel the individual toward the creation of defensive compromises. Terrifying as it is, the loss of the penis is still only a loss of a part of oneself, a relatively small loss compared with the still-active fears of pre-Oedipal total annihilation. What is observed later as castration anxiety is often a desperate attempt to 'escape forward,' as it were, to more advanced levels of representation, escaping from the more primitive and frightening versions of narcissistic threat.

As I have tried to indicate, no one has conceived of development without the emergence of some hierarchy of fears. Clinically, disentangling those portions of the individual's personality organization that have been constructed for the specific purpose of avoiding fantasied fears, or for the purpose of actualizing masochistically sought fearful fantasies, assumes a major portion of our therapeutic effort. Defense against the disorganizing qualities of these primitive fears as they emerge toward consciousness is a matter of highest psychic priority. If the defenses are successful, what were originally defenses against fears often achieve secondary autonomy and are experienced as if they were wishes of the most powerful sort, the patient being totally unaware of the underlying or originating fears. It is important to recognize that these defenses against fears may themselves be fears, although fears at a higher level of organization, less frightening and tolerable in consciousness, and at times not consciously acknowledged as fears. Castration anxiety, terrifying as it may be, is one of those higher-level fears, organized at a time when structuralization through verbalization and cognition is more advanced, and therefore it may serve as a defense against more primitive, cognitively chaotic, and disorganizing infantile terrors. Castration anxiety, conscious or close to consciousness and therefore allowing real or symbolic preventive actions to be undertaken, affecting a body part rather than the whole self, is defensive against those earlier, more fantastic fears.

The following is a brief clinical vignette, illustrating the complex intertwining of castration anxiety with other fears.

Clinical vignette

History

A 40-year-old research scientist, Mr A, presented for treatment stating that he was suicidally depressed. He felt this was largely a consequence of his increasing conviction that he was a hopeless failure. The patient was a highly intelligent, cultured man of unremarkable appearance, who had been married since age 31 to a woman he liked but who seemed even less interested in sex than he. They had had a few wonderful sexual experiences before marriage and had then settled into being good friends.

He described himself as having been a fearful child, unathletic, afraid of bodily injury, especially disturbed at his having to wear glasses, for which he was teased. His father was an affable man, pleasant and passive at home, and physically powerful and athletic. He was friendly to the patient but took no special interest in him or in his academic achievements.

155

His mother was a powerful figure, self-important, fashionable, seductive, contemptuous of her husband's relative lack of success. She was quite paranoid and talked often of how neighbors were trying to pry into the household secrets. Though without real interest in what her son's talents might be, she regarded him as special and different from other children since he belonged to her. She insisted that he be well dressed, learn how to eat properly in restaurants, and be as ostentatiously bourgeois as she tried to be.

The patient's paternal grandmother was a significant figure who visited a number of times a year, lived with his family during his fourth year, and was lively, loving, and unselfconscious. His most vivid childhood memory was of jumping into his grandmother's bed in the morning and having a tickling session with her, with both of them laughing as hard as they could. This was in dramatic contrast to the mother who, the patient insisted, literally never touched, fondled, or played with him, and attempted to interfere with any of his spontaneous pleasures.

The patient recalls being attracted to the girls in his class in grade school, high school, and college but having no idea how to go about making any contact, convinced he lacked any qualities that would attract a woman. In short, he was a well-integrated, severely narcissistic character, convinced that he was a psychopath, which he was not, and without borderline features. At the time he entered treatment he maintained the firm belief that were he ever to attempt intercourse with a woman other than his wife, who was as sexually frightened as he, she would treat him with such contempt and scorn that he would be crushed for life. He had a significant success phobia, certain that in any comparison with another man, he would be found wanting and would be humiliated. At the same time, he was secretly scornful of everyone, including me.

Course of treatment

For the sake of brevity, I will mention only a few significant foci of Mr A's preoccupations in sessions early in the fourth year of his analysis and will recount a series of dreams that relate to the nature of his complicated anxieties.

In extended associations the patient described himself as made of shit. Napoleon's description of Talleyrand as 'shit in a silk stocking' accurately described his self-image. He perceived his body as a soft shit phallus, constantly endangered by women or stronger men. At the start of treatment he spoke of his penis as too small, soft, and unattractive but at the time of the dreams I will relate he felt his penis was at least adequate, and perhaps even beautiful, especially if erect. At this time in the analysis there had been a profound change in his capacity for healthy assertiveness and he seemed to have overcome his fear of success. He remained terrified of women, their bodies, their parts, their 'cutting'

156

behaviors, their fantasied humiliation of him. Female genitalia seemed 'spooky' to him, and he mildly depersonalized if he tried to look at his wife's genitals. He remained literally terrified of the idea of being in bed with a woman other than his wife, whom he regarded as nonsexual.

Despite giving vivid descriptions of his mother's insensitivity and somewhat bizarre behavior, several years of treatment passed before he began to be aware of his feelings that she had not always been a good mother, and he was angry with her.

It was late in the treatment before he could acknowledge the beginnings of any sense of relationship and possible attachment to me. He preferred to view me as a technician with a job to do. Underlying this was the certainty that I could have no interest in someone made of shit. This view also served to ward off regressive and frightening pre-Oedipal transferences in which I would emerge as the terrifying mother of infantile fantasy. The dreams I will report occurred during a two-week period in the fourth year of treatment, after the following changes had taken place in the treatment and in his life. His relationship within the transference had become distinctly more positive. He felt an identification with my kindness toward him and began to see himself as basically a kind person. He resumed a hobby that he had always loved but never pursued because his mother ridiculed it when he was a boy. He found himself hugely attracted to a woman he met at work. During the two weeks prior to the dreams I will report, he had a number of dreams affirming his fantasy that his body substance consisted of shitty fluids from his mother, as part of his anal birth.

Dream 1

I've read of a new procedure for curing cross-eyes. You make three surgical cuts around the eye, two on the outside of the eye and one on the inside. It releases lots of fluid. It works. No one knows why. I feel that I've lagged behind in my knowledge. I must do it. It's simple and rapid. I'm in an operating room. There are parts of equipment that I've never investigated, and I don't know how to handle them. I become unsterile, I touch something. I'm too embarrassed to tell anyone. A doctor there, a man older than me, knows all the parts of the machine.

Dream 2

There's a woman in a grave somewheres buried. The woman is a distant relative. They couldn't embalm her properly. We had to be sure she was totally embalmed. I asked, 'So what if she's only half embalmed?' They say,

'Cockroaches will eat her body. It's a state law to prevent that.' There are photographs around the grave. I think it must have a personal meaning for the family.

Associations

I know I'm afraid of exploring a woman's body. I know you think that the eye has something to do with female genitalia. I always feel so unappetizing. I can't see how anyone can be attracted to me as a sexual object. Seeing my mother in the bathroom always scared me. I remember the first time my wife had a vaginal discharge. It was a creamy, fetid fluid like spoiled rotten milk. It was a milky discharge, maybe poisonous milk. I've always had a fantasy of being preoccupied with fluids building up in cavities of my body and having to be released. I had the notion that if women can't give milk with their breast the pressure has to be released and it comes out as a discharge through the sexual orifice. I really believed that. I'm not sure that I still don't. I always had the feeling that the buildup of fluid requires an immediate release. Like feces. If I have to go I have to go right on the spot. If I have an urge to ejaculate, I have to do it. The thing about the eye, I was reading in the newspaper about a new cure for some eye disease where they put in botulinus toxin to paralyze the muscle of the eye. It poisons the muscles and temporarily cures the disease. In the dream it seemed terribly important that you didn't have to cut muscles. You'll probably say I'm afraid of anything to do with cutting because I'm not sure that my penis is firmly attached.

I don't know what the cockroaches are about. I'm comfortable in disgusting situations. As a child, I would think of disgusting things coming out of my mother's bottom. I saw rust stains on towels and assumed it must be something from her that was very disgusting. I think of vaginas as a disgusting sort of place. If I have to put my penis into it, I want to get it out fast. I remember as a child seeing my mother's breasts. I called them fat bellies. She got very angry. I didn't know that breasts made milk. I really thought it was milk coming out of my wife's vagina the first time I saw that milky discharge. As a child, it never occurred to me that milk came out of breasts. Breasts were always frightening, and they were always hidden. I was absolutely astounded by the idea of children being fed by breasts. My mother never told me anything about women. I remember my baby sister's pussy was pretty. It was pink and hairless. Women's parts are bizarre like moon creatures. I hate pussies with lots of hair. I remember looking at pictures of female anatomy once and looking at the cervix. I loved the picture of the cervix. It seemed like a cute button, maybe a little mouth, an end to the passageway or a little nose. I remember thinking that it is the mouth to the uterus and sad that it was covered with all that milky stuff.

The patient continued to discuss these dreams with a powerful sense of sadness interlaced with an even more unusual optimism that he need not continue to maintain such distorted and self-destructive fantasies.

Two days later he had the interesting experience of suddenly recalling several satisfactory sexual affairs that had taken place during his early twenties. Mr A said, 'I'd completely forgotten these. I'm amazed to remember them. It's hard for me to believe that I put my penis into the womb.' He was unaware that he had said womb for vagina. He then went on to speak of how seductive his mother was. 'She wore beautiful black dresses with her breasts exposed. She had huge breasts. Like my mother, I look best in black.'

He reported the following dream the next session.

Dream 3

I'm in the kitchen of our apartment with my wife. I suddenly see three or four brown, flat snakes on the floor moving very fast like cockroaches. They are brown, the color of earth or bugs or feces. I run into the next room for a bug spray. I am frantic. The bug spray is in a jar labeled with a chemical name. I run back, my wife is frantic too. The snakes have found their nest; a large bloated thing with fur on top of it. It's a dead cat. The white fur is being lifted off the body of the dead cat. It's disgusting. I spray, but I feel I can't kill them. There's a plastic bubble around it. We put it in a garbage bag. The big garbage bag is on the street. I have missed the pickup of the garbage. This ominous-looking bag with the thing in it has to sit in our garbage room, which is painted bright red. I write garbage on the bag so that no one will open it. I notice that garbage is the name of the bag maker. I write 'trashe' on the bag. I see that I've misspelled it. I cross out the 'e.'

Associations

I always thought sex was dirty. Taking advantage of poor girls, hypnotizing them, sticking my penis where it didn't belong. From the first time I heard that men put their penis in the vagina, I was repelled. When a kid said that my mother – I mean father – sticks his penis in mother, I was revolted. That whole area is dirty. The dead cat bloated like shit. The snakes rapid as roaches. There was a roach here, there are roaches in my apartment, I was masturbating and saw a roach. The flat snakes wriggling is like a disgusting part of my life, like sudden roaches that panic you. I think the dream is about me as disgusting and rotting. It's odd that I dreamed that I'm disgusting after talking of successful sex with women.

It's odd. Maybe I think that I'm a female. I feel like the image in the dream, distended and round. The snakes are soft brown penises. They have a homing propensity to this large, dead cat. It's a nest in plastic. A large balloon with fur on it. Then I can see that it has feet and paws. The dead cat in the state of decomposition. I always thought the womb was an unhealthy place. It had acrid odors. That the womb sheds its lining means that it's a cavity that rots. The sexual parts of the woman are frightening. You never know what will come out of it: liquid, farts. It's like going into a cavern with stalagmites and stalactites. You could get lost in there.

I will end the report of the clinical material at this point. The patient's fantasies and their elaboration are dense, and I can only give a hint of their character in this presentation. A theoretical proposition cannot be 'proved' by the presentation of complex clinical data. I hope only to indicate that the point of view I am putting forth provides interesting new ways of thinking about and integrating the clinical material.

Discussion

It is my suggestion that we can describe multiple intertwining fears in this patient, none of them fully subsumed under others, giving rise to versions of castration anxiety. There are fears of the female genitalia as a poisonous sewer emitting rotten milk and feces, attended by fantasies of his body and penis as weak and useless by-products of this birth canal, all made of shit. There are fears of the female person as overwhelming, disappointing, castrating and controlling, accompanied by fears that his penis is small and soft and will be swallowed or bitten off or corroded by the vagina. In fact, he prefers to think of the smaller cervix as the vagina. There are fears of the female breast as a squashing, enormous, unattainable symbol of power, with the anxiety that by comparison his penis is a pitiful object of ridicule to any woman, incapable of creating the fluids that connote sexuality. There are fears of the male as hard, castrating, retaliatory, with the consequent fear of exposing his penis in a murderous competition that he must lose. There are fears that his own body is a derivative of his mother's genitalia, disgusting and unacceptable, and unable to support his ideals and ambitions. Furthermore, there are fears of acknowledging the difference between the sexes – in numerous parapraxes, penises and vaginas switch gender and gender is grossly confused. For example, when describing his first ecstatic sexual encounter with his wife, he said, 'It was beautiful. She was very wet. I just slid into her penis.' The very existence of the sexual difference implies terrifying consequences – mother can make new babies, steal his penis, swallow him into her huge cavity, and more. This fear-induced confusion leads to defensive wishes to have mother's more powerful breasts and genitalia, or to endow her with a penis, or to shed his penis so she won't be envious and so on. I could expand this list of pre-Oedipal fears and their attendant representations in forms of castration anxiety.

The underlying terrors described are terrifying in their own right, and not primarily because they arouse the fear of loss of the penis; rather they are frightening because they arouse the terror of being overwhelmed, they damage the capacity for activity and awaken the threat of being driven back into helplessness and passivity. The new and strange perceptions of infancy, whether of the strange genitalia or of the primal scene, for example, shake existing cognitive schemata and threaten to extinguish the reassuring power to anticipate, thereby giving rise to potent new anxieties. The fear of castration, as it appears in the oedipal phase, may be relatively *de novo* in some instances, but in the more usual characterologically disturbed patient it represents the arousal of earlier fears of which the fear of castration is the tolerable close-to-consciousness compromise representation. Giving up a narcissistically endowed part is preferable to giving up the narcissistic self. Castration anxiety may not in itself simply subsume and replace the earlier fears; rather it indicates an attempt to disguise and escape from them. Even under the best of circumstances, the earlier infantile sense of inadequacy is revivable and feeds the terror underlying the defense of the penis. In cases such as my patient, where development does not proceed relatively undamaged, a veneer of castration anxiety hides the fact that the patient is only too willing to forgo penis narcissism and concede the inadequacy of his penis, expanded to include his entire self-image, in order to assure himself that his rage and envy at his mother need not elicit retaliation and annihilation from her and that he still merits her care. Simultaneously, in a bitter irony, he unconsciously demonstrates masochistically what it was that she did to him – destroyed him as a person; castration is only one portion of that.

Summary

Psychoanalysts, following Freud, have generally emphasized that castration anxiety is the central fear, for which pre-Oedipal fears represented an evasion through regression. It is my suggestion that, at least in the patients with character pathology who are seen in analysis today, castration anxiety serves to defend against more primitive pre-Oedipal terrors, still active unconsciously and readily activated in the analytic situation.

I have tried to show, with the aid of a hugely condensed clinical vignette, that the clinical presentation of the castration complex may productively lead to a search for underlying fears. These more elemental fears, threatening the narcissistic integrity of the individual, are often masked by a façade of conspicuous castration fears. In these cases the castration anxiety is best understood as a less frightening defensive compromise in which the individual is willing to imagine the loss of a prized possession, however painful that may be, in order to maintain a semblance of wholeness and the assurance of survival.

THE UNCONSCIOUS CORE OF PERVERSION*

It is characteristic of psychoanalysis today that concepts that once seemed clear and precise are now, in our pluralistic theoretical framework, diffuse or expanded, often beyond definition, although analysts continue to speak and write as if we all know what we are talking about. It would be surprising if the idea of perversion did not show some of these attributes, since perversion not only is one of the earliest analytic concepts but is highly bound both to theory and to cultural norms. I will begin by giving some samples of attempts at definition that may illuminate the domain of our interest, omitting some major contributors as I illustrate the shifting meanings of perversion. I will then discuss the core conflict of passivity and the three fantasies that are always present in perversion, the male–female difference in perversion, and a bit about perverse play and the range of perverse life.

In the 'Three essays on the theory of sexuality,' Freud announced a number of the themes that concern us here. He began with a clear sense of what should be called perversion: 'Perversions are sexual activities which either (a) extend, in an anatomical sense, beyond the regions of the body that are designed for sexual union, or (b) linger over the immediate relations to the sexual object which should normally be traversed rapidly on the path towards the final sexual aim' (Freud 1905b: 150). He formulated perversion as the primacy of a partial sexual instinct, and neurosis as its negative (p. 165). We might note the ambiguity that cultural inventiveness has created concerning what the regions designed for sexual union are and what constitutes lingering rather than rapid traverse. Freud

---

* An early version of this paper was presented a a symposium on 'The Perversions of Everyday Life' sponsored by the Association for Psychoanalytic Medicine, New York, 1989. A later version was presented as the William F. Orr Lecture at Vanderbilt University Medical Center in Nashville, TN, 1989. It was published as Cooper (1991b) 'The unconscious core of perversion', in *Perversions and Near-Perversions in Clinical Practice*, eds G.I. Fogel and W.A. Myers. New Haven, CT: Yale University Press.

stressed this point when he said, 'The most striking distinction between the erotic life of antiquity and our own no doubt lies in the fact that the ancients laid the stress upon the instinct itself, whereas we emphasize its object. The ancients glorified the instinct and were prepared on its account to honor even an inferior object; while we despise the instinctual activity in itself, and find excuses for it only in the merits of the object' (p. 149). In this footnote, added in 1910, not only does Freud emphasize the looseness of the ties of the sexual instinct to the (expected) sexual object, but one might, reading between the lines, suggest that he considered the ancients as having the better of the argument from the viewpoint of pleasure. (Norman O. Brown took this comment of Freud's seriously; in *Life Against Death* (1959) he argued that humans would be better off with instinctual freedom from society's guidance – that is, with freedom for perversion.) Freud went on to emphasize the role of disgust in determining what it is that we choose to call perverse (p. 152), and the need for shame and disgust to constrain the sexual instincts within bounds considered normal (p. 162).

Simultaneously, he held that perversion is the base for the most valued human constructions:

> What we describe as a person's 'character' is built up to a considerable extent from the material of sexual excitations and is composed of instincts that have been fixed since childhood, of constructions achieved by means of sublimation, and of other constructions, employed for effectively holding in check perverse impulses which have been recognized as being un-utilizable. The multifarious perverse sexual dispositions of childhood can accordingly be regarded as the source of a number of our virtues, insofar as through reaction-formation it stimulates their development.
>
> (Freud 1905b: 238)

Perversions – disavowed or repressed, or, perhaps most important, suppressed – were surely part of everyday life, and it is clear that, for Freud, defenses against perverse impulses were a bedrock of human civilization.

Finally, it may be worth reminding ourselves of Freud the moralist who, when discussing '"Civilized" sexual morality and modern nervous illness' in 1908, expressed some views that he never changed – on the one hand, the relentless antagonism between the demands of culture and those of the sexual instincts, and on the other, his own view of the true aims of sex. Referring to the perverse versions of intercourse, he said, 'These activities cannot, however, be regarded as being . . . harmless . . . in love-relationships. They are ethically objectionable, for they degrade the relationships of love between two human beings from a serious matter to a convenient game, attended by no risk and no spiritual participation' (Freud 1908: 200). Freud was serious in claiming love as a criterion of normality, and the perverse is objectionable – or the perverse is perverse –

because it trivializes or degrades love. He objected to masturbation, for example, because it made it too easy to obtain sexual pleasure and because it led to an excessive and facile idealization of the love object without its being measured against the struggle of obtaining satisfaction within the limitations of real people.

Laplanche and Pontalis echo Freud, adding, 'In a more comprehensive sense, "perversion" connotes the whole of the psychosexual behavior that accompanies such atypical means of obtaining sexual pleasure' (1973: 306). They also make the very important point that 'in psychoanalysis, the word "perversion" is used exclusively in relation to sexuality. Where Freud recognises the existence of instincts other than sexual ones, he does not evoke perversion in connection with them' (p. 307). Today some of us consider aspects of aggressive and narcissistic activities as the major source of behaviors we would label perverse. Focusing on the inherent problems of conceptualizing perversion, Laplanche and Pontalis attempt to find the guiding normative principle for Freud in his concept of sexual development and its completion only in the genital phase, but they acknowledge the many difficulties with this view.

Laplanche and Pontalis sound old-fashioned, perhaps, and we might be tempted to think of the *Diagnostic and Statistical Manual* (American Psychiatric Association 1987) as its polar opposite. The difference is surprisingly small, however, and resides more in the details of social politics than in principle. Having abolished the term *perversion* in favor of *paraphilia*, the manual says, 'The Paraphilias are characterized by arousal in response to sexual objects or situations that are not part of normative arousal–activity patterns and that in varying degrees may interfere with the capacity for reciprocal, affectionate sexual activity' (p. 279). The authors' morality is precisely the same as Freud's, but they differ in not attempting a developmental or structural understanding of the phenomenon. The manual continues, 'The essential feature of disorders in this subclass is recurrent, intense sexual urges and sexually arousing fantasies, generally involving either (1) non-human subjects, (2) the suffering or humiliation of oneself or one's partner (not merely simulated), or (3) children or other non-consenting persons. The diagnosis is made only if the person has acted on these urges, or is markedly distressed by them.' It has never been a secret that the manual's view of perversion, right or wrong, was powerfully shaped by the politics of gay liberation, which in turn has influenced analysts' ideas of the everyday perversions.

The effort to escape from the uncomfortable idea of perversion as cultural deviation is well illustrated by Stoller. In an important paper in 1974 and in a major set of works since then, he stressed that everyone is more or less perverse (Stoller 1974: 432), and he distinguished 'perversion' as a diagnosis applied to a personality dominated by a sexual fantasy versus 'perversion mechanisms' universally applied in the attempt to preserve sexual gratification against trauma; the difference is quantitative. Perversion consists of the pursuit of gratification through hostility and vengeance designed to deny and defend against the frightening sexual curiosity, mystery, and danger that surround the traumatic attachment to mother. And very importantly, he suggested that 'in men, perversion may at bottom be a gender disorder,' reflecting the difficulty for men in establishing masculine identity after their primary feminine identification with their mothers (p. 429). Stoller emphasized that without the energizing force of hostility, we are in the realm of mere deviance.

Stoller's work is especially important because it melds concepts of sexuality and the older emphasis on castration and fetishism in forming a perversion with newer concepts derived from the understanding of pre-Oedipal narcissistic and safety needs and the problems of separation and individuation. He also touches on the idea that the male–female perversion difference derives from these earlier states rather than from the anatomical difference alone.

Person and Ovesey (1983), in a series of careful and penetrating studies of gender differentiation, have shown that normal core gender identity is a function of sex assignment and rearing, basically non-conflictual. Gender-role identity, however, is a product of many conflictual issues, involving problems of separation–individuation, complex body perceptions, and all the conflicts of the Oedipus phase. They reject Stoller's concept of primary femininity and stress that where core gender identity of the male is tenuous as a result of disturbances of separation, there is a greater incidence of some forms of perversion. Discussing transvestism, they emphasize that this perversion 'is not simply a sexual disorder, but is best understood as primarily a disorder of the sense of self' (Person and Ovesey 1976: 219). They demonstrate that this disorder of the self is a result of an ego split of male and female gender identities secondary to unresolved separation anxiety occurring during infantile separation–individuation. Person and Ovesey emphasize 'that gender precedes sexuality as in development and organizes sexuality, not the reverse' (1983: 221).

Khan went further in taking the definition of perversion away from the sexual and toward the object-relational. He said, 'The pervert puts an *impersonal* object between his desire and his accomplice: this *object* can be a stereotype fantasy, a gadget or a pornographic image. All three alienate the pervert from himself, as, alas, from the object of his desire. Hence the title of the book, *Alienation in Perversions*' (Khan 1979: 9).

Another step leading analysts far from their original definitions of perversion is illustrated in Arlow's 1971 paper 'Character perversion.' Briefly, he described individuals with an original perversion or tendency toward perversion who replace the symptomatic activity with a character trait. For example, he described characters whose capacity for everyday reality testing was damaged secondary to defenses against voyeuristic and fetishistic perverse needs. Arlow emphasized that in these male patients the root trauma involved exposure to the female genital and consequent discovery of the missing phallus. Here, then, in the concept of perverse character, we have come the full distance toward the idea of perversion as a mechanism without a symptom.

166

I will mention only two more workers in tracing the changed ideas of perversion. Chasseguet-Smirgel has been influential in understanding perversion as a magical attempt to deny the inevitable infantile traumas to omnipotent fantasy in the discovery of the difference between the sexes and the difference between the generations. This disavowal is achieved by the creation of an anal–sadistic universe in which distinctions are erased (penis = feces = child), differentiation from mother is unnecessary, father is nonexistent, pregenitality is idealized, and sublimation is impossible and unnecessary (Chasseguet-Smirgel 1984: 141). In this view, although the psychodynamic premises could not be more different from Kohut's, perversion is an attempted repair of a narcissistic pregenital injury, probably reflecting significant failures in maternal care.

Finally, McDougall describes the neosexualities, emphasizing the desperate inventiveness that characterizes perversion. She stresses that 'the leading theme of the neosexual plot is invariably castration . . . the triumph of the neosexual scenario lies in the fact that the castrative aim is only playfully carried out . . . [Perversions] are all substitute acts of castration and thus serve to master castration anxiety in illusory fashion, at every conceivable level' (McDougall 1985: 252). She also emphasizes that in the neosexualities the patient is unendingly involved in hatred and envy toward the breast-mother while attempting to idealize a maternal image that allows no place for the difference between the sexes (p. 249). 'Neosexualities, then, serve not only to maintain libidinal homeostasis but narcissistic homeostasis as well' (p. 251).

Let me briefly summarize this summary. Over time analysts have changed both their definition of perversion and their theories of perversion. The original definition referred to a sexual action carried out with the wrong body parts (not heterosexual genitalia) and with the wrong sexual ideas (not heterosexual adult loving union). The definitions today vary. Some would retain the original definition intact while others would modify it 'slightly' to permit the use of same-sex genitalia. Another group would stress the contamination of the sexual act, however it is carried out, by rage and hostility; still others would see the essence of perversion in the mode of sexual fantasy, which may be expressed in character traits regardless of the form of sexual action. There is no agreement on whether they should be defining a disorder or a universal psychodynamic mechanism. For the sake of brevity I am omitting a largely nonanalytic group who would maintain that the essence of the definition involves labeling for the purpose of social control.

Theories of perversion today reflect the multiple psychoanalytic points of view – ego psychological, object-relational, and self psychological – that must be considered in describing a complex psychological construction such as perversion. As a result, the universe of the perverse has expanded enormously. Once simply unrepressed or undeveloped pregenital activities, the perverse now includes elaborate fetishistic constructions for healing castration anxiety, attempts to cope with the stresses of gender differentiation, failures to overcome severe narcissistic injury involving generational and sexual difference, failure to separate from early terrifying maternal representations, the characterologic expressions of perverse desires, and expressions of rage and vengeance via sex. Analysts emphasize the fear and aggression, with primitive splitting mechanisms or overdimensional castration fears and disorganizing rage, that derail the capacity for benign object ties. Following the hint of Laplanche and Pontalis (1973) when they spoke of Freud's not evoking the concept of perversion in connection with nonsexual instincts, many later workers have seen perversion primarily or equally as a miscarriage of narcissistic development and consequent aggression, rather than as a primarily libidinal deviation. Within this multiplicity of views, there is remarkable agreement among analysts on the psychodynamics of perversion, focusing on issues of narcissism.

In elaborating this view of the narcissistic base of perverse development, I want to emphasize that the core trauma in many if not all perversions is the experience of terrifying passivity in relation to the pre-Oedipal mother, perceived as dangerously malignant, malicious, and all-powerful, arousing sensations of awe and the uncanny. The development of a perversion is a miscarried repair of this injury, basically through dehumanization of the body and the construction of three core fantasies designed to undo the intolerable sense of helpless passivity. Stoller (1974) and Khan (1979) have taught us about dehumanization in perversion and its relation to fetishism, and I will briefly elaborate their themes. Dehumanization is the ultimate strategy against the fears of human qualities – it protects against the vulnerability of loving, against the possibility of human unpredictability, and against the sense of powerlessness and passivity in comparison to other humans. In every perversion there is the interposition of a nonhuman quality in the otherwise human loving relationship; this may be a fetish object, a rigid routine not subject to emotional influence, or a demonstration of the inhumanity of the seemingly human. The hostility that Stoller correctly identifies as a core of perversion is an aid to the maintenance of dehumanization, not its cause. All attempts to abolish difference – whether of gender, physical size, maturational level, developmental level, power and control, and so on – have dehumanization, the absence of individuation, as one of their goals and consequences.

The attempt to dehumanize is carried out through the use of three specific fantasies. Regardless of which perverse role is adopted in action or conscious fantasy, the perversion is always a result of mixtures of three key unconscious fantasies constructed in the perverse defense against fears of passivity when confronted with maternal malevolence. These fantasies are all efforts to deny the experience of being the helpless, needy baby at the mercy of a frustrating, cruel mother. First fantasy: 'I need not be frightened because my mother is really nonexistent; that is, she is dead or mechanical, and I am in complete control.' Second fantasy: 'I need not be frightened because I am beyond being controlled by my malicious mother because I am myself nonhuman – that is, dead and unable to feel pain – or less than human, a slave who can only be acted upon rather than act.' And third: 'I triumph and am in total control because no matter what cruelty my squashing, castrating, gigantic monster mother-creature visits upon me, I can extract pleasure from it, and therefore she (it) is doing my bidding.' Differing mixtures of these three unconscious fantasies account for different presentations, but they are always present in perversion. They erase passivity by denying human maternal control of oneself as human, by defensively converting active to passive, and by extracting pleasure out of being controlled. These three fantasies deny that mother has hurt or can hurt the child. In effect the infant says, '(1) She doesn't exist, (2) I don't exist, (3) I force her – now a nonhuman "it" – to give me pleasure.' Regardless of whether sexual pleasure is consciously an aspect of the activity and regardless of the prominence of the fetish object, the perversion dynamic is in action whenever the body is treated as not human and mixtures of these three fantasies are present. I will illustrate these themes with two examples from fiction.

The Secret History of the Lord of Musashi by Tanizaki (1982), an eminent contemporary Japanese writer, provides a vivid and deep description of the development of a perversion (I am indebted to Dr Theodore Shapiro for telling me about this book). At the age of six, young Lord Musashi was sent as a hostage to the home of a superior lord who brought him up, part prisoner, part noble. When he was 12, the castle in which he lived was under siege, and though he was too young to be involved in the battle, he was emotionally caught up in it. Young Musashi is befriended by an older woman who says that she has been close to battle, and she agrees to permit him secretly to view how the women attend to the enemy heads taken in battle. The women's nightly task after the day of battle is 'dressing' the heads – cleaning them, arranging the hair, touching up the dye on the teeth, applying some light cosmetic to make the heads presentable, and generally making them look as if they were alive. The primal scene aspects of Musashi's curiosity are powerfully conveyed as the author describes how, while the castle sleeps, he and the woman creep silently through the dark chambers: the woman leading him 'no longer looked like the refined, warmhearted matron that he was used to seeing by daylight. The deep shadows in her sunken flesh gave her the haggard look of a demon mask . . . The night light made . . . the old woman's face so unearthly' (p. 22). He is terrified. He is then led to the room where the women are working. Musashi 'riveted his eyes on the most terrifying objects in the room, determined to let nothing frighten him . . . The heads themselves did not make a strong impression, but the contrast between the heads and the three women awakened a strange excitement in him. Compared to the pallor of the lifeless heads, the women's hands and fingers looked strangely vital, white, and voluptuous . . . They worked mechanically and impassively, their faces as cold and unfeeling as stone. But somehow their impassivity was different from that of the heads. The one was hideous, the other sublime' (pp. 23–24). The fantasy of the female with total power, handling the

169

passive dead male head, the fetishistic object, becomes exciting. Beauty equals cruelty. He finds it all 'alluring' (p. 25).

The youngest of the three women – she is 15 or 16 – is described as having a natural charm; 'as she gazed at a head an unconscious smile would play about her lips. It was this smile that attracted [Musashi] to her. At such moments, a guileless cruelty showed in her face. And her hands were more supple, more graceful . . . To [Musashi] she was irresistibly beautiful' (p. 25). Musashi realizes 'he had witnessed an extraordinary scene . . . To a boy of twelve, it must have seemed that a separate, hidden world had unfolded before him for a moment and then abruptly disappeared' (p. 26). The next day he is not certain that it was not all a dream, but he cannot free himself of the images of the night, and he feels himself falling in love with the young woman. 'Hers was a bewitching beauty, spiced with the bitterness of cruelty.' He 'envied the head placed before the beautiful girl. He was jealous . . . He wanted to be killed, transformed into a ghastly head with an agonized expression, and manipulated in the girl's hands. Becoming a severed head was a necessary condition. He found no pleasure in imagining himself alive at her side; but if he could become such a head and be set before her in all her charm, how happy he would be!' (p. 30). This is obviously the core of perversion – to become the passive, manipulated, dead, and deformed object of the malicious female.

As he discovers these feelings in himself he realizes that something diseased and malignant is going on in him; contrary to his outward boldness, bravery, and aggression, he has discovered his inner passivity in the identification with the mutilated, dead object of his passion. These strange feelings reach a climax on the third night of watching, when the girl he is in love with has before her the head of a young samurai whose nose has been cut off, a so-called woman-head. 'As a result the face was uglier and more comical than those of ordinary ugly men. The girl . . . as she always did, gazed at the center of the face where the nose should have been and smiled. Juxtaposed with the mutilated head, the girl's face glowed with pride and joy of the living, the embodiment of flawless beauty and her smile, precisely because it was so girlish and unaffected, now appeared to be brimming with the most cynical malice and provided the boy with a wheel on which to spin endless fantasies . . . The fantasies it inspired were inexhaustible and before he was aware of it had lured his soul away to a land of ambrosial dreams where he himself had become this noseless head and was living with the girl in a world inhabited only by the two of them' (p. 33). The double castration and the sense of womanly malevolence arouse him to heights of masochistic pleasure.

Thinking to please the girl, and wishing to again have the pleasure of watching her with a 'woman-head,' he tries to capture one himself but is unable to sever the head of his enemy, managing only to sever the nose, which he carries around with him, not knowing why. The 'secret paradise' of his perversion has been discovered (p. 54).

Later, as a young samurai, Musashi learns that the wife of his lord is the daughter of the man whose nose he cut off. She believes the deed was done by her husband and has asked an admirer of hers to cut off her husband's nose as a humiliating vengeance. Musashi, discovering a woman with such capacity for cruelty, falls instantly in love with her. Her husband, comically, is bit by bit deformed by partial castrations – the loss of an ear and of a part of his lip as a result of arrow wounds from the eager-to-please suitor, who keeps just missing his target, the nose. Musashi establishes forbidden contact with his love by hiding in the shit pit of her toilet, climbing in through that tunnel to her room. The anality of perversion is made literal. Musashi plots with her to cut off her husband's nose, since he is eager to see another noseless head beside the woman, and he accomplishes this deed. The full-fledged perversion that emerges later involves Musashi's need to threaten violent castration (cutting off the nose) of a man in order to achieve arousal. But the author makes clear that the aggression masks the masochistic identification with the castrated object. His secret desire is to be the victim of the woman's cruelty. 'His secret desire is to see the noseless husband beside his incomparably beautiful wife' (p. 101).

The novel contains all the elements of the development of a perversion: parental abandonment, exposure to violence during childhood or adolescence and reexposure as a young adult, confirmation of the fantasies of the cruelty of women, a lost struggle against his own castration fears and terror of passivity, the equation of beauty with lust and cruelty, and the inability to maintain asexual self-representation apart from the representation of the male as the victim of female cruelty. Incidentally, I find that this is the case in all sadistic perversions. In sadistic perversion, the perverse sadistic humiliating act conceals the underlying masochistic identification. All three of the fantasies I described – mother is not human, I am not human, I enjoy torture – are illustrated in Musashi's perversion. The female is demonic, the man is a fetish object, and being tortured by the demonic mother is an exquisite pleasure. These fantasies are the bedrock out of which the perversion is formed. This novel portrays the child's awe of the mysteries of mother and the arousal of the sense of both beauty and the uncanny, what Freud described as 'that class of the terrifying which leads back to what is known of old and long familiar to us' in the perverse. The experience of awe and the uncanny, so common in perversion, is, of course, part of the construction of art and literature, and its exploration is one of the paths Freud alluded to when he spoke of the perverse as the stimulus for our virtues. Beautiful objects are perhaps created in part to allay the fear of passivity – the object of art is not alive. But that is another topic.

The Piano Teacher, a novel by Elfrieda Jelinek (1983/1988) illustrates some of the differences between male and female perversion. Erica Kohut, a 35-year-old piano teacher who failed to make it as a concert pianist, is totally and hopelessly enmeshed in her dependency on and rage against a ferociously intrusive narcissistic controlling mother. She is friendless and sexless but harbors secret fantasies.

171

Periodically she buys extravagant, wildly colored outfits that she doesn't wear; many nights she walks in the park observing and disturbing sexual couples, and she participates in a peep show along with the male voyeurs. She is secretly exhibitionistic, overtly voyeuristic. She is also a secret cutter. 'She sits alone in her room . . . She gingerly tests the edge; it is razor sharp. Then she presses the blade into the back of her hand several times but not so deep as to injure tendons. It doesn't hurt at all. The metal slices her hand like butter . . . She makes a total of four cuts. That's enough, otherwise she'll bleed to death' (p. 43). Erica is frigid, feels nothing sexually. Her life is dedicated to appearing superior and sabotaging those of her students who might be successful. She places broken glass in the coat pocket of a young woman flutist who shows great promise, is the pride of the school, and is about to give a recital. When the young musician puts her hand in her pocket, she is badly cut and unable to perform. Erica, incidentally, breaks the glass while she is in the toilet, again the anal theme. The hatred motivating Erica to such perverse violence is, it is clear, the consequence of her inability to separate herself from the feeling of total control by her mother. 'Her mother demands obedience. If you take a risk, you perish. That advice comes from mother too. When she is home alone she cuts herself, slicing off her nose to spite other people's faces . . . She sits down in front of the magnifying side of the shaving mirror, spreading her legs, she makes a cut, magnifying the aperture that is the doorway into her body. She knows from experience that such a razor cut doesn't hurt . . . Her hobby is cutting her own body' (p. 86).

A young student of hers, a narcissistic body-builder, forms a plan to seduce her, and she becomes interested. She sends him a letter telling him what he must do in order to possess her. The letter is an elaborate, detailed, obsessive description of the forms of bondage and beating and torture that she wants him to put her through, including when and at what commands he is to perform which acts. He is completely repelled by her assuming control over his seduction and is made impotent by her demandingness and provocation. Their mutual perversions finally take the form of rape. He, to recover his potency, becomes enraged and beats her, breaking her nose and ribs, bloodying her, and penetrating her with a triumphant erection. She, in response to the rape, is briefly angry, takes her razor to pursue him, and ends up cutting herself again, somewhat depersonalized.

In this novel, issues of conquest and control have totally replaced anything resembling human love, and perversion is one aspect of the heroine's pathology. We have here a different arrangement of the core fantasies. Never having separated from mother, she manages to avoid total passivity by hating all living creatures, manifested partly in her self-mutilation, and dehumanizing her mother and herself. Still merged with the mother, she proves by a single act – cutting without feeling – that both mother and child are nonhuman. Remnants of sexuality are used defiantly, and the masochistic pleasure she pleads for from her would-be lover is denied her in the form that she demands – with herself in control of her victimization – and is instead carried out with herself totally passive. One might note that in both novels, the perverted characters are concerned with beauty – Erica is a serious musician, although we never learn that she has been moved by music.

The differences between Lord Musashi and Erica Kohut lead us to a difficult theme – the male–female differences in perversion, Most authors who have written about perversions seem agreed that 'the leading theme of the neosexual plot is invariably castration' (see McDougall 1985: 252).

In an earlier paper (Chapter 13 of this book) I noted that the seemingly central role of castration anxiety in male character and symptom formation most often disguises underlying pre-Oedipal anxieties of the loss of narcissistic well-being, as represented in feelings of safety, adaptive organization, and continuing attachment to mother (Fogel *et al.* 1986). Castration anxiety, I tried to demonstrate, represents an escape to a cognitively more organized fear – fear of the loss of a body part – that displaces an unbearable tension of annihilation or disorganization. Person has emphasized that before castration anxiety appears, the boy's inability to secure his mother's love and prove adequate to her are predisposing narcissistic traumas that heighten later castration anxiety (Person 1986: 20). It is McDougall's view also that the evils of maternal attachment are condensed in the castration anxiety involved in perversion, and she emphasizes the narcissistic as well as libidinal trauma in perversion.

The assumption that castration anxiety is a façade may help us understand why women seem less involved, or at least less overtly involved, in sexually perverse activities. In the absence of the direct symbolic castrative object, as embodied in the creation of the fetish, women's perversions take more subtle forms. Although women are not usually accused of perverse exhibitionism, much of women's fashion and the peek-a-boo game that is played with the breast are, for certain women, an opportunity to enact a female version of the 'flasher.' It may be that it is women's perversions, not their superegos, as Freud thought, that lack crispness and definition because of their attenuated castration anxiety. The perverse exhibiting woman uses her capacity to excite a male by the sight of her breast or body to overcome her own sense of smallness and unfemininity compared to her mother, as well as to demonstrate the greater power of her breast or whole body compared to the male penis. The sexual excitement she experiences in this triumph involves dehumanization of her own body and the male's and murder of the mother. The fetishistic object is not a phallus but a breast. In fact, one can raise the question whether fantasies of the huge breast do not underlie the fantasies of the phallus in fetishism. A homosexual patient described that he would much rather caress a man's penis than a woman's breast because the penis was larger. When asked to describe how he was conducting his measurements, he explained that he was comparing the nipple of the breast to the entire penis, a clear denial of the full breast. Another homosexual male speaks of his requirement that his pick-up partner have 'perfect good looks, be like a perfect meal or a great wine.' The oral reference is not accidental.

We also are quite unknowing, I believe, of the extent of female perverse activity. Late-night television and dirty-talk telephone numbers indicate that some women seem quite eager to tease men with their exhibitionistic activities. The classic striptease represents an exhibitionistic frustration and the teasing, not the gratification, of male voyeurism. Intermittent homosexual relations are carried out by women far more casually than by men, and vibrators and dildos are common apparatuses of many female sex lives. Many women reveal during the course of an analysis that they routinely check men's crotches, becoming aroused by looking at the outline of the genitals. Adolescent girls, however, seem not to spend the hundreds of hours that adolescent boys devote to trying to glimpse the mysterious forbidden body of the opposite sex. Numbers of normally functioning women periodically prefer intercourse tied spread-eagle to the bed or wish to be slapped on the buttocks. Some of the recent sex scandals that have emerged in nursery schools indicate that women also seem involved in a variety of pedophiliac activities. Which of these activities should be considered perverse is answerable only by knowing the extent to which they dehumanize actual relationships. Although female perversion is certainly present, it may be quantitatively less of an issue either because of the constancy of gender identification, as Stoller has indicated, or because of the greater difficulty the male experiences in gender-role establishment.

The point I want to stress is that female perversion may show less fetishistic focus and clearer central emphasis on struggles over passivity and control. Women are perhaps at less risk for the violent terrors the boy experiences as he realizes his need to establish masculinity. The female inability to separate from the mother is the entirety of the rage, whereas for the male that rage is compounded by the need for male gender definition in face of the awe and wonder excited by the sense of the mother as different, alien, as well as proof of the reality of castration. Much of the history of Western culture and religion includes the relentless effort of the male to tame, control, and demystify the female to relieve his anxiety.

Finally, I want to stress the difference between perversion as play within the culture and perversion as pathology. As play, perversion carries into life some of the spice of the forbidden, the mysterious, and the dangerous in forms allowed by society although not always recognized as perverse. Freud took it for granted that remnants of infantile sexuality can always be found in adult life, and we would surely consider that ordinary rather than pathological. I take it for granted that each of us has secrets, that some secrets relate to the perverse, and that they help provide us with individual boundaries and identity. The question is never whether but how much. Fashion provides one example of perversion as play, creeping into the forms of daily life. Transvestism, a recognized paraphilia in the *Diagnostic Manual*, has clearly been a major theme of fashion and of rock musicians in recent years. This play with sexual ambiguity, combined with a spirit

174

of aggression and potential violence, fits very well into the scheme of the perverse attempt to erase difference and to dehumanize. Similarly, the popularity of films like *Blue Velvet* or *The Night Porter* demonstrates that the ordinary citizen is pleased to have a chance to play with perversion and enjoy its forbidden fruits without having to be perverse. Reading or viewing porn is another instance of playing with perversion, and the apparently common practice of couples using porn movies on the VCR to assist in increasing sexual excitement can also be considered the playful use of perversion. In these senses we may view our society as dedicated to playing with perversion. But we may not be different from other societies in the past. From the point of view, for example, of the exhibitionistic need to show something and the voyeuristic need to be frustrated in the desire to see something, it probably matters little whether the game is being played with an ankle or a breast or the genitalia.

The severe inhibition of these forms of play – the inability to engage in the touchings and suckings and odd kissings of foreplay, or the inability to tolerate perverse play in society – is another outcome of conflict over perversion. Individuals in whom the shame and disgust needed to overcome perverse impulses are so overwhelming that they are forced to regard the body as humanly unacceptable and beyond human play are thereby paradoxically succumbing to the perverse need to dehumanize.

In between play with perversion and obligatory perversion we can place the facultative, or occasional, pervert. The majority of perverse individuals, which may be the majority of people, feel the pressure for perverse action primarily when there is an additional stress to their narcissistic well-being. Beginning a creative work, preparing for an examination, being away from home and spouse, are typical occasions for perverse actions – masturbation with pornographic movies or magazines, calls to porn hotlines, visits to homosexual bars, dealings with prostitutes. Some men report compulsive masturbation after seemingly satisfying sex with their wives; some others report that their sex lives are entirely satisfactory – provided that there is no demand on them for any kind of tender or affectionate interaction, or provided that the routine never changes. In all these instances, fears of ultimate passivity are aroused by the task or by the absence of a supporting selfobject or by the evidence of the woman as independent, with a capacity to make demands and to have her own feelings. These perverse acts deny the woman's existence and the man's need for her. Again, these acts seem more prevalent among men than women, but we may know less about the female versions.

Perversion has become somewhat like masochism and narcissism in that the term needs to be described in each usage if we are to understand each other. I have stressed the common psychological mechanism at work in all those situations in which, however briefly, the body is dehumanized and in which mixtures of three defensive fantasies – mother is not human, I am not human, and I enjoy victimization – are constructed in the effort to avoid the fear of infantile passivity. I have taken a dimensional rather than a categorical view of perversion. Within that broad spectrum it remains important to specify our quantitative differences. As with all aspects of character, playing games with perverse mechanisms, stopping short of serious damage to the object or the relationship, needs to be sharply distinguished from malignant sexual perversions that destroy the object. A quantitative assessment of the extent of perverse encroachment on all aspects of character function is essential. The overt obligatory pervert is hugely different from the playful pervert, but realizing what they have in common will help analysts both to better understand and to empathize with the severely ill pervert and to recognize the amount of perverse activity in everyday lives. At certain points quantitative differences lead to qualitative distinctions, and we need different names for the different activities; but my aim, at this moment, is to stress the psychodynamic commonality of our perverse activities.

The perversion dynamic is present whenever an action or fantasy is dominated by the denial of unconscious passivity through the triple fantasies of dehumanizing the object, dehumanizing the self, and securing masochistic pleasure. This dynamic is universal, with huge and important quantitative differences in individuals and in the same individual in different circumstances. Differences between male and female perversion may reside in the diminished awe and castration anxiety experienced by the female in gender definition and separation–individuation. Understanding the ubiquity of perversion ought to help analysts empathize with very damaged perverse patients and to understand the role in everyday life of the perverse aspects of our psychic structures.

14

PARANOIA

A part of most analyses*

Franz Kafka (1923), an expert on paranoia, gave a vivid description of some of the characteristics of the paranoid personality in his story 'The burrow.' The story is written in the first person by some unidentified creature describing the construction of his hidden underground burrow. I shall quote some excerpts from the beginning of the story:

> I have completed the construction of my burrow and it seems to be successful. All that can be seen from outside is a big hole. That, however, really leads nowhere . . . True, some ruses are so subtle that they defeat themselves. I know that better than anyone . . . but you do not know me if you think I am afraid or that I built my burrow simply out of fear . . . Someone could step on the moss or break through it and then my burrow would lie open and anybody who liked – please note, however, that quite uncommon abilities would also be required – could make his way in and destroy everything for good. I know that very well and even now, at the zenith of my life, I can scarcely pass an hour in complete tranquility . . . All this involves very laborious calculations and the sheer pleasure of the mind in its own keenness is often the sole reason why one keeps it up . . . For despite all my vigilance may I not be attacked from some quite unexpected quarter? . . . I certainly have the advantage of being in my own house and knowing all the passages and how they run. A robber may very easily become my victim and a succulent one, too . . . And it is not only by external enemies that I am threatened, there are also enemies in the bowels of the earth . . . But the most

* This paper was first presented at a symposium on 'Paranoia: New Psychoanalytic Perspectives' sponsored by the Association for Psychoanalytic Medicine, New York, in 1991. It was later published as Cooper (1993b) in *Journal of the American Psychoanalytic Association*. Reproduced with permission.

beautiful thing about my burrow is the stillness. Of course, that is deceptive. At any moment it may be shattered and then all would be over.

(Kafka 1923: 325–327)

The creature describes the center of his burrow, the Castle Keep, the room where everything is stored and everything is absolutely in order. He says:

The soil is very loose and sandy, and had literally to be hammered and pounded into a firm state to serve as a wall for the beautifully vaulted chamber, but for such tasks the only tool I possess is my forehead, so I had to run with my forehead thousands and thousands of times for whole days and nights, against the ground, and I was glad when the blood came for there was a proof that the walls were beginning to harden; and that way, as everybody must admit, I richly paid for my Castle Keep . . . It is not so pleasant, however, when as sometimes happens, you suddenly fancy, starting up from your sleep, that the present distribution of your stores is completely and totally wrong, might lead to great dangers, and must be set right at once, no matter how tired or sleepy you may be. Besides, it is stupid but true that one's self-conceit suffers if one cannot see all one's stores together and so, at one glance know how much one possesses.

(Kafka 1923: 327–330)

No, if one takes it by and large, I have no right to complain that I am alone, have nobody that I can trust. I certainly lose nothing by that and probably spare myself trouble. I can only trust myself and my burrow.

(Kafka 1923: 338)

The troubled beast describes the impossibility of achieving any sense of safety, endlessly imagining outside creatures that threaten to enter his burrow. Each new security measure leads to new possibilities of hazard in endless sequence, and he experiences increasing frenzy and disorganization as he is unable to quell his conviction of possible unknown attackers who may be intruding on his space. He experiences the gradual collapse of his defenses.

This is a good description of the paranoid character as it appears in many analyses – rather more complete, but entirely consonant with the DSM-III-R description (American Psychiatric Association 1987). (1) At almost every moment one's very life is at stake. (2) One's entire psychic life is devoted to defense against imminent attack, and endless anxious vigilance is required. No space or energy is left for pleasure. Peace or certainty lasts only a moment. At the same time fear and passivity are ferociously denied. (3) The surface is all façade; the real life is underground, secret, not available to scrutiny. There is enormous pride in the capacity to disguise intentions, hide meanings, keep secrets. (4) There is great pleasure in feeling that one is smarter than one's

enemies. Keenness of mind is valued for its own sake. (5) Murderous oral canni-
balistic thoughts, eat or be eaten, are omnipresent. However, every aggressive
intention feels as if it were only defensive. (6) Enemies are outside and inside.
(7) The edifice of defense and attack is constructed entirely with the efforts of
one's mind, the forehead. The achievement is solely one's own; no one else has
helped. (8) The life is totally isolated, but malignant others are constantly
imagined. (9) No defense feels adequate. Inner reproach cannot be laid to rest,
and failure and danger are always imminent. (10) Obsessional defenses bolster
paranoid construction (as Melanie Klein (1932, 1935) pointed out). (11) There
is a bittersweet pleasure in the feeling of enforced isolation. (12) Finally, one
would conclude that the paranoid life is a hard one.

Psychoanalytic views of paranoia

With this view of paranoia in mind, I would like to place paranoid defenses
within the context of our growing knowledge of pre-Oedipal object relations,
infantile narcissistic needs, and masochistic defenses, and to show how aspects
of paranoia are important parts of most analyses, often requiring specific address.
Meissner (1978, 1986), particularly interested in processes of internalization,
advances similar views in considerable detail, with a perspective on the manifestation of the paranoid process through the life cycle.

It is part of the history of psychoanalysis that clinical characteristics studied
originally for their pathological meanings and consequences were later restudied
with an emphasis on their role in normal development and their functioning
as an aspect of health. Narcissism has most recently received this revision,
due in large part to the work of Kohut (1977), who gave special emphasis to the
healthy aspects of narcissism. Brenner (1959) and a succession of later workers
on masochism, including myself (Cooper 1984b, 1988a, 1989a), have established
masochistic tendencies also as an aspect of ordinary, i.e. healthy or normal,
characterologic functioning. Not only are masochistic tendencies ubiquitous,
but masochistic defenses regularly serve important purposes in character formation. Obviously, the same can be said for all of the characterologic disorders
and traits – histrionic, obsessional, etc. In these discussions we sometimes
blur whether we are talking about precisely the same mechanisms in differing
degrees or whether we are merely noticing similarities of some of the outer
manifestations of different internal structures. When we label people histrionic,
do we mean that they always have both exhibitionistic tendencies toward
outward affective display and a tendency toward the defenses of repression
or dissociation, or do we mean only the former? Similarly, when we discuss
obsessional tendencies, do we mean only orderliness, stinginess, and stubborn
control, or do we also mean the internal struggle over defiance and passivity?
I suggest that the dynamics, as well as the phenomenology, are present even in

the mild cases. Like any other character trait, paranoid mechanisms are ubiquitous, serve important adaptive functions as well as being a source of pathological
distortions, and in the course of analysis they come to the forefront of attention.

There is no need here to review Freud's ideas on paranoia in detail. I shall
mention a few papers of Freud and others to emphasize something we all know
today – that Freud later held a view of paranoia quite distinct from that presented
in the Schreber case (Freud 1911). In 1931, many years after Freud wrote his
analysis of Schreber's book, he wrote his ground-breaking paper 'Female
sexuality,' in which, for the first time, he acknowledged the critical role of pre-
Oedipal development and conflict in understanding the psyche. Freud stated:

> Our insight into this early, pre-Oedipus, phase in girls comes to us as a surprise
> . . . *that in this dependence on the mother we have the germ of later paranoia in women.*
> *For this germ appears to be the surprising, yet regular, fear of being killed (? devoured)*
> *by the mother.* It is plausible to assume that this fear corresponds to a hostility
> which develops in the child towards her mother in consequence of the
> manifold restrictions imposed by the latter in the course of training and bodily
> care and that the mechanism of projection is favoured by the early age of the
> child's psychical organization.
>
> (Freud 1931: 226–227; emphasis added)

Later, in his 'New introductory lectures' he expanded this insight and, writing
on 'Femininity,' said, 'we discover the fear of being murdered or poisoned, which
may later form the core of a paranoia illness, already present in this pre-Oedipus
period, in relation to the mother' (Freud 1933a: 120). While Freud conservatively
confined his considerations to women, today we recognize this conflict as an
aspect of every individual's psychic organization. This is also, of course, the nidus
of Melanie Klein's constructions, which were being elaborated at the same time
(1932, 1935). Because her work on paranoid formation is so well known, I shall
assume its presence in this discussion and will briefly mention some parallel
contributions.

Ferenczi (1988), in his *Clinical Diary*, entry of 10 April 1932, made a similar
point. Under the heading of 'Erotomania as the basis of all paranoia,' he tried to
understand grandiose delusional formation as a narcissistic defense against the
traumatic loss of the love object. He wrote:

> Being loved, being the center of the universe, is the natural emotional
> state of the baby, therefore it is not a mania but an actual fact. The first
> disappointments in love (weaning, regulation of the excretory functions, the
> first punishments through a harsh tone of voice, threats, even spankings) must
> have, in every case, a traumatic effect, that is, one that produces psychic
> paralysis from the first moment. The resulting disintegration makes it possible
> for new psychic formations to emerge. In particular, it may be assumed that

a splitting occurs at this stage. The organism has to adapt itself, for example, to the painful realities of weaning, but psychic resistance against it desperately clings to memories of an actual past and lingers for a shorter or longer period in the hallucination: nothing has happened, I am still loved the same as before (hallucinatory omnipotence). All subsequent disappointments, later on in one's love life, may well regress to this wish-fulfillment.

(Ferenczi 1988: 83)

In other words, all losses revive the trauma of original narcissistic loss and awaken reparative regressive revivals of the state of narcissistic blissful grandeur, but now in the form of paranoid grandiosity.

Fairbairn, writing in 1941, further diminishing the centrality of the Oedipus complex in psychic development in favor of pre-Oedipal development, proposed that the Oedipal situation is primarily sociological rather than psychological, and that all psychopathology results from the hazards of the unconditional dependent identification of the infant with the object, and the life-and-death choice involved in coping with frustrations by the object. He saw paranoia not as a stage of fixation, but as a technique characterized by externalization (excretion) of the internalized object, not just of inner impulses. At the end of his paper Fairbairn states, 'even the most "normal" person must be regarded as having schizoid [i.e. paranoid] potentialities at the deepest levels' (Fairbairn 1941: 101).

So much for history. I obviously have selected my few authorities to make a point. Viewed in the light of the emphasis on the critical nature of the pre-Oedipal phase in psychic development, and the shift in Freud from a psychology of impulse to a psychology of object-relations, we may suggest (and I have done that in an earlier paper (Cooper 1986c)) that in paranoia, underlying the original emphasis on the projection of unacceptable homosexual wishes and castration anxiety of the Schreber analysis, we find: (a) terror over inner passivity, stressed particularly in 'Analysis terminable and interminable' (Freud, 1937a: 252; Cooper 1991d); (b) terror and fury over the loss of narcissistic intactness occasioned by perceived loss and failure of perfect mothering, and consequent fears of loss of capacity to maintain self-esteem; (c) terror of the building murderous rage that accompanies these fears; and (d) the defensive projection of this rage onto the external world, beginning with the mother. Freud, Abraham, Klein, Ferenczi, Fairbairn, Bergler, Bak, Kernberg, Blum, Meissner, myself, and many others have seen paranoia as a part of the responses to the inevitable mortifications to the narcissism that sustains infantile self-esteem. If this is the core of paranoia, as this reading of Freud suggests, then of course we shall find the mark of these conflicts in every variety of character formation, but especially in the narcissistic–masochistic character (Cooper, 1988a). What gives a particular conflict or character its paranoid flavor is not the content alone, but also, as Kafka (1923) and Shapiro (1965) have described, the extent to which certain specific

181

cognitive styles and uses of projection shape the defenses against the narcissistic hurt and masochistic guilt. Paranoid thinking implies a fixed preconception of the malevolent nature of the world and its objects, or at least of specific objects, and an intolerance for personal responsibility; faults and imperfections are always the result of the malign activities of others.

While we know astonishingly little yet about the specificity of choice of neurosis, Westen (1990), in an important paper on empirical research on the theory of borderline object-relations, makes several points about our knowledge of development that are germane to an understanding of paranoia. As Emde (1981) and others have done before, Westen suggests a 'new look' to our psycho-analytic understanding of all psychic functioning, one that I endorse. Research suggests the following.

1. We have underrated the role of cognitive style and cognitive deficits in understanding character development generally and specifically the 'splitting' or 'lack of capacity to tolerate ambivalence' so characteristic of both the border-line and the paranoid. These are best understood as results of the impact of deficits in affect regulation on cognition – specifically, deficits in the control of the impact of high affective arousal on cognitive processing. While these deficits arise at a variety of developmental junctures from infancy through adolescence and beyond, nonetheless, 'The affective quality of the object world and the capacity to invest in other people are fundamentally shaped in the preoedipal years, so that disruptive or abusive attachments are highly pathogenic' (Westen 1990: 689). Borderlines and paranoids do not develop the cognitive abilities to counteract dysphoric affects with positive cognitions, e.g. the ability to tell themselves that all is not lost after a bad event. In my view, the paranoid pervasive sense of calamity is also sustained by the grandiose and masochistic conviction that each bit of injustice that befalls one is specifically meted out by a cruel object to torture the innocent individual who would be perfectly, autarchically self-sufficient without this malign interference. This affective, object-relational origin of the paranoid's rigid, blaming, distorted, causal cognitive style becomes fixed, secondarily autonomous, and in adult paranoid behavior it represents a deficit, not simply a conflictual compromise, and is not responsive to inter-pretation alone. Change requires the full weight of prolonged transferential experience with the uniquely persistent and consistent analyst, and the eroding effects of cognitive dissonance within the safety of the analytic setting, as well as the structural and motivational shifts occurring in the course of analysis.

2. According to Westen (1990), object-relations are the result of a number of separate and distinct developmental lines, e.g. specific and generalized self-representations and object representations, representations of social interactions, understanding of social causality (that is, what causes people to think, feel, and act as they do), capacity for mature cathexis or emotional investment in the self and others. The cognitive, affective, and motivational processes that constitute object relations are at least partly independent, and pathology may

exist differently in each mode. Paranoids, for example, may have highly distorted object representations, accurate representations of social interactions, and inaccurate understanding of affective meanings. The patients under discussion are, at particular times and under particular circumstances, also paranoid; it is not their primary character trait.

3. Systematic child observation requires that we abandon our traditional global view of developmental stages, as well as the idea that infantile stages could be reconstructed from adult treatment – a point also strongly made by Emde (1981, 1988). In this view, borderline object-relations are not identical to the object-relations of toddlers, and adult paranoid syndromes are not identical to infant or child projections. Whether we are viewing narcissistic, masochistic, paranoid, or borderline pathology, we are not in the presence of an arrest of normal growth – either simple fixation or regression – but we are observing the outcome of pathological growth. No matter how primitive wish–fear–defense–affect–cognition–structural configurations may appear to us, they are never simply infantile.

For example, Rorschach research indicates that borderlines, in contrast to depressives and normals, make their most cognitively advanced attributions of intention on figures regarded as malevolent rather than benign. Malevolence of this degree of complexity of form is not simply a pre-Oedipal issue, but requires development well past latency. I suspect this finding on borderlines would apply equally to the more severely narcissistic patients using paranoid defenses. Unlike borderline patients, these patients clearly separate self and other, do not have identity diffusion, and maintain a far greater degree of object constancy; but while the malevolence of the object is fixed, maturation confers greater complexity and conviction to the object-relation.

This fine dissection of the complexity and individual variability of the object-relational, cognitive, and affective deficits we encounter clinically helps us to understand the various levels of paranoid functioning, its waxing and waning under varied conditions of psychic stress, and the compatibility of primitive affective and cognitive features with high-level social functioning. Paranoia as it appears in ordinary analyses is not a constant, but is a quality that appears under specific conditions of conflict for that patient. I shall try to illustrate some of these points with a clinical vignette.

Clinical illustration

A highly successful professional man in his late thirties began analysis because he was not getting anywhere in his desire to be married, and did not know what the trouble was. He had seen another analyst for two months, but quit when he concluded the analyst was cold, stupid, and sadistic, and he could not stand the withholding and the demand that he speak.

He described his family as close, loving, and completely ordinary. He expressed fear that he might fail in analysis because analysis was supposed to make him hate his mother and he was not sure he had any reason to do that. He was an only child of middle-class parents, the father a successful business-man, the mother a housewife. He was the apple of their eye, and was expected to be perfect. He had no difficulty describing that the mother was expert at suggesting that any misbehavior on his part would lead to her death. When, in his early teens, she developed a carcinoma of the breast and required a mastectomy, he was convinced he was to blame, a conviction he still retained. The father, less overt in his guilt induction, shared with his son the feeling that the mother was fragile and great care should be exercised to be sure she was never upset.

After several preliminary interviews, I recommended analysis, and he thought I might be smarter or livelier than his previous analyst and he was willing to go ahead. He expressed his conviction that because he was so bright, he would figure it out quickly, and he would set a record for speedy analysis. On the other hand, he voiced deep concerns that he would turn out to be hopelessly psychotic and untreatable. Asked about his fear of psychosis, he could not elaborate, other than to say that he must be crazy if he had not been able to figure out his life better than he had. He wanted to be a person with a wife and family, so why wasn't he? He described himself as a worrier as a child. He remembered feeling anxious and telling his parents, perhaps as young as four or five, 'I'm worried.' And indeed worrying was a major part of his personality, as it was of his mother's. 'Worrying,' an acceptable adult family trait, was a tolerable substitute for acknowledging that he was frightened. He was exceptionally bright as a child, had friends, but preferred to be alone. He described trying to get his mother to make excuses for him when the other children called and asked him out to play, but denied any fears of the other children.

He was pleasant, friendly, likeable, had a lively sense of humor. In fact, he went out of his way to be sure that I knew he was witty, was successful in his work and well-liked, and that he had a circle of friends that dated back to childhood, about whom I never learned any details for almost two years of analysis. It emerged over time that no one knew him intimately. At considerable incon-venience, he lived in a neighborhood close to where he had grown up, and where his parents still were.

The first sessions on the couch were striking. He lay down, changing his position frequently in almost convulsive jerky movements, issuing bark-like sounds as he began to say something, and withdrew his beginning commu-nication. He was acutely uncomfortable, with a paralyzing inability to permit himself to make a coherent communication to me. Inquiry as to what this was about revealed that consciously he either had several topics in mind and could not decide which was more worthy of my attention, or the things that came to mind were not appropriate topics – too trivial and nothing that I would be interested in – or he was thinking about problems he had left behind at work and that surely was not a topic, or he could not find a way to phrase his communication in a sufficiently literary style. He prided himself on being articulate, and he was angry with himself whenever he spoke an ungrammatical sentence, or felt the grammatical construction was ungraceful. It was clear that he was unable to muster the degree of trust and control that would allow him to drop some of his critical faculties. Lest there be doubt about at least one level of his conflict, he came in one session, threw himself on the couch, fell into his barking, squirming routine, and said, 'You'd think after I come in bursting to get something out and plop myself down like that I'd come out with something big and juicy rather than the piddling little stuff I have.' When I said that sounded as if he were talking of a bowel movement, he gave a great guffaw, enjoying my absurdity, but relaxed a little and seemed relieved to be understood.

Aware that he had left one analysis because he could not tolerate the anxiety of the analytic setting, I was careful not to let a silence go on very long, and not to leave him with a feeling of losing the power struggle he was creating. Although my interventions were seen as my one-upping him, this was not as anxiety-provoking as the helplessness he felt if a silence continued. For patients of this type, the analytic setting itself seems almost ineluctably designed to excite paranoia. The analyst is out of the patient's line of sight behind his defenseless back, not answering questions, and the patient is in the impossible position of being asked to trust the good intentions of someone unknown and invisible. Paranoia in the analytic situation confronts the analyst with a delicate balance. Any abrupt attempt to interpret a defense arouses all the prior conviction of the imminence and inevitability of attack, and the defenses are paradoxically strengthened, since the patient's fantasy of attack has now been substantiated. Secret-keeping is a routine aspect of paranoid behavior, representing the shame the patient experiences about so many aspects of his inner life, the malevolence he expects from the analyst, and the aggressive attempt to tease the analyst and frustrate him, trying to goad him into attack, and thereby proving the a priori truth of the analyst's malignancy. Considerable patience is required in the face of this hostile teasing, since almost any premature activity on the part of the analyst confirms the patient's aggressive projections. This man withheld important information about sex, self-image, feelings about his body, and feelings toward me. Again, I want to underscore that this outwardly friendly, gregarious man would not have been diagnosed paranoid or borderline by any nosologic system. The analytic situation brought out prominent paranoid defenses that were otherwise well contained.

Over the next several months he relaxed somewhat, his movements on the couch diminished markedly, and he could begin to tolerate silences. At one point he said, 'To me it's obvious that if two people are in a room and not talking to each other they are angry at each other. I'm an outsider in your room – I don't share your thoughts and activities. Things that interest me I'm sure don't

185

genuinely interest you. I can't believe that anyone would actually feel as I do and share my interests. I'm self-centered, and I'm lonely.' He revealed how impossible it was for him to conceive of intimacy with other human beings; he could only hope to appease them, but they could never enter his world. The patient was an unusually able, dedicated, and caring professional, but inwardly he felt that his concern for his clients was indistinguishable from his need to control them, and the conviction that if they did not do well, it was a scheme to make him guilty and anxious. Later in the analysis he said, 'It's a terrible thing for me to realize that I'm not so dedicated to my clients, but only to my not being embarrassed. If I'm on a holiday and a colleague of mine screws up with one of my clients, I'm relieved and I don't feel bad about the client at all. I'm only worried that I shouldn't be shamed.'

The patient had been a humanities scholar before beginning his professional training, and had a lively interest in drama. Despite his subtle appreciation of literature, he was entirely unable to tolerate any ambiguity or ambivalence in himself or in his relationships, insisting that they be black or white. Also, his belief in magic and superstition was prominent. It was difficult for him to talk about anything bad – e.g. sickness or accidents – because talking about it would make it come true. He literally had to find a piece of wood to knock on if we mentioned a possible misfortune. These clearly obsessional devices covered the more primitive aspects of his paranoid fantasy.

He lived in a crude, split, inner world of good and evil. If he revealed a negative thought to me, he was absolutely certain that I would retaliate ferociously and instantly. He thought that was an evidence of his craziness, but he also believed it to be true. He was convinced that if we ever found out what he was really like, I would give up the analysis, unable to 'stomach' him, and he would have to leave because he would turn out to be psychotic. It was a year and a half into the analysis before he could let me know that he had fantasies of my dropping dead in my chair and his having to administer CPR. He could tell me this only after a colleague of his, also in analysis, told the patient that he had those fantasies and had told his analyst. Having told me, he said, 'Don't take it to heart, I don't mean it,' and 'maybe I should leave now, because you certainly won't be in a very good mood toward me for the rest of the session. Who could stand someone who had those thoughts about him? What do you need that for?' This was a rather precise mirror of his view that he could tolerate no attack upon himself and therefore needed to hold everyone at bay lest they find out who he was really, and attack him.

At the same time that he seemed concerned with pleasing me, he engaged in multiple minor provocations. For example, he had great difficulty paying my bills. In an almost comic routine, he described writing the check and not being able to find it five minutes later, writing another one and putting it in his shirt pocket, and then sending the shirt to the laundry, writing a check while sitting in the waiting room, but on finding that my secretary was not there, deciding

186

not to give it to me despite my suggestion that he pay me directly – too crass – and of course he forgot to give it to her later, and so on. He described doing this in every area of his life, pushing his defiance of rules to the brink and counting on 'magic' to rescue him from evil consequences. 'I'm always innocent. But one day my luck will run out, and you will rise in anger against me, maybe because you're starving because I didn't pay you, and you'll demand payment. I can't imagine that the rules are enough reason to insist on my doing something. So what if the check is late! But if you need it, I'll get it to you.' I said, 'You are above the rules and give crumbs to helpless people. All the power lies with you.' 'Exactly,' he replied.

This mixture of paranoid, narcissistic, masochistic, and obsessional features is a common presentation of analytic patients. The extent of paranoid suspicion and rage is often underestimated, comingled as it is with the patient's narcissistic fears of humiliation, and obsessional defenses designed to control and hide the extent of his malignant expectations. Warfare is usually carried on at the level of guerilla resistance rather than nuclear explosion, although occasional cold paranoid fury would burst through. Later in the analysis, after a relatively silent session in which he lay motionless on the couch, he said, 'You did what you wanted. You beat me. Satisfied? It won't happen again.' Paranoia in these patients is not a pathological island in a sea of healthy function. Rather, it represents an available defensive mode that can appear in varying degrees of intensity, whenever there is a threat to higher-level narcissistic defenses. In this patient the relatively polite, ironic, aggressive style that only occasionally broke into overt rage reflected his mother's masked, martyred, relentless aggressive demand that he be an endless source of satisfaction to her – and nothing else. Oedipal conflicts were also apparent. For example, without my knowledge, he began to use the telephone in the resident mailroom near my office to make business calls if he was early. One day there was a notice on the mailroom door that the room was to be kept locked, and he was convinced that I had had that notice put up just to keep him out. He said, 'I don't blame you. Next thing I would have had my feet on your desk and you would have thrown me out.' When I asked him if he thought I was afraid to tell him directly if I did not want him using the mailroom telephone, he said, 'Why would you want to create such a frightening situation?' After a moment's pause he said, 'You mean maybe I provoke frightening situations,' and then said, 'You think it's not so frightening.'

However, the deeper, less available target of his anger and source of his fear was the female. During the early part of the analysis he complained endlessly about all the women calling him for dates, none of whom he was interested in. He dated someone nearly every weekend, angry, but afraid to say no to them, and believing that somehow I thought it would be good for him. When he realized that I did not require that he make dates and was interested mainly in his feelings of victimization by these women, he stopped dating. Subsequent inquiry about masturbation led to a slightly surprised and offended air – clearly that was none of my business – and no reply. He knew that I meant to shame him, and his paranoid defenses hardened.

Telling me a masturbation fantasy was far more difficult than telling me a dream in which a man and woman are going to have a physical fight. She's tough and wiry, the man is ordinary. The woman is the odds-on favorite to win. They go into a closed room and the man emerges, looking bloody and battered, but when they look in the room the woman is dead. It is clear that she was beaten unfairly – she has been bludgeoned with a lead pipe. Furthermore, there has been some kind of torture – a rope with knots has been passed from her mouth and out of her anus. She is hoisted on the rope and left to die – murdered and mutilated. He says images of mutilation have appeared before. 'It makes me a little shaky, says something about me – something nasty.' He adds, 'I felt nauseated yesterday [before the dream] and was embarrassed by my mother's excessive concern. I was empathic with the man in my dream who was doing the bludgeoning. I knew he planned to mutilate her. How did I get so crazy?' While the patient identified overtly with the victorious man in the dream, it became clear that he saw himself as my feminized victim, as well as the victim of any woman close to him. Being closeted in a room with me required that he be always on guard against my perverse and spiteful 'tricks' and power. The patient then discussed his analysis and his original expectation that there would be a catharsis that would cure him. He now felt he was getting in deeper and deeper and maybe he was really crazy. In fact, he was not at all psychotic, but being crazy, although terrifying, was an acceptable, because blameless, explanation for fantasies and behaviors he could not alter, explain, or accept.

Discussion

While projected rage is always present, projection for the everyday paranoid has less to do with emptying the self of unacceptable contents than with explaining away to a ferocious superego the reasons for one's weaknesses and failures. Someone to blame is a critical requirement for these patients. One can hear the child's cry, 'It's not my fault. It's your fault. You made me do it.' The paranoid object for the less severe paranoid is primarily the projection of a desired, fantasied but unattained, powerful, destructive self-representation, combined with the primitive distorted malignant internal objects whose creation probably begins early in life as rationalization for why one is not able to avoid all frustration. Narcissism is salvaged in the form of blame. 'I'd be fine if that monster, wizard, evil genius were not out to get me. If I were up against an ordinary human being, I would win.' This defensive tendency of the frustrated baby coming to grips with the limits of its autonomy becomes the claim of the narcissistic–masochistic character explaining before accusing inner conscience why he is not meeting the standards of the ego ideal. This blaming defense easily blends into magical thinking. Only secondarily in these patients is the paranoid object either the repository of bad inner contents or the projection of an unassimilated internal object. The relentless harshness of the superego's shaming accusations is projected onto an external world in which one is innocent victim and masochistic provocateur. All masochism has a paranoid element to it, with the conviction of being the victim of another person or of a malignant fate aimed at oneself. Blaming may be the universal paranoid mechanism.

In paranoia, in contrast to borderline personality disorder, the paranoid object relation does not rupture. The self and the object are stable, and identity, rather than diffused, is maintained through the relation to the powerful object. The self is defined by the enemy, giving it its substance and importance, and providing the hostile object-relation that, no matter how frightening, is still less dangerous than either the intrusion of intimacy or the horror of inner, empty isolation. The full extent of this patient's paranoid isolation, well hidden by his bonhomie and social façade, was not appreciated by me until well into his analysis. He truly lived in his burrow. The developing transference, of course, both provoked the paranoid fear of intrusion and provided the beginning confidence to be able to risk exposure. The need of patients at some points in the analysis to feel that the analyst is malignantly withholding, or torturing, or controlling, represents attempts to experience themselves as powerful enough to be yielding only to an object of such grand dimensions, to assure themselves that the external world is exactly as predicted, and to protect a fragile self from the hazards of intimacy. It is at these times that the analyst is likely to experience countertransferential boredom, withdrawal, counterattack, inadequacy, blame.

I have tried to demonstrate that paranoid defenses are a very common part of the structure of character pathology generally, and especially prominent in narcissistic–masochistic character pathology. Paranoid constructions may be a minor or major part of the patient's character, and our treatment strategies will differ accordingly, but it is useful to recognize how common they are, how intimately connected with narcissistic and masochistic pathology, and how enticing paranoid challenges are to countertransferential counterattack.

The full acceptance of paranoid defenses as a significant, although sometimes subtle, aspect of the defensive structure in character pathology will better attune us to the ways in which paranoid processes influence the presentation of the patient's suffering, the transference, and our responsiveness.

PART IV

The analyst at work

15

SOME LIMITATIONS ON THERAPEUTIC EFFECTIVENESS

The 'burnout syndrome' in psychoanalysts*

While most analysts are aware of the attractions and pleasures of our profession, we also like to characterize ourselves as members of an impossible profession, taking pride in the idea that we do something that is extraordinarily difficult. Clearly, we don't think it is impossible, but it is worthwhile attempting to catalogue some of the realistic difficulties of analytic work, because there is a group of analysts that do not tolerate well the long-term strains of doing analysis, losing their zest, their skill and their confidence over the course of their career – who 'burn out.' I shall try to catalogue some of the sources of difficulty in analytic work, along with their serious consequences for a group of analysts, and to suggest some remedies. I shall largely confine this discussion to personal issues, rather than the social and professional problems that are inimical to pleasure in the work.

Long experience with psychoanalysis seems to teach that most analyses, although not all, go best over the long run if the analyst maintains an attitude that, paradoxically, includes both therapeutic fervor and therapeutic distance. In gloomy moments it has sometimes seemed to me that the life course of too many analysts begins with an excess of curative zeal and proceeds in the latter part of their careers toward excessive therapeutic nihilism. Both are serious handicaps to therapeutic effectiveness. The task is to extend the period of more or less ideal balance.

The peril of an excess of *furor therapeuticus* is that it places the analyst in the parental position. The patient's failures become personal failures for the analyst,

* This paper was presented at the Baltimore–Washington Psychoanalytic Society in Washington, DC in 1982. It was first published as Cooper (1986a) in © *The Psychoanalytic Quarterly*, 1986, 55: 576–598.

who demands that his patient get well. This, in turn, creates an irresistible unconscious temptation for the patient to manipulate this powerful control over the analyst. The patient's knowledge that he can torture his analyst for all the old real or imagined crimes of parents creates a therapeutic impasse. It is a necessary piece of the analyst–patient relationship that both parties, at some level, are aware that although the analyst's dedication to his patient may be total, his emotional involvement is limited. That is, he will make his utmost effort to do everything to help the patient but should he fail, the analyst may be sad, will examine his responsibility for the failure, may mourn, but he will never feel as if it were his child whom he had lost. The patient is one of many; the analyst will go on doing his work, temporarily sadder and perhaps permanently wiser. Analysts cannot carry out good treatment if they have the same sleepless nights over their patients that parents may have over their children. Simultaneously, the analyst cannot do his job well if he is not basically optimistic and dedicated to the work he is conducting with his patient. One aspect of therapeutic efficacy arises from the patient's perception that an analyst will not easily be discouraged, is extraordinarily persistent, will stick by the patient almost no matter what, and really believes the seemingly bizarre or stupid interpretations he keeps insisting upon. Since analysis is not always rewarding, either immediately or in the long run, the dangers of therapeutic discouragement or disillusionment are great and occur with considerable frequency. The analyst who no longer believes in the efficacy of his methods, who is bored with his patient, who no longer listens carefully or puzzles over his patient's communications, cannot provide the basic elements of the therapeutic situation that are required for optimal treatment.

The suggestion that optimal therapeutic efficacy depends on maintaining a stance that includes both zeal and distance, both devotion to the patient and exclusion of the patient from one's personal life, leads to the self-evident conclusion that this optimal stance will be difficult to maintain. Maintaining the balance of therapeutic determination and remoteness, of deep empathy and emotional detachment, of shared responsibility between patient and analyst, of therapeutic persistence and willingness to let go – it is these difficult balances that give rise to appropriate therapeutic modesty. It is wise to be aware of how easily we can become de-skilled and of how difficult it is for us to maintain an optimal balance as analysts.

Another set of therapeutic limitations involves the relationship of the analyst's character to the treatment situation, as I have discussed earlier (Cooper, 1982d). A purpose of the analyst's analysis is to enable the analyst to be aware of his range of responsiveness, even if he cannot change it. I will not enter into an extended discussion of character, but in a psychotherapeutic era in which we all acknowledge the emotionally interactive nature of the therapeutic process, it is clear that the analyst has an obligation to know a good deal about what frightens him, what makes him angry, what seduces him, what brings out his sadism, and what lulls his interest. We all know analysts who seem reluctant ever to let a patient go, and we all know analysts who seem unable to retain certain kinds of patients in treatment. Winnicott (1960) wrote about analyses that were false because the analyst never engaged the true self of the patient, and a potentially endless charade was carried out between the two. We also know analysts who cannot abide severe obsessionals or who hate to treat manipulating histrionic patients. It is not always clear, however, whether these kinds of situations should be labeled technical, i.e. better training would enable the analyst to overcome them, or whether they are, at least for certain analysts, characterologic and are not alterable by education: rather, they require a characterologic change in the analyst.

Waelder (1960: 245) once wrote of the impossibility of analysis for certain kinds of revolutionaries because the analyst's ego ideal and the ego ideal of the patient were too far apart. He implied that the analyst's empathic capacity would inevitably fail under such circumstances. I would suggest that Waelder was describing a special case, true for him, of the more general proposition that psychoanalysis will fail if the analyst cannot find points of empathic contact with his patient. I think I am more likely to have difficulty with a child abuser than with a revolutionary. In discussing the complex issue of the limitations of the analyst's character, I would like to separate several dimensions: character, values, theory, rules of technique, and analytic style. These characteristics of the analyst are not clearly separable but it may be useful to discuss them separately.

We usually mean two different things when we talk about character. We say admiringly of someone that that man or woman has character and pejoratively that he or she lacks character. When we say someone has character, we imply that there are qualities of perseverance, a capacity to endure, a core of belief that does not readily change, perhaps an ability to sacrifice for beliefs, and a consistent identity. It is important to recognize that a person can, in this description, be a person of character and yet be someone we detest, if in our opinion his or her beliefs are detestable. No one ever suggested that Charles de Gaulle lacked character, but not everyone found him an admirable person.

We also speak of persons having good or bad character, depending on whether they have attributes such as honesty, loyalty, industry, respect for culture, and so on. We expect of analysts both that they should be persons of character and that their character should be good. Our demands are rather heavy. We expect the analyst to be empathic, benevolent, reliable, dedicated, steadfast in his analytic endeavor, flexible, and so on. It is unlikely that many of us have either as much or as good character as we would like.

I am convinced that any long-time analysis reveals the analyst's character to the patient. However, character is, fortunately for our patients and ourselves, not a simple fixed quality. Rather, it is state-dependent. Many of us are much better persons with more reliable and more desirable character traits in the analytic situation than outside of it. The analytic situation is so constructed that the analyst's safety is assured – we need not answer embarrassing questions, we need not speak when spoken to, and our quirkiness is hidden behind our technique. In this atmosphere of safety and limited responsibility – we ultimately give the patients responsibility for their lives – we have every reason to be good characters. Many of us know that we can be more empathic, forgiving, benevolent, and consistent toward our patients than we can be toward our families.

However, basic characterologic flaws will show through in the analytic situation and will seriously handicap analytic work. Psychoanalysts with sociopathic or severe narcissistic tendencies are likely unconsciously to communicate these characterologic deficits and will deprive the patient of opportunities for idealization, core identifications, and the firming up of consistent superego qualities. I believe, however, that this situation is rare. A larger danger comes from the analyst's inability to be adequately alert to his own core characterologic make-up. The analyst's analytic ego must allow him to see the interactions of his own characterologic qualities and his patient's behavior and to use these as the engine of the treatment. Transference emerges most usefully in the gap between the patient's correct observation of our character and his distortion of that observation. We must be able to acknowledge, at least to ourselves, the correctness of the patient's observation if we are to be able most effectively to point out the distortions.

Those of us with more than our due share of narcissistic needs or anal, controlling, sadistic qualities or characterologic reaction formations – the list is endless – will find ourselves with certain patients with whom we are periodically enjoying the treatment too much or not enough. We look forward to the hour, or dread it or forget it. I believe the issue is not one of characterologic match or mismatch – should sadists treat masochists or vice versa – but rather the specific modes with which any patient of any character manages to carry out resistances by consciously or unconsciously fitting or thwarting the analyst's characterologic needs. Our job is to know how and when this is occurring, and when we are out of our depth. Clearly, we cannot treat patients we dislike. Equally clearly, we cannot treat patients whom we love too much.

An analyst's value systems, usually interwoven with his character, are a more likely overt source of therapeutic difficulty. Which of us has not had to bite his tongue when hearing a patient proclaim political views that make us see red? While the situation has changed dramatically in the last decade, it is still not uncommon to discover analysts, both male and female, with value systems concerning the feminine role that they unhesitatingly urge upon their patients in the name of therapeutic help.

We analysts may be blind to our value systems or may be unable to maintain therapeutic neutrality in the face of a challenge to our value system. It was, after all, only a few decades ago that analysis was held to be a value-free enterprise (Hartmann 1960: 20–21), and not all of us have rid ourselves of that illusion. The blend of values and characterologic needs is deep and may be subtle. Helping a passive masochistic male to understand his pathology may easily blend into expressions of macho contempt from the analyst, who is defending against recognition of his own passivity. The harsh unfriendliness of a competitive female patient toward her young male analyst may expose him to narcissistic castration anxieties which lead to his angry exposition of his patient's phallic competition and create a silent, angry, therapeutic stalemate. The analyst, however, thinks he is helping his patient become more 'feminine.' I know of several instances in which analysts inadvertently, or casually, revealed their contrary views about a political issue or an issue of social values to masochistic patients who were secretly hurt and enraged but too intimidated to work through what, for them, was a traumatic event. Rather than being a minor difference of opinion it was, for these patients, an actualization of a narcissistic, mocking parent contemptuously dismissing the opinions of a child. These kinds of situations, often transparently clear to a consultant or supervisor, can be completely masked by the pseudotherapeutic zeal with which the analyst protects his values, which serve important defensive functions.

The analyst's character inevitably relates to his version of psychoanalytic theory. In the United States today, significantly different theories are being advocated and advertised, and analysts have a choice. We must choose whether we wish to be so-called 'classical,' object-relational, self psychological, Kleinian, interpersonal, and on and on. It is obvious that after discounting the effects of specific training and indoctrination, and without clinical data that clearly support one theory over another, analysts will choose the theory that best fits their character and value systems. While all self-respecting theorists claim, perhaps correctly, that their theory allows for a full range of flexible therapeutic attitudes and behaviors, it does seem to be the case that, in practice, different theories coincide with particular therapeutic attitudes and behaviors. It is also the case that therapeutic flexibility is a quality with which not all analysts are equally endowed. Let me give an example: Kohut (1977: 249–261) claimed that there is a group of patients with narcissistic character disorders and damaged selves who require the analyst's vivid presence and activity to help counteract the early lack of mirroring and the withdrawn qualities of their internalized objects. He derived this therapeutic recommendation from his theory and explicitly stated that the classical technique of muted responsiveness, derived from the classical theory, was the wrong treatment for these patients. It is my impression that, regardless of any intrinsic merit, Kohut's theoretical position appealed to analysts who were eager to interact with their patients and who welcomed a theoretical justification. I believe it is also the case that numbers of analysts, while overtly rejecting Kohut's theory, accepted his permission for a more interactive stance. Conversely, I suspect that one bit of the more violent response to Kohut came from those who could not tolerate the prospect of a requirement for personal liveliness in the conduct of treatment.

Even where theories do not clearly dictate a set of treatment attitudes, they surely indicate the content of interpretations. Unless one believes that interpretations are merely metamessages through which patient and analyst establish a mode of discourse, and that the actual content of the interpretation is not important, then theories will powerfully influence what we do. If we subscribe to Kernberg's (1975: 241) view of pathological narcissism, we are likely to interpret the patient's rage early. If we believe Kohut's (1977: 92) view, we will bypass the rage and examine the enfeebled self. Some analysts are more comfortable dealing with rage, and some are more comfortable dealing with victimization, and this must influence one's choice of a theory.

In a field in which every communication from the patient is so filled with meanings, in an era in which alternate theoretical claims are actively competing, and without experimental data to demonstrate the correctness of a theory, there can be a great comfort in adhering tightly to a single theory that provides a consistent explanation of phenomena and justifies our personal needs. We may even continue to cling to our theory although the patient seems to fit it poorly or not to be benefiting. No one can operate without theory. It is desirable that we know what our theory is, how it suits our character, and how each theory limits us in some direction. I am quite certain that the universal theory that will supply correct meanings and attitudes for all treatment events is not yet at hand.

Technical rules come in two forms: there are rules that are clad in theoretical language and rules that speak directly to clinical behavior. An example of the former is the rule of technical neutrality – the analyst maintains a stance equidistant from ego, id, and superego. An example of the latter is that the analytic situation requires the use of the couch. Both types of rules present problems. The rules cast in theoretical language are subject to multiple clinical interpretations. Fairbairn (1958), for example, as he developed his object-relations theory, became convinced that the use of the couch represented a reproduction of the infantile trauma of maternal separation and deprivation and, therefore, was not technically neutral. In the name of technical neutrality, he decided toward the end of his career that his analytic patients would sit up and be able to face him. The peril of rules that dictate clinical behaviors is that they may not permit the full range of therapeutic behaviors that suit a particular patient.

Rules of both kinds are necessary, and, like all rules, they can be broken. The experienced analyst breaks them, but, one hopes, not unknowingly, unwittingly, or without having made the decision to break the rule. Certain gifted analysts have always been able to fly by the seat of their pants and define the rules later. For most of us, it is better to know what we are doing. Less able analysts are likely to cling to rules blindly or to flout them without knowing that they are doing so. Anyone who has ever taken tennis lessons knows the difference between trying to think of how to make the stroke – keep your eye on the ball, bring your racket back, turn perpendicular to the net, shift your weight, etc., etc., etc. – and having mastered the stroke. With mastery, one does more or less what the rules indicate, but one adapts to the needs of each situation and the rules are broken whenever necessary. Rules get people started, impose outer limits on behavior, but fade in importance as each analyst develops his own integrated technique. It is to me an astonishing failure of our education of young analysts that silence, or support, or any other activity, is so often believed to be a core behavior rather than a technical device in the service of one's deeper goals. We all know the plight of the analytic candidate with his first analytic case, sitting silently behind the couch, unable to help his patient explore the new, strange situation in which the patient finds himself or herself, because the budding analyst is afraid that breaking his personal vow of silence will mean that he is not doing analysis (Cooper 1985c).

In discussing theories and rules, we are, of course, aware that not only will analysts choose the theories and rules that already suit their characterologic needs, but a major purpose of theories and rules is to provide analysts with assistance in curbing their nontherapeutic characterologic tendencies.

It is all too rare that we have the chance to actually observe analysts at work. When we do, we often discover that they have analytic styles that we might not have predicted from knowing them outside of the analytic situation. Many people, when they are being analysts, speak in a different tone of voice, abruptly change their level of vivacity, change their facial expressions, and so on. Under optimal circumstances, this therapeutic style represents the integration of character, theory, values, rules, and experience. It is the way in which the analyst is comfortable performing the task he has set for himself. Style, in my view, is generally the least important aspect of the analyst's behavior, although for the patient it is likely to be the aspect of the analyst of which he is most conscious. I have been impressed that successful analyses are carried out in circumstances in which the patient feels his analyst was not all that bright, or had terrible taste in furniture, literature, or clothes, or spoke bad English, or lacked a sense of humor, or was too bourgeois, and so on. All of these opinions provide grist for the analytic mill and are not in themselves significant difficulties.

Two situations involving the analyst's style do, however, present serious problems. One is when the analyst cannot tolerate the harsh critique of his style by certain astute patients, especially if they are also able mimics. The second is when the analyst's personal style is congruent with a traumatic aspect of the patient's difficulties and the actualization of a past trauma becomes so vivid that opportunities for analyzing it are seriously handicapped. When the patient says he does not like something or other about an analyst, it may be extremely difficult to know whether the patient's complaints about the analyst really represent a mismatch or are analyzable and unavoidable aspects of the transference. In general, I would suggest that patients who respond initially to their analyst with powerful negative feelings that cannot be understood and moderated within a few sessions are probably well advised to find another analyst with whom they feel more comfortable.

The paucity of reliable research data is a significant source of the anxieties and of the limitations upon the analyst, which tend to erode our confidence and enthusiasm. Three kinds of data are needed: data supporting theoretical propositions, psychoanalytic outcome data, and psychoanalytic process data. I shall discuss them briefly.

I indicated above that we are now in an era of competitive theoretical claims and that theories are not trivial since they significantly influence the regulation of the psychoanalytic situation. To my knowledge, despite vast clinical experience, subject, of course, to vast error, we are without reliable data indicating that any one theory is superior to another. Any analyst's choice of theory probably reflects some combination of his assessment of the intellectual depth of the theory, its accord with his character and values, and its political and social status. Because it is difficult to affirm the correctness of any of our theories through research, we are prone over the course of time to various defensive behaviors. We may cling too rigidly to theoretical beliefs and make a dogma out of a theory. We may become disillusioned with all theory and pretend to be theory-free, or pick up bits and scraps eclectically without having a coherent theory, or we may run to the latest fashion and adopt last week's new theory. Each of these tendencies will hamper our clinical work in obvious ways.

The issue is further complicated by the fact that anyone who finds a new theoretical proposition interesting may have great difficulty testing it. Kohut (1977: 88), for example, recommended that in the case of certain narcissistic personality disorders the first several years of the treatment should be devoted to a non-interpretive phase in which transference regression and idealizations occur. Specific content interpretations should be carefully avoided. It is hard to imagine how an analyst could carry out this recommendation over several years of treatment as he watched all sorts of aggressive and sexual conflictual material cross his path, unless he already had a powerful belief in the correctness of Kohut's point of view. But how is one to obtain that strong belief in advance of the experiment? The paradox defeats us.

The issue of the experimenter's beliefs is significant in all forms of experimental work. It is particularly germane in the conduct of psychoanalysis where the complexity of the enterprise is such that every analyst is sure to defeat his own effort if he is consciously or unconsciously opposed to the method being suggested. It is a common experience with young analysts in training that when, for whatever reason, their own resistances to analysis are strong, they are likely to find the ways to provide their patients with the opportunity to defeat analytic endeavors.

The absence of outcome data creates an increasingly serious handicap for the psychoanalyst. I will not review in detail the current status of outcome studies. The research does demonstrate that overall, psychotherapies have a positive effect (Smith *et al.* 1980), but the studies shed little light on the relative effectiveness of different treatments or on the therapeutically effective components of treatment. The best-studied therapies are the short-term therapies. The least data is available for long-term psychotherapy or psychoanalysis. Twenty years ago we were all reasonably comfortable in shaking off the lack of information concerning our efficacy. We were all convinced that we did good, and, besides, nothing else was available. That blind confidence is now eroded or gone. We know that there are effective biological, short-term, and behavioral treatments, and we know that some forms of depression, panic, phobia, and obsession yield to medication. We cannot comfortably prescribe a long and expensive treatment if an effective alternative is available. Furthermore, we are not the only ones uncomfortable about our lack of outcome data. Government agencies and insurance companies are pressing us for evidence of our efficacy if we wish them to fund our activities.

Increasingly, the lack of outcome data will inhibit our willingness to press for the most intensive therapies for those patients who would benefit from that treatment. Lacking the data to make the best discrimination for treatment decisions, we are liable to be excessively timid. Already one sees patients in second or third treatments whose earlier therapists failed to press for full analysis when, retrospectively, that was the treatment of choice. If therapists hesitate to recommend psychoanalysis except as the treatment of last resort for the sickest patients, then the consequent decline in good treatment outcome will even further damage our confidence.

I believe that the data absence has already led to a change in the profession. Many talented therapists now seek analytic training primarily for what it adds to their overall clinical skill, but without conviction concerning psychoanalysis itself. As all of medicine has begun to develop effective treatments, psychoanalysis, probably effective, will have to prove that it is in fact effective or that its effectiveness can be studied if it is to continue to attract the brightest minds into the field. Faith alone will not sustain the profession.

Not only are we without confirmation of our long-range effectiveness, but also we lack good methods for monitoring the patient's treatment progress. We lack process measures. For example, as the patient enters a severe transference regression, are we really sure he is not just getting worse? Sometimes we are, and sometimes we are not. Or the patient may for long periods show little change. Appointments are kept, the patient talks, the analyst clarifies or interprets, but there is no movement and no excitement. Is this an unavoidable phase of resistance or working through, or has the analyst lost empathic contact with the patient and entered a stalemate? It may not be easy to tell. We have all seen examples of unconscionable prolongations of stalemated treatments. The common experience of presenting our own case material or reviewing another's case and hearing vastly different views of the treatment situation does not add to our confidence that we are not missing something vital.

Our lack of process measures contributes to another paradox of the analytic situation. With the exception of certain specific time-limited brief psychotherapies, 50 years of advances in psychoanalytic technique have led to an enormous lengthening of treatment and a lessening of clear positive results. In the early

201

days of analysis our goals were modest – symptom relief or the elucidation of the Oedipus complex – and these goals seemed to be achieved in relatively short periods. As our sophistication grew and we learned more about what we were doing, our goals became more ambitious; we sought deep structural change. The more we learned about the psyche, the more deeply we sought to probe, and, whether in actuality or in our perception, our patients simultaneously changed from simple neurotics to those having complex and severe character disorders.

These changes in our view of the analytic process and our uncertainty concerning our appropriate goals are further confused by differing views concerning therapeutic intent. Where Freud, early in his therapeutic career, suggested that analysis could enable one to exchange neurotic misery for ordinary human unhappiness, Kohut (1977: 44–45) more recently has suggested that analysis can enable the patient to achieve a life of joy and creativity. The difficulty of knowing the proper end-point of treatment, which Freud pointed to in 'Analysis terminable and interminable' (1937a) half a century ago, is still with us. Without clear guidelines, overly zealous analysts are unwilling to free their patients to pursue their own growth, and overly modest analysts hesitate to battle the patient's resistances to achieve the fullest therapeutic effect.

In a culture that contradictorily demands both immediate gratification and the achievement of perfection and happiness at whatever cost or effort, we analysts are properly confused concerning what constitutes a therapeutic aim and what constitutes a social gratification. Given all these difficulties with monitoring the analytic process, our profession undoubtedly uses consultation too seldom. We would benefit enormously from freer exchange of material and more frequent use of consultation when an analysis seems chaotic or flat.

I will add yet one more difficulty in the area of the data deficit. By and large, we analysts work with a paucity of data concerning the patient's real-life non-analytic situation. For many purposes this absence of data has advantages – we see the world through the patient's eyes and understand the difficulties as the patient understands them. However, whether this is always the best therapeutic environment is subject to doubt. Family therapists have long spoken of the enormous advantage of knowing the patient's actual interpersonal environment. Some analysts, professedly orthodox, believe in seeing a spouse at some point in the course of the analysis. All of us have had the experience of discovering that we had grossly underestimated or overestimated our patient's ego assets. While the discovery of this misperception is a significant treatment event permitting important treatment interventions, there are cases where more accurate information, available earlier, would have been of great help to the conduct of the analysis. I know that some analysts have ended treatment with a wildly inaccurate view of the patient's actual talents, environmental advantages or obstacles, and psychological resources. While this misperception reflects the patient's deep resistances, the analyst may have been more effective with the aid of additional information. The excessively data-free field that I have been describing is a potent source of difficulties, and only partially intrinsic to our work.

I would like, finally, to address a peril of the profession – the 'burnout' syndrome as it appears in psychoanalysts. Freud unhesitatingly identified psychoanalysis as one of the impossible professions, along with teaching and government. I have discussed a number of hazards of our field. Let me describe them in a slightly different light.

First, analysts operate in a climate of extraordinary isolation. (a) The full-time analyst suffers the loneliness of social isolation. He is likely to spend a full day seeing no one but his patients and sometimes, literally, not even seeing them. While this social withdrawal is a comfort for some analysts, it is, for most, a terrible strain. (b) As I have indicated, we operate isolated from data. We require strong belief systems in order to maintain the vigor that our work requires and this, historically, has led to certain intellectual perils. The isolation from scientific data has cost us dearly. (c) With rare exceptions, we are isolated from outcome knowledge of our own patients. Few of us are likely to have significant contact with many of our patients after the completion of treatment. Having been intensely involved for many months or years, convinced or hoping that the result has been a good one, we may never again hear from the patient and cannot accumulate either the confidence that our work was well done or the knowledge that would come from a careful review of our errors. Our separation from our patients' futures is another significant isolation.

Second, analysts carry on their work with very little opportunity for the usual rewards present in the healing arts. Most psychoanalysts see very few patients in their lifetime. Our emotional investment in each of our patients is large, our propensity for disappointment is great, and our opportunities for reward are deliberately limited. Not only do we not continue to see our grateful patients, as does the internist, for example, but the treatment situation is designed to inhibit the patient's tendencies to reward us except through fees. In general, we do not receive gifts, we do not become social friends with our patients, and we do not enjoy the atmosphere of continuing idealization from our patients, either in analysis or after it, as most other healers do.

Confronted with the many difficulties and strains of doing psychoanalysis that I have described, it is not surprising that burnout syndromes are liable to appear in analysts and constitute serious limitations on our doing our best work. I shall describe two manifestations of the burnout syndrome: masochistic defenses and narcissistic defenses.

The masochistic defenses to which analysts are prone appear as discouragement, boredom, and loss of interest in the psychoanalytic process. Self-reproaches are translated into projected aggression against the analytic work. The various tensions, uncertainties, and sources of self-doubt that plague every analyst are, for these masochistically inclined individuals, an unanswerable source of inner guilt and self-recrimination, as well as an unconscious opportunity for adopting the role of victim toward their patients and their profession. Faced with these inner accusations and masochistic temptations, these analysts are unable to maintain their self-esteem and cannot sustain their claim that they are doing all that any analyst can do – i.e. to try his best to help his patient with the theories and skills available to him. For combinations of reasons related to character and to training, they cannot produce inner conviction that what they are doing in the conduct of analysis is sufficient for a clear conscience. It is an evidence of both the attraction of masochistic victimization and the harshness of the superego of the analysts involved that they are willing to doom themselves to a relatively pleasureless professional existence, for the sake of the deflection of the inner reproach against their talent or skill. Feeling helpless against their inner conscience which charges them with not helping their patients, they say, 'Don't blame me, blame psychoanalysis.' The cynicism that may be part of this defense can be startling in its depth. I know analysts who have refused to permit members of their own family to enter analysis because they did not regard the treatment as helpful. Obviously, anyone going through the motions of a treatment in which he lacks faith has lost the power to maintain his own self-esteem. Conscious self-pity over the difficulty of the work or the shortcomings of psychoanalysis is matched by unconscious acceptance or even welcome of the opportunity to enact an endless infantile drama of being unloved or unappreciated or overwhelmed. Depression is always on the horizon for these analysts, apparent in their lack of pleasure in their patients or in the profession of psychoanalysis, both of which have let them down by not adequately protecting them from their unconscious conscience.

A corollary of this discouragement is boredom. Boredom is an affect of which we are all capable and is probably a part of every treatment. In itself, it is a valuable clue to transference and countertransference events. What I am speaking of here, however, is chronic boredom. I have heard analysts say that all patients seem the same to them, the patient's story lacks interest, struggling to unravel meanings seems either too difficult or unchallenging, and the analyst struggles through his patient's sessions unstimulated and uninterested. Clearly, treatment cannot be optimal under such circumstances. The odd thing, however, which raises questions about the therapeutic factors in the treatment situation, is that certain patients seem to get better even under these conditions. Some patients are self-healing and seem not to require very much from the analyst. This knowledge is a useful check on therapeutic hubris.

A consequence of discouragement and boredom is, of course, loss of inventiveness. The analyst, frightened of not succeeding, discouraged in advance by the harshness of his superego reproach that it is grandiose for him to think that he can help someone else understand his unconscious desires and conflicts, especially when he is aware of his own neurotic shortcomings in the conduct of the treatment, gives up his active inquiring role. The analyst no longer puzzles, plays with the data, tries out interpretations, finds excitement in deciphering new meanings of old data and new connections that previously had escaped him and his patient. Playful inventiveness is a necessary part of the analytic dialogue, and its loss deadens treatment. These secretly frightened, consciously bored analysts may resort to stock answers, bullying patients with what they were taught were correct interpretations, often unconsciously parodying their teachers in secret vengeance. They find it difficult and threatening to maintain close contact with the patient, whom they perceive primarily as a source of inner reproaches for their professional incapacity.

Finally, these masochistic defenses of the discouraged analyst lead to chronic anger at his patients, his profession, his colleagues, and himself. The patients of these analysts, when later they see someone else, sometimes report an analytic atmosphere of sarcasm, denigration of the patient, devaluation, and lack of appreciation. This pairing of masochistically angry, discouraged analyst and masochistic patient may last for many years.

It has long been my view that narcissistic and masochistic pathology are closely intertwined, representing two different defensive faces of the same constellation. The narcissistic defenses of the burned-out analyst take a different form. The image of the great analysts of the past, or even of the imagined present, is often a significant factor in the ego ideal of these analysts. However, lacking adequate capacity for sustained positive identification, or unable to sustain genuine efforts at emulation that do not provide rapid affirmation or gratification, they seek other means of narcissistic comfort to avoid the humiliation they experience if they have not met their unrealistic perfectionist goals. Convinced they cannot be as creative as Freud, they can only carry on a secretly ironic imitation of the analyst ensconced in their ego ideal.

Unable any longer to restrain his narcissistic needs in the isolated, unrewarding setting he experiences analysis to be, the narcissistic analyst abandons efforts toward neutrality and increasingly uses charismatic behaviors to elicit the patient's overt admiration. These analysts intrude into the patient's life, give guidance and advice, are grossly directive and paternalistic, and attempt to maintain the patient in childlike devotion. Should the patient be famous or rich or live an interesting life, these analysts are liable to attempt to enliven their own inner deadness by living through their patient's success or fame. They are prone to lure the patient into amusing and interesting them and to abandon discretion and confidentiality in social situations. The tales of the success or glamour of their patients give the analyst a sense of a richer life than in fact he has. These analysts are also prone to use the profession as a badge of social distinction, allying themselves with groups or theories for the sense of narcissistic power such alliances may provide. Because their beliefs and identifications are often shallow, based on narcissistic need rather than on intellectual and emotional conviction, any challenge to their professional role produces severe defensive responses. In narcissistically threatening situations they are prone to respond with attitudes of superiority and superciliousness, toward both their patients and their colleagues.

I assume that all of us are subject to one or both of these tendencies during the course of a given treatment or during a given period in our careers. The tendencies are self-observable markers for attending to our psychoanalytic well-being, continuing our efforts at self-analysis. When they become chronic, however, it is obviously time for a return to analysis. It is to the credit of the profession that many analysts do exactly that. Sadly, however, some do not.

Good psychoanalysis involves many paradoxes. We must maintain therapeutic fervor and therapeutic distance. We must maintain belief in our theories and an experimental attitude. We must be firm in our character and flexible in our therapeutic approach. We must believe in our therapeutic effectiveness and be prepared to admit therapeutic defeat and to suggest that someone else might do the job better. We must obtain satisfaction from the work while labeling as exploitation the usual modes by which healers obtain satisfaction from their patients. Indeed, this is an impossible profession. But I have been discussing only the difficulties; I could write at even greater length about the gratifications of the profession. Many of us are unable to imagine anything else as interesting, exciting, important, challenging, or gratifying. No other profession provides us the opportunity to know human beings so well, to touch their suffering so closely, to have the opportunity to help. To realize that we have at least been a factor in bettering lives and perhaps releasing creativity and joy where none existed before is a great satisfaction and privilege. There is even the opportunity to add to the sum of human knowledge. I also believe that doing psychoanalysis is good for the mental health of the not-too-neurotic psychoanalyst.

We surely need research to strengthen our enterprise. We cannot be self-satisfied about our own assessment of our own activity. Studies are needed for our well-being and for our patients' well-being. But I think we are fortunate in being analysts at this time. Not since the earlier days of psychoanalysis has our field been so exciting. Theories compete, theorists are boldly breaking out of old molds and making suggestions that are productive and interesting and would not have been seriously considered two decades ago. Psychoanalytic research is achieving new levels of productivity and sophistication. The data from infant observation have begun to penetrate our clinical theories, and productive ferment surrounds us. We have every reason to believe that our knowledge and effectiveness will vastly increase in the future. It has been my hope that by considering some of the difficulties and perils of our professional lives, we will be better prepared to overcome them. I am optimistic that we will shortly be in a position to prove Freud wrong. We will discover that our profession is not impossible; merely difficult.

16

DIFFICULTIES IN BEGINNING THE CANDIDATE'S FIRST ANALYTIC CASE*

I suspect that in most institutes, there is a common observation of beginning analytic candidates with their first cases. A young physician or other professional, with considerable psychotherapeutic experience, generally sensitive to his patients' affective state, reasonably alert to the interaction between himself and his patient, although often ineffectual in attempting to alter that interaction, now has reached a landmark in his training. He is about to place the patient on the couch.

Depending upon a variety of extraneous circumstances, he may have had up to six or a dozen previous meetings with the patient to assess the patient's suitability for analysis, and he has had some advice from his supervisor as to how to begin the first session on the couch. That advice varies among supervisors but often includes such pearls as suggesting that some description of the analytic process be given to the patient, not to wait until late on a Friday afternoon before telling the patient that he will be on the couch Monday morning, how the invitation to use the couch should be extended, and so forth. Finally, the moment arrives. The patient is on the couch, the budding analyst is seated somewhere to the rear, ready to take notes, and a remarkable transformation instantly occurs. This astute and responsive young therapist, previously able to ask appropriate questions, raise an issue for clarification, ask for an expansion of a hinted-at feeling or poorly suppressed desire or anger, is now struck dumb. He has begun a new career as a psychoanalyst, and this, for him, most important moment becomes a moment of signification, and the signifier he chooses is that in order to be an analyst he must remain silent.

* This paper was first presented at the 40th Anniversary of the William Alanson White Institute, New York. It was published as Cooper (1985c) in *Contemporary Psychoanalysis*, 21: 143–150.

This previously empathic healer now expects that his patient, who is in a strange position, with a unique form of communication with another human being, should be expected to adapt instantly to these jarring circumstances. Where once this young therapist would have wanted information about how it feels to be on the couch, what had been the fantasies since the question of the couch was raised, is the patient's evident discomfort on the couch, or glaring evasion of even mentioning the couch, something that the patient might want to discuss; now the budding analyst sits silent. None of the missing content emerges. If the patient should comment, the former therapist, now analyst, is likely to sit stonily, 'allowing the material to develop.' Clearly, this experienced therapist has a model in his mind for what psychoanalysis is or should be; he has a conviction that it is a technique requiring new skills and that the acquisition of these new skills requires abandonment of some of his old ones. In his uncertainty about his new profession, the only certainty seems to be that one must not talk. Where do these ideas come from, and is our young analyst-to-be correct in his assumption?

The first and most obvious source of these sets of beliefs is, of course, ourselves, their teachers. Through numerous debates in the analytic literature, and through many education committees, the claim has been asserted that the distinctions between analysis and therapy are sharp and represent distinct entities rather than dimensions of a single type of activity. The distinctness of psychoanalysis has been ascribed to the use of the couch, to the use of at least four sessions per week, to the systematic analysis of the transference, to the induction of maximal regression in the transference neurosis, to the neutrality of the therapist in terms of therapeutic goals or values or even therapeutic intent, to the therapist's neutrality as a provider of gratification, to the emphasis on interpretation as the sole or at least one major instrument of therapy. I could expand that list. Of course, these discussions about the distinctiveness of analysis are so recurrent because it is not so clear that the analysis/therapy distinction is as clear as some would wish it to be. Some would argue that all of these measures, and others, are part of psychotherapy as well as analysis, and the differences are quantitative rather than categorical. Furthermore, it is clear that few, if any, analyses are purely analytic. Suggestion, supportive measures, encouragement, unanalyzed bits of transference are always present. The analyst is never as neutral as we once thought or hoped, and the curative elements of the analytic situation are more complex than is included in interpretation alone.

Nonetheless, most analytic theory and most observers agree with our naive young student that analysis is somehow different from therapy, even if we cannot clearly specify that difference. Most analysts would probably be saddened, might even perceive it as a considerable narcissistic injury, if we did not believe that analysis is something other than just more or better psychotherapy. So, we convey the idea to our young candidate that he is about to do something he has not done before, and that idea may not be wrong. Of course, few of us would agree on where the difference lies, or whether it lies in the simple fact of not talking, but the student must begin somewhere, and that may not be the worst place, although sometimes it is. Our teaching of our theory and technique, therefore, both inspires and misleads our young analyst.

The second spur for our student to abandon his former skills can be considered psychosocial rather than theoretical, and lies in his conviction, again fostered by us, his teachers, that the new analyst is about to enter the mysteries: to join a cult to which he has not had previous access. These magical and infantile idealizing and voyeuristic fantasies, the emphasis given to his now focusing on exploring rather than curing, sitting behind the patient and looking without being seen, are powerful sources of regression and grandiosity. The entry to student life at a late point in one's career and the extraordinary effort that is now to be expended on this additional training create powerful narcissistic desires for the candidate to share with us our belief that what he is now learning is unique and separates his from his fellow practitioners.

The third, and perhaps most important, source of the peculiar de-skilling of the young analyst comes from his misunderstanding of his own analytic experience. Most candidates in analysis have every desire to cooperate with the analytic process. They enter it knowing something of the method, knowing that their futures are connected with their own success as patients, and fully aware of the status difference between student and master. Few, if any, analytic candidates would think of objecting to the use of the couch and while they may hate the analyst's withholding of gratification, they are likely to believe that it is a necessary part of the process, being done for some important good, even if that good cannot yet be perceived. At the very least, they perceive it as an initiation rite. It seems extremely difficult for candidates to put themselves in the place of the ordinary patient who may know nothing of analytic theory, have no reason to trust this strange procedure, no reason to trust the analyst, no background that can ease the pain of the initial frustration of the analytic situation, and no reason at all to believe that any of that process makes any sense. I am sure that our beginning analysts know all this, and yet it is hard for them to behave differently with their patients than their analysts have behaved with them. Contrary to their clinical knowledge, they expect their patients to act like themselves. Is this positive identification with their analysts a mimicry of an idealized analyst? Or is it ironic mockery of their analyst's painful behavior toward them, or an identification with the aggressor? Perhaps one or all of these and more. Whatever the reason, it is clear that the young analyst feels permitted to do only what his own analyst did, or more likely what he perceives that his analyst did by way of depriving him. It is often said of the tripartite structure of analytic education that it is the analyst's own analysis that is the most important element in it. I am suggesting that though it is a most important element, it also can be hugely misleading to the young analyst.

Finally, I will suggest that in thinking about the learning behavior of the candidate, we must acknowledge the candidate's feeling that since a supervisor sits behind him, silence may be the better part of valor; it is better to be quiet than to seem stupid.

Whatever the reasons, it is clear that the young analyst feels permitted to do only what his own analyst did, and he will not step out of that role. Faced with our candidate's difficult-to-alter conviction that being an analyst means adopting a ritual silence as the main therapeutic activity, should we try to do something about it? And if so, when? And how vigorously? Analysts will differ in the degree to which they are themselves silent, and there are important arguments on the question of gratification within the analytic situation. The key question, however, returns to where our young candidate began. Is analysis really different from therapy? If it is, and I believe it is, at least dimensionally different, then it may be good pedagogy for the student to put aside much that he has previously learned and to try to learn a new technique from the beginning. Many supervisors are concerned that the already skilled therapist may use his skills to inhibit analytic regression, to ward off the more threatening transference responses of the patient, and so to smooth or flatten the therapeutic relationship, preventing the affective storms that might otherwise occur.

There is a general concern that the experienced therapist will convert what should have been analysis into what is usually referred to as 'merely' psychotherapy. Let me give an example of the problem. A candidate beginning a first case forgot an appointment with the patient. At their next scheduled appointment, the angry and confused patient asked what happened. The embarrassed and equally confused candidate said nothing and continued to say nothing through a session of mounting frustration and despair on the part of both patient and doctor. In discussing the episode in supervision, the candidate stated that had this been a therapy case, he might have asked the patient what his feelings and fantasies were when his therapist didn't appear. Or he might even have apologized for his behavior. He feared, however, that any intervention in analysis would disrupt the development of his patient's full transference response. In a sense, he is right, of course, except that he is failing to distinguish spontaneous transference regression from induced transference regression. The candidate has, at any rate, through his behavior, had an experience of remaining unsupportive through a powerfully demanding, guilt-inducing session with his patient.

I have tried to show that these kinds of errors are to be welcomed as possible indicators of the seriousness of the enterprise to the candidate. While, inevitably, they may be harmful in some respects, they must be monitored and should change in the course of education and experience. The development of analytic skills requires experimentation with uncomfortable and unnatural ways of thinking and behaving.

Is there a better way to each analytic technique? I have several suggestions.

The iconography of psychoanalysis – the innumerable cartoons of the analyst sitting behind the couch, paper and notebook in hand – certainly affect both patient and analyst. This iconography is encouraged by our official organs. The newsletter of the International Psychoanalytic Association has for many years featured a series of photographs of the psychoanalyst's furniture – photos of the couch and chair of analysts around the world. The pictures of Freud's office are known to every analyst. The couch has become the signifier of the psychoanalyst in the way that the stethoscope once was of the physician. Unfortunately, this couch symbolism, like the cross in Christianity, has come to represent the core of the belief system, rather than a possible mechanical convenience in service of analytic goals. Budding analysts are, they feel, being inducted into a mystery, rather than being educated in a depth psychology and its derivative therapeutic techniques while simultaneously being encouraged to question the enterprise, perhaps even developing research programs.

Most analytic institutes currently encourage candidates to begin the first case as early in their analytic training as possible. I believe, however, that very few institutes provide specific instruction to their students about the special emotional responses of an unsophisticated analytic patient being inducted into an analytic process. There is a great deal of discussion of analyzability, of the distinction between psychoanalysis and psychotherapy, of converting psychotherapy patients into analytic patients, but none of these courses directly address the experience of the first analytic session. Students need specific help in understanding the distinctions between their experience beginning analysis and what it is that their patients are likely to experience.

Finally, I would suggest that much more needs to be done to bring the budding psychoanalyst into contact with the larger body of his profession. Until quite recently, many analytic societies around the world did not welcome beginning candidates into all of their clinical meetings, and it is still the case that few analytic institutes have ongoing presentations of clinical material by faculty members to which candidates, including the very beginning candidates, are invited. We still tend to maintain barriers between the students and the faculty – barriers that exist in no other educational enterprise. Clearly I am echoing the plea of many others as we move away from seminarian or trade school practices towards genuine graduate education (Kernberg 1986).

17

CHANGES IN PSYCHOANALYTIC IDEAS

Transference interpretation*

Psychoanalysts, since the earliest days of the studies on hysteria, have always given special attention to the transference and to the interpretation of transference, believing it to be central in our theory and technique. While there has never been a lack of interest in transference interpretation, it has recently become a particular focus of study and discussion. It is not clear why this is so, and the reasons may vary in different parts of the international psychoanalytic community. In America, at least, Gill's (1982) recent and somewhat radical presentation of transference interpretation has surely helped to grab our attention. I believe another reason for our intensified interest in transference interpretation is the opportunity it provides for discussion of the full panoply of diverse analytic theories and techniques that today compete for our attention and allegiance. In this respect transference interpretation seems to have replaced self psychology as the encompassing topic that allows analysts of varied persuasions to discuss almost every aspect of psychoanalysis.

Despite the diversity of analytic views that abound today, analysts seem to agree on the centrality of the transference and its interpretation in analytic process and cure, differing only in whether transference is everything or almost everything. This somewhat unusual degree of agreement may be aided by our inability to give a clear definition of what transference is.

Laplanche and Pontalis (1973), in their dictionary, write, with some sense of despair:

* This paper was presented as the 28th Sandor Rado Lecture sponsored by the Association for Psychoanalytic Medicine and the Columbia University Center for Psychoanalytic Training and Research, 1985. It was published as Cooper (1987c) in *Journal of the American Psychoanalytic Association*. Reproduced with permission.

212

The reason it is so difficult to propose a definition of transference is that for many authors the notion has taken on a very broad extension, even coming to connote all the phenomena which constitute the patient's relationship with the psychoanalyst. As a result the concept is burdened down more than any other with each analyst's particular views on the treatment – on its objective, dynamics, tactics, scope, etc. The question of the transference is thus beset by a whole series of difficulties which have been the subject of debate in classical psychoanalysis.

(p. 456)

Sandler (1983) has discussed how the terms 'transference' and 'transference resistance', as well as other terms, have undergone profound changes in meaning as new discoveries and new trends in psychoanalytic technique assumed ascendancy. He said, 'major changes in technical emphasis brought about the extension of the transference concept, which now has dimensions of meaning which differ from the official definition of the term' (p. 10). I am not sure there has ever been a simple official definition of the term. While a certain flexibility of definition makes conversation possible in a field of diverse views, that we may never be clear on what any two people mean when they use the term is a significant handicap to our discourse.

With this in mind we might review one of Freud's last comments on transference. In 'An Outline of Psycho-Analysis' (1940), published posthumously, he wrote of the analytic situation:

> The most remarkable thing is this. The patient is not satisfied with regarding the analyst in the light of reality as a helper and advisor who, moreover, is remunerated for the trouble he takes and who would himself be content with some such role as that of a guide on a difficult mountain climb. On the contrary, the patient sees in him the return, the reincarnation, of some important figure out of his childhood or past, and consequently transfers on to him feelings and reactions which undoubtedly applied to this proto-type. This fact of transference soon proves to be a factor of undreamt-of importance, on the one hand an instrument of irreplaceable value and on the other hand a source of serious dangers . . . The analyst may shamefacedly admit to himself that he set out on a difficult undertaking without any suspicion of the extraordinary powers that would be at his command . . .
>
> Another advantage of transference, too, is that in it the patient produces before us with plastic clarity an important part of his life-story, of which he would otherwise have probably given us only an insufficient account. He acts it before us, as it were, instead of reporting it to us.

(pp. 174–176)

Freud saw the transference interpretation as a method of strengthening the ego against past unconscious wishes and conflicts:

It is the analyst's task constantly to tear the patient out of his menacing illusion and to show him again and again that what he takes to be new real life is a reflection of the past. And lest he should fall into a state in which he is inaccessible to all evidence, the analyst takes care that neither the love nor the hostility reach an extreme height. This is effected by preparing him in good time for these possibilities and by not overlooking the first signs of them. Careful handling of the transference on these lines is as a rule richly rewarded. If we succeed, as we usually can, in enlightening the patient on the true nature of the phenomena of the transference, we thus shall have struck a powerful weapon out of the hand of his resistance and shall have converted dangers into gains. For a patient never forgets again what he has experienced in the form of transference; it carries a greater force of conviction than anything he can acquire in other ways.

(p. 177)

While Freud at one time or another entertained almost all possible views of the transference, I believe these statements at the end of his career give a clear sense of where he stood. He believed that the transference represents a true reconstruction of the past, a vivid reliving of earlier desires and fears that distort the patient's capacity to perceive the 'true nature' of the present reality. The analyst is a wise guide who already knows the path, and the task of the transference interpretation is cognitive 'enlightenment' that carries the emotional conviction of lived experience, while preventing excessive emotional regression.

Although it is a vast oversimplification and the division is not sharp, I shall suggest that there have been two major ideas about the transference and its interpretation during the history of psychoanalysis. One is explicit in Freud, as I quoted him above; the other is implicit. The first idea, close to Freud, is that the transference is an enactment of an earlier relationship, and the task of transference interpretation is to gain insight into the ways that the early infantile relationships are distorting or disturbing the relationship to the analyst, a relationship that is, in turn, a model for the patient's life relationships. I shall refer to this as the historical model of transference, implying both that it is older and that it is based on an idea of the centrality of history. The second view regards the transference as a new experience rather than an enactment of an old one. The purpose of transference interpretation is to bring to consciousness all aspects of this new experience including its colorings from the past. I shall refer to this as the modernist model of the transference, implying both that it is newer, in fact still at an early stage of evolution, and that it is based on an idea of the immediacy of experience. I would like to distinguish this discussion of models of transference and transference interpretation from the debate on the 'here-and-now' interpretation that Gill has brought to the fore. Gill is primarily interested in issues of technique, and both models that I will discuss lend themselves to interpretive work in the here and now. These two models are not

214

entirely mutually exclusive, but they do imply significant differences in basic assumptions and in treatment goals. Although the historical view is clearer and prettier, I believe that the modernist version of transference interpretation is more interesting and more promising.

In the first, historical, view, the importance of transference interpretation lies in the opportunity it provides in the 'transference neurosis' for the patient to re-experience and undo the partially encapsulated, one might say 'toxic,' neurosogenic early history. In the second, modernist view, the purpose of transference interpretation is to help the patient to see, in the intensity of the transference, the aims, character, and mode of his current wishes and expectations as influenced by the past.

The historical view is more likely to regard the infantile neurosis as a 'fact' of central importance for the analytic work, to be uncovered and undone. The modernist view regards the infantile neurosis, if acknowledged at all, as an unprivileged set of current fantasies rather than historical fact. From this modernist perspective, the transference resistance is the core of the analysis, to be worked through primarily because of the rigidity it imposes on the patient, not because of an important secret that it conceals.

Similarly, it is a corollary of the historical conception to view the transference neurosis as a distinct phenomenon that develops during the analysis as a consequence of the expression of resistance to drive-derived aims that are aroused toward the analyst. Those holding the modernist view, much more influenced by object-relational ideas of development, are likely to blur the idea of a specific transference neurosis in favor of viewing all transference responses as reflecting shifting self-representations and object representations as they are affected by the changing analytic relationship, and significant transferences may be available for interpretation very early in the analysis. There is no doubt that the modernist view also reflects the scarcity of the once classical neurotic patient.

The historical view is more likely to see the analyst as a more or less neutral screen upon which drive-derived needs will enact themselves. He is observer and interpreter, not coparticipant in the process of change. The person of the analyst is of lesser importance. Those taking the modernist view hold that the analyst is an active participant, a regulator of the analytic process, whose personal characteristics powerfully influence the content and shape of the transference behaviors, and who will himself be changed in the course of the treatment.

The historical view emphasizes the content and precision of the transference interpretation, especially as it reconstructs the past. The modernist view, at least in some hands, is likely to de-emphasize reconstructive content and see the transference interpretation as one aspect of the interpersonal relationship in the present, acting as a new emotional and behavioral regulator, when past relationships have been inadequate or absent. Incidentally, this concept of a relationship as an organismic regulator is consonant with current research on grieving men and motherless mice and monkeys, in all of whom a missing relationship creates vast neuroendocrine and emotional consequences.

The increasing influence of the modernist version of transference and its interpretation represents an adaptation to several long-term philosophical, scientific, and cultural shifts we can now recognize. This changing view of transference is also the most visible emblem of the deep changes in psychoanalytic theory that are now quietly taking place, and of the theoretical pluralism that is so prevalent today (Cooper 1984c).

One of these long-term changes in the climate in which psychoanalysis dwells results from a large philosophical debate concerning the nature of history, veridicality, and narrative. Kermode (1985) has written of the change during this century in our modes of understanding and interpreting the past and the present:

> Once upon a time it seemed obvious that you could best understand how things are by asking how they got to be that way. Now attention [is] directed to how things are in all their immediate complexity. There is a switch, to use the linguists' expressions, from the diachronic to the synchronic view. Diachrony, roughly speaking, studies things in their coming to be as they are; synchrony concerns itself with things as they are and ignores the question how they got that way.
>
> (Kermode 1985: 3)

This distinction, put forth by de Saussure (1915), has achieved philosophical dominance today and is the clear source of the hermeneutic view so prevalent in psychoanalysis, proposed by Ricoeur (1970). From here it is a short distance to Schafer (1981), or Gill (1982), or Spence (1982), who in varying ways adopt the synchronic view. In this view, the analytic task is interpretation, with the patient, of the events of the analytic situation – usually broadly labeled transference – with a construction rather than a reconstruction of the past. In effect, while there is a past of 'there and then' it is knowable only through the filter of the present, of 'here and now.' There is no other past than the one we construct, and there is no way of understanding the past except through its relation to the present. I would emphasize that psychoanalysis, like history but unlike fiction, does have anchoring points. History's anchoring points are the evidences that events did occur. There was a Roman empire, it did have dates, actual persons lived and died. These 'facts' place a limit on the narratives and interpretations that may seriously be entertained. Psychoanalysis is anchored in its scientific base in developmental psychology and in the biology of attachment and affects. Biology confers regularities and limits on possible histories, and our constructions of the past must accord with this scientific knowledge. Constructions of childhood that are incompatible with what we know of developmental possibilities may open our eyes to new concepts of development, but more likely they alert us to maimed childhoods that have led our patients to unusual narrative constructions in the effort to maintain self-esteem and internal coherence. A second, far less secure, anchor is the enormous amount of convergent data that accumulate during the course of an analysis, which are likely to give the analyst the impression that he is reconstructing rather than constructing the figures and the circumstances of his patient's past. While a diachronic view may no longer suffice, it may also not be fully dispensable if our patients' histories are to maintain psychoanalytic coherence, rooted in bodily experience, and the loving, hating and terrifying affects accompanying the fantastic world of infantile psychic reality. Not all analysts are yet as ready as Spence, for example, to give up all claim to the truth value or explanatory power of the understanding of the past, even if it is limited to knowing past constructions of the past. Nevertheless, the change in philosophical outlook during our century is profound and contributes to our changing view of the analytic process as exemplified in the transference and its interpretation.

Approaching the same issue from an entirely different vantage point, Emde (1981), speaking for the 'baby-watchers' and discussing changing models of infancy and early development, details a second source of the major change of climate to which I refer. He writes:

> The models suggest that what we reconstruct, and what may be extraordinarily helpful to the patient in 'making a biography,' may never have happened. The human being, infant and child, is understood to be fundamentally active in constructing his experience. Reality is neither given nor necessarily registered in an unmodifiable form. Perhaps it makes sense for the psychoanalyst to place renewed emphasis on recent and current experience – first, as a context for interpreting early experience and second, because it contains within it the ingredients for potential amelioration . . . Psychoanalysts are specialists in dealing with the intrapsychic world and in particular with the dynamic unconscious. But we need to pay attention not only to the intrapsychic realm, conflict-laden and conflict-free, but also to the interpersonal realm.
>
> (Emde 1981: 217–218)

He concludes: 'we have probably placed far too much emphasis on early experience itself as opposed to the process by which it is modified or made use of by subsequent experience' (p. 219). This view of psychic development, discarding the timeless unconscious and so powerfully at odds with the views that were held by psychoanalysts during the time when most of our ideas of transference interpretation were formed, clearly suggests the modernist model of transference interpretation.

A change in the cultural environment of psychoanalysis provides a third source for the changing model of transference interpretation. Valenstein (personal communication) describes oscillations in psychoanalytic outlook between an emphasis on cognition at one end, and on affect at the other. One might see these as differences between old-fashioned scientific and romantic world views. Surely the period of ego psychology, perhaps reflected in the English translation of Freud, and certainly reflected in the effort to insist on the libidinal energic point of view, represented the attempt to see psychoanalysis as Freud usually did, as an objective science in the nineteenth-century style, with hypotheses created out of naive observation. It accorded with that view to see the transference as an objective reflection of history. We are currently in one of our more romantic periods. It is consonant with that view to see transference as an activity – stormy, romantic, active, affective – a kind of adventure from which the two individuals emerge changed and renewed. In this romantic view, interpretations of the transference are intended to remove obstacles interfering with the heightening and intimacy of the experience, with the implication that self-knowledge and change will result from the encounter. As romantic figures, the patient and analyst set forth on a quest into the unknown, and whether or not one of them returns with a Holy Grail, they return with many new stories to tell and a new life experience – the analysis. Gardner's (1983) book, *Self Inquiry*, epitomizes this romantic view of analyst and patient as a poet-pair engaged in mutual self-inquiry. It is clear that many analysts would rather be artists than scientists. By contrast, the older, cognitive view of the transference is of an intellectual journey, emotionally loaded of course, but basically a trip back in history, seeking truth and insight.

Finally, our newer ideas of transference interpretation come from the rereading and reinterpreting of Freud that necessarily accompany the changes in outlook that I have been describing. Corresponding to the swings of analytic culture between classical and romantic, there were swings in psychoanalytic technique from Freud's actual technique, as reconstructed from his notes and the reports of his patients, to the so-called 'classical' technique that held sway after Freud's death, and again to the currently changing technical scene. Lipton (1977) has insisted that in the 1940s and 1950s the so-called 'classical' technique replaced Freud's own more personal and relaxed technique, probably in reaction to Alexander's suggestion of the corrective emotional experience. It was Lipton's view that the misnamed 'classical' technique, in contrast to Freud's, emphasized rules for the analyst's behavior and sacrificed the purpose of the analysis. Eissler's 1953 description of analysis as an activity that ideally uses only interpretation became the paradigm for 'classical' analysis. It was, Lipton says, a serious and severe distortion of the mature analytic technique developed by Freud. Freud regarded the analyst's personal behaviors, the personality of the analyst, and the living conditions of the patient as nontechnical parts of every analysis, as exemplified for Lipton in the case of the Rat Man. The so-called 'classical' (and in his view non-Freudian) technique attempted to include every aspect of the analytic situation as a part of technique and led to the model of the silent, restrained psychoanalyst. Lipton's argument is persuasive.

These two different models of technique have obvious implications concerning the transference and its interpretation. Unless we believe in an extreme version of the historical model, we must expect that the silent, restrained, nonparticipatory psychoanalyst will elicit different responses from his patient than will the vivid, less hidden, more responsive analyst. The range of personal behaviors available to the analyst before we need be concerned that the analyst is engaging in activities that are excessively self-revelatory or that force the patient into a social relationship is probably much broader than we thought a few years ago. But we also know that almost any behavior of the analyst, including restraint or silence, immediately influences the patient's responses. In these newer views of the analytic situation it is not easy to know what in the transference are iatrogenic consequences of analyst behaviors rather than intrapsychically derived patient behaviors.

It is evident today that psychoanalysts, under the sway of their theories and personalities, differ greatly concerning matters to which they are sensitive, and, of course, we can interpret only the transferences we perceive. Despite this limitation, a review of the literature reveals, along with the usual rigidities, a laudable tendency to describe one's experience as fully as possible, without heed to how it contradicts belief, often blurring over when experience and theory do not match. However, we have always been better at what we do than at what we say we do. This is exemplified in Heimann's (1956) paper, 'Dynamics of transference interpretation.' Speaking from a modified Kleinian perspective, and holding the historical theory of transference interpretation, Heimann managed 30 years ago to describe vividly and to support passionately much of what today is under discussion as the modernist version. That her positions were contradictory bothered her not at all. While many of us prefer to think we are following our theories, like all good scientists, good psychoanalysts, beginning with Freud, have always seen and responded to far more than our theories admit. When we have seen too much, we change our theories.

I have spoken of long-term trends in philosophy, child development, cultural attitudes, and psychoanalytic techniques that have influenced the development of psychoanalysis during the last half of this century. I will not discuss here how these trends, as well as our ever-increasing knowledge and our increasing distance from Freud's authority, have led to specific theoretical developments (Cooper 1983b, 1984c), many of them inferred in the newer transference model. Our current pluralistic theoretical world, in which almost all analysts are working, wittingly or not, with individual amalgams of Freud's drive theory, ego psychology, interpersonal Sullivanian psychoanalysis, object-relations theory, Bowlbyan or Mahlerian attachment theory, and usually smuggled-in versions of self psychology, lies at the base of the newer ideas and disagreements concerning transference interpretation. Although the historical definitions of transference and transference interpretation have the merit of seeming precision and limited scope, they are based on a psychoanalytic theory that no longer stands alone and has lost ground to competing theories. Of necessity, the historical definition is being replaced, or at least subsumed, by modernist conceptions that are more attuned to the theories that abound today. In this hodge-podge setting, it might help us both in our thinking about transference interpretations and in our understanding of the theories we hold, if we discuss a few of the sharper alternatives that are now available; indeed, that confront the psychoanalyst. I shall present a brief vignette to illustrate some of the issues. It will become apparent that in my conception of the modernist view, we have not abandoned the historical perspective; rather, it has become a component part of a larger, more complex conception.

A woman in the second year of analysis says, 'This treatment is all flattened out. It's like everything else in my life. It goes on, but nothing comes of it, certainly nothing good.' Suddenly the patient begins sobbing uncontrollably and says, 'You never give up on me. You keep thinking there's hope.' And then, after a pause, for the first time in her adult life, she vividly and movingly recalls the detailed circumstances of her father's leaving her mother and herself when she was five years old.

Let me begin by pointing to the obvious. I made no interpretation and yet a long-repressed memory emerged to consciousness with full affective coloring. Why did this happen? The feeling that nothing was happening was frequent during the treatment, often felt by me as well as by the patient, as I was the target of her projections. These complaints were usually accompanied by her insisting that she could not understand why I bothered to treat her when surely I had more worthwhile patients. I had made many interpretations relating these feelings about the two of us to her feelings about a father who had abandoned her, and she had regularly responded with polite boredom.

There were a number of converging reasons for a new memory to emerge at this point in the analysis: she wanted to be sure that I would remain hopeful and not give up on her; she was giving me a gift for showing an interest in her; furthermore, my interest in her confirmed her self-pitying view that her parents had never been interested; she felt guilty for obstructing my efforts, etc. More than anything else, though, she was responding to mounting anxiety over an impending disruption of our appointments. Whereas in the past, such anxiety regularly led to depressive anger, a sense of rejection, and impending panic, this time, in response to a new and growing conviction that I would not abandon her, this new memory allowed her to emphasize the difference between her father and me, thus partially relieving her anxiety. The earlier transference interpretations relating to her disappointing father, combined with the actual safety and reliability of the relationship with me in the analytic setting, had eventually led to a changing perception of me that could no longer be denied by the patient. This created a changing intrapsychic balance.

Under these new circumstances, inner conscience increasingly became the ally of the analyst, as the patient began to experience the growing discrepancy between her developmentally derived internalized expectations of me and the predictable actuality of that relationship. In effect, the voice of conscience, ever on the attack, found a newly accessible failing and said, 'Feel guilty for not letting him help you and for insisting on continuing your masochistic disappointments.' The new memory enabled her to make a new compromise: 'Even though I admit that my analyst is different from my father, my father was just as bad as I claimed, and I'll now prove it. I also feel safe enough now to revive those old and terrible memories.' Later in the treatment, she will even remember good times with her father. In one important aspect, the analytic situation acts as a Proustian madeleine. It awakens sweet resonances of the sense of childhood security and safety, whether actual or fantasied, and thus allows the release of memories, even painful memories. This portion of the transference is usually interpretable only in retrospect.

At the risk of further complicating this little vignette, I will try to summarize what I have described. A recovered memory, an important event marking a change in the analytic atmosphere, was the result of a number of interacting factors. (1) There was a background of specific old-fashioned transference interpretations – in effect, 'you think I am your father, but I am not.' Many of these interpretations related to the missing memories. (2) These interpretations were made in the here and now – when the patient felt angry and rejected, I talked about how she was actually making a statement about me; that I was, in her opinion, just like her father, and I encouraged her to talk about how I was like him, or why she was now frightened of me or angry at me. (3) While the analyst was, of course, often the object of projections of representations of the past, I played an equally important role as the necessary background of safety for the patient's experimentation with new self-representations and object representations. Projections onto the analyst may occur during this experimentation, but those experiments are going on everywhere in the patient's life, and the analyst may not always be the center of interest. (4) A change in intrapsychic balance occurred, with the need for new compromises, because of increasing unconscious cognitive dissonance and new alignments of guilty feeling. A mismatch of internal representations and new perceptions is never tolerable, and in neurosis we rearrange our perceptions to suit our rigidly held internal expectations. The persistence, constancy, and facilitating qualities of the analytic environment, including the transference interpretations, not only provide a background of safety, but lead to a new psychic reality of greater tolerance for shameful and frightening unconscious fantasies. Paradoxically, they also create increasing guilt over maintaining old grievances in a new environment. (5) This led to a need for a new adaptation to an old danger – the impending disruption of the sessions – because the old adaptation had become too conflictual. Inner conscience would no longer permit simple enactments of the old fantasy of abandonment. (6) Finally, the outcome of all these ingredients was the need for a new intrapsychic compromise formation. To achieve this, a memory was recaptured (incidentally, confirmed by her mother). The memory, whether created or recaptured, was important in helping the patient to organize a new transference relationship with the analyst, more clearly distinguishing him from the damaging remembered father, and in helping her to restore a more satisfactory arrangement with her altered superego. She could begin to accept her anger at the father of childhood without quite so much need to justify and enact it in the present. The historical view of the transference interpretation – the analyst as abandoning father – has played a part in this transference reorganization, but only one part. The modernist version of the transference interpretations urges us toward a richer and more inclusive understanding of the transference events. The patient is changing, indeed, in response to the analyst's transference interpretations; but she is changing in the course of a relationship with the analyst. In this relationship, transference interpretation has played a vital role not only in helping her to gain insight, but also in helping her to regulate her feelings and her relationship with me, as well as mine with her. Her expectations of me have changed. We have attained better empathic contact. It is here that what I referred to above as the 'romantic' and intersubjective emphasis of the modernist view becomes apparent, in the effort of two people to connect affectively.

When we speak of transference interpretations, it is probably wise to include also those that are silent – the many interpretations we entertain but never utter to the patient. These silent transference interpretations – hypotheses about what is happening in the analysis – are crucial for the analyst's conduct of the treatment, influencing the way he listens and intervenes, and leading to many subsidiary interpretations. These unspoken interpretations deserve to be considered in any narrative of the analytic process, even though they may achieve utterance only later in the analysis. Their absence is at least one reason why recorded analyses often sound stilted.

The modernist view also stresses the open-endedness of the analytic situation. The new experiences of the interpretations and the facilitating environment of the analytic setting force significant alterations of internal representations, structures, and conflicts. This changing intrapsychic balance leads not only to alterations in the transference, but, far more important from the patient's point of view, it leads to changes in extratransference relationships as well. These changes outside the analysis may then facilitate new experiences in the analysis. In fact, one of the significant elements in the background of our vignette was the patient's greatly improved relationship with her husband. Psychoanalysis is not a closed system of an intrapsychic world impinging on a single target.

I would like to stress two of the points that have already been implied in what has been said. The first pertains to the relative roles of intrapsychic and interpersonal perspectives. Since Freud's discovery of psychic reality, it has been part of the historical conception to focus primarily on the intrapsychic life of the patient, the psyche being conceived largely as driven toward objects, rather than formed and constantly reforming in relation to objects. Analysts holding this view (Curtis 1980) of course acknowledge the interpersonal aspect, but they are likely to see it as a part of the surround rather than a part of the core of analytic work. They believe that the intrapsychic realm is the only one to which analytic expertise applies, and that any emphasis on the interpersonal is liable to lead to dilution of analytic work, excessive intrusion of the analyst into the patient's life, or a shallow corrective emotional experience. All these dangers are real, and have occurred in the history of psychoanalysis, but I believe, with Gill and Emde recently and Sullivan long ago, that we cannot fully interpret transference resistances without acknowledging their interpersonal quality. There has been a mistaken tendency to equate psychic reality with the intrapsychic, and to neglect the contribution of interpersonal interaction to the creation of new psychic reality.

Freud (1905a), in the postscript to the Dora case, made this point when he wrote:

> I ought to have listened to the warning myself. 'Now,' I ought to have said to her, 'it is from Herr K. that you have made a transference on to me. Have you noticed anything that leads you to suspect me of evil intentions similar (whether openly or in some sublimated form) to Herr K.'s? Or have you been struck by anything about me or got to know anything about me which has caught your fancy, as happened previously with Herr K.?' Her attention would then have been turned to some detail in our relations, or in my person or circumstances, behind which there lay concealed something analogous but immeasurably more important concerning Herr K.
>
> (Freud 1905a: 118).

While Freud was interested in the hidden motive, he recognized that the route to it was through the interpersonal connection. Although he spoke of the transference from Herr K. onto himself, he implied that it could not have occurred unless the patient had seen something about him that made such a concordance of perception possible. Schwaber (1983) has emphasized this point. Of course, the patient needs to match the interpersonal world to his intrapsychic world, and to achieve this he or she uses all available data, no matter how one-sidedly perceived – the analyst's silences or his talkativeness, attitudes, tastes in art, manner of dress, speech habits, etc. The analyst who cannot tolerate this close scrutiny of himself and denies the veracity of his foibles that are included in the patient's transference is unable to interpret the transference fully and is encouraging deceit in the analytic relationship. At the same time, the analyst must be able to discover how his foibles and failures are being used in the service of the patient's neurosis, as well as to distinguish the misperceptions that patients create to suit their needs. Otherwise, indeed, the patient's neurotic defenses are strengthened.

223

This touches on the issue of 'distortion' in the patient's communications to the analyst. Schwaber (1983) and Gill (1982), from somewhat different perspectives, have both suggested that the analyst is in no better position to know the patient's 'truth' or the correctness of his perceptions than is the patient. They maintain that both parties' views of the transference are valid, and it is a failure of logic to think of transference interpretations as 'correcting' distortions. Schafer (1985) criticizes Gill's view as removing the gradients of expertise, of need for help, of closeness to conflict, etc. that characterize the different responsibilities of therapist and patient in the analytic situation. I would go further and suggest that the concept of defense, central to the idea of transference resistance, carries with it the clear implication that the patient, in the neurotic areas of his psychic functioning, has to some degree unconsciously constricted, distorted, and rigidified his perceptual, affective, and cognitive capacities. We know that all historians are biased, and we have every reason to be alert to the unconscious sources of bias in the histories constructed by our patients.

It behooves the analyst to know not only the content of his patient's narrative, but the needs that compel its construction, the elements that must be a part of any human history that are missing in the particular history, and the effect of the shared experience of analyst and patient in creating new histories, often quite different for each of them. When the patient in our vignette says everything is flattened out, it would not be unreasonable for the analyst to suspect that exactly the opposite was the case. The purpose of the analyst's alertness to distortion is not to correct his patient, but to allow him to understand the needs that are dictating the patient's construction.

I shall give another vignette to illustrate my view of the problem. A woman in her last months of analysis said, 'I never wanted to say thank you to my mother. That would have meant to be chained to her . . . It's terrible, but to feel free I had never to be spontaneous with my mother.' I said, 'It's been very difficult for you here to feel that you could be entirely spontaneous and trust me not to make you feel guilty or dependent.' The patient became silent for a time and went on, 'It makes me very angry to hear you say that I didn't trust you. It isn't that I didn't trust you, it was that whatever you said invoked in me a reaction like my mother had said it. As a child I was always uniform, balanced, defended. If I thought I mistrusted you how could I keep coming here? If I kissed my mother goodbye before going to school and at the same time thought that I wanted her to be dead, I'd be terribly guilty. It's hard to accept that you could allow me to have both feelings toward you.'

The patient felt accused over the matter of trust, explaining that it had nothing to do with the analyst, but was a reaction to her mother. She sharply differentiated (some would say split) between the analyst she trusts enough to keep coming, and the analyst–mother whom she mistrusts. One of the aims of interpretation is to develop the capacity to bring these different representations closer together with less anxiety and guilt.

This dialogue had been preceded by years of work on her feelings about both the analyst and her mother. Initially, her mother was simply absent from her childhood description, dismissed as a bland, not very intelligent woman, who played no part in her upbringing; in fact, the patient from earliest years recalled that she was the one who took care of her incompetent mother, and she had no memories of ever being cared for. From the analyst's perspective, it is essential both to understand what the patient believes and to hypothesize about how that belief came about. We know that childhood could not have been as the patient recalled it; her mother did care for her as a little girl, even though the patient is also telling us that she felt inadequately cared for. It wounds her narcissism to have to admit that she was not always the independent Oedipal victor she later became. Distortions of history have been elaborated, and the analyst will try to understand the psychological circumstances, intrapsychic and interpersonal, that led this woman to erase any evidences of infantile helplessness, to eradicate her mother's essential caretaking, and to adopt her thinly disguised hostile attitude toward a fantasied helpless mother. The analytic aim is not to contradict the patient's view; rather it is to be alert to predictable reactions that will arise in the transference with a patient who holds such beliefs (e.g. her fear of attachment and dependency, her mistrust of the analyst's capacity to tolerate her murderous competitiveness) and to be ready to assist the patient in her struggle to come to grips with internalized versions of her mother and herself that she has not been able to entertain consciously. For example, during years of analysis, this woman insisted that everything I did was guided entirely by my need to obey the rules of my profession, and had nothing to do with her personally. She also maintained she did not in any way know me or anything about me. These beliefs can be clearly regarded as transference distortions by means of which the patient attempted to maintain her original repression both of her attachment to her deeply depressed and disappointing mother, and of her mother's interest in her child, however faulty that interest was. In fact, when she was ready to know what she knew, she knew an enormous amount, both about me and about her mother. Until then, as far as she was concerned, it was an honest statement. The concept of distortion neither demeans the patient nor implies a single correct truth.

The transference and its interpretation are at the center of all considerations of analytic theory and technique. Freud, throughout his life, seemed astonished by the power of transference, and we are no less so. The concept was relatively simple when we understood persons as in the grip of their drives, and the purpose of the analysis was the expansion of consciousness. Today, the idea of transference has become so complex that we are no longer sure what in the analysis is not transference, and if it is not, what it is. Our loss of innocence is part of a large change in world view concerning history and truth. Major philosophical, scientific, and cultural movements, as well as our own researches, have led to a new and desirable situation of theoretical pluralism in psychoanalysis, although at the price of the loss of a great overarching theory. As a result, our once straightforward historical understanding of transference interpretation has yielded to a more polymorphous and confusing, but more interesting modernist view. This modernist view has raised our awareness of elements of the transference that were previously neglected, and has opened the way for experimentation and reconsideration of many old problems.

— 18 —

SOME THOUGHTS ON HOW THERAPY DOES AND DOESN'T WORK*

It is consonant with our newer view of psychoanalysis that we cannot at this time give a very satisfactory answer to the question of how therapy works. Psychoanalysis and, by implication, dynamic psychotherapy now rest upon a series of interlocking partial theories involving drive theory, object-relations, self-development, structural organization, interpersonal interactions, and narrative construction, at least. Where we once enjoyed the luxury of a single overarching theory that undertook to explain all, or nearly all, of psychic life, we now struggle with competing theories, none of which has yet demonstrated sufficient power or has mustered enough evidence to compel anyone to give up his favorite point of view. While this situation may be distressing to theorists, I believe it is advantageous to clinicians, because it permits, in fact requires, that we examine more carefully what we are doing, under what theoretical aegis, and to what end. This is, therefore, an excellent time to examine what are the active and necessary ingredients of the complicated action called psychotherapy, aware that it is highly unlikely that any single element will be able to claim primacy. I shall, perhaps controversially, treat psychotherapy as a derivative of psychoanalytic theory, employing more openly and in different proportions a large range of technical procedures that are present but muted in psychoanalysis. My perspective is that psychoanalysis and psychotherapy exist on a continuum, clearly distinguishable at the ends of the spectrum and blurred in the middle (see Chapter 8).

Freud's views on the source of therapeutic efficacy changed progressively throughout his lifetime. At various times he held that therapeutic efficacy was a

---

* The earliest version of this paper was first presented as 'Some thoughts on how therapy works' at Michigan Psychoanalytic Society in 1989. This version includes some of what was previously published as Cooper (1988e) in © The Psychoanalytic Quarterly, 1988, 57: 15–27, and Panel (1992).

result of making the unconscious conscious, or of abreacting strangulated affects, or of reconstructing the buried traumatic sexual past, or of replacing aspects of the id with the ego, or of re-experiencing infantile traumas within the transference and thereby learning to master them and more. These techniques were aimed towards the recovery of preexisting capacities, or towards the resumption of thwarted lines of growth. All of these conceptions were in the service of the underlying idea that the resolution or mastery of unconscious conflict – the triad of wish, defense and resulting compromise – was the key to therapeutic success, a mastery achieved through the affective re-experience of conflictual derivatives brought to awareness by regression and interpretation within the transference. I will, for brevity's sake, omit a review of the literature on how analysis works, but in general our literature today emphasizes the centrality of the patient's experience of himself and the analyst within the transference and the crucial impact, positive and negative, of the analyst's empathic registration of and responsiveness to his patient, generally guided by his attunement to his own countertransferential arousals. Analysts differ in their emphases and theorists of therapy may be broadly divided among those who emphasize insight over new and corrective experience, or those who emphasize structural change over narrative reconstruction, or those who emphasize deficit repair over conflict resolution. One could add to this list. It is more important to stress that these are not mutually exclusive points of view. Newer ideas and concepts have been additive rather than alternative, and any therapeutic encounter involves multiple elements in differing proportions. While our literature has tended to emphasize *the* source of therapeutic action of psychoanalysis, it is my thesis that it is now more useful to recognize that we carry out a large array of activities during analysis or therapy, each subject to technical variation, all of them necessary but none of them sufficient to account for the therapeutic action of our treatment. This makes for a very uncomfortable therapeutic world, lacking the clear guidelines that most of us would like to have. The history of our understanding of therapeutic efficacy reveals that few if any of our ideas have been wrong. Rather, they have been partial.

With a century of psychoanalytic experience behind us, we need no longer share Freud's concern over maintaining the purity of psychoanalysis uncontaminated by elements of psychotherapy. For one example, Freud worried that if he admitted elements of suggestion into psychoanalysis he would be subject to the charge that psychoanalysis was nothing other than suggestion, but today we know enough about the power of psychoanalysis as a map of the mind, a method of investigation, and a mode of therapy that we can adopt a much broader view of the psychoanalytic process and its essential interactional constitution, in which suggestion is inevitable, in contrast to Freud's use of surgical metaphors to describe what we do. Our contemporary concern lies with how to do analysis best, rather than with stereotypes that attempt artificially to separate psychoanalysis from other therapies. If we view psychoanalysis as the

228

effort to conduct the deepest possible exploration of psychic function and to open the maximal opportunities for restructuring and altering psychic structure and content, with the aim of enhancing the range of autonomy and choice, then everything that contributes to that process must be considered psychoanalysis.

A bit of history may help us to understand the issue. In 1953 Eissler published his paper on 'The effect of the structure of the ego on psychoanalytic technique.' This paper may serve as a marker for the quiet revolution that has occurred in psychoanalysis. Eissler's paper was, in a way, the Maginot Line of 'orthodox' technique, an unassailable structure designed to defend psychoanalysis as it had been up to that time, but facing in the wrong direction and designed to fight the wrong war. Even while Eissler suggested that psychoanalysis was a largely completed enterprise, advances in psychoanalytic theory and technique were being put forth in many quarters. Alexander's advocacy of a flexibility in the analytic setting and of the corrective emotional experience, unfortunately describing it as artificial conduct on the part of the analyst rather than as an automatic and necessary component of a well-conducted analysis by a humane and empathic analyst, was apparently the catalyst for Eissler's paper. At about the same time, Rado and Kardiner were advocating the abandonment of libido theory and the structural point of view and their replacement with the concept of an action-self. Glover, in 1955, pointed out that the classical technique was inappropriate for the vast majority of analytic cases who had deformed, or in Eissler terms, modified egos. Bowlby's work on the child's tie to the mother and on separation anxiety, published during the 1950s, had profound new implications for the role of the actual environment and experience of the child in later development of psychic structure. Loewald was urging an object-relational point of view including a personal loving parental attitude of the analyst toward his patient. Leo Stone, in 1961 in *The Psychoanalytic Situation*, vividly described psychoanalysis in terms of the interaction between two people changing each other, abandoning the metaphor of a surgeon operating on the presumably passive mind. Stone rather remarkably said: 'It is one of the paradoxes of the position of psychoanalysis . . . that, having brought the concept of the whole and living person vividly to the attention of clinical medicine, it does, nevertheless, in fulfilling its paradoxical scientific destiny, often treat the living and indeed waking patient . . . somewhat as a patient in anesthesia' (p. 65). British object-relations theory was being brought to these shores and carried a description of the analytic process quite different from the American tradition.

The death of Hartman, ego psychology's major proponent, and the acceptance of Kohut into the realm of analytic discourse rapidly accelerated the shift of analytic views. One may ask retrospectively why Eissler's paper and the so-called 'orthodox' point of view held power for so long. I think the clarity and authoritative tone of the paper and its scientistic aspect were and are attractive to many analysts. Eissler defined analysis as a procedure using only questions and interpretation. Any other action is a 'ruffle' of the analytic process, a 'parameter' in his odd language. To qualify as psychoanalysis, 'the final phase of the treatment must always proceed with a parameter of zero.' The paper gives the impression that analytic technique can be assessed with the same assurance as a surgeon's aseptic technique. How much all of us in the middle stages of difficult analyses wish that we had clear guideposts, knew where we were heading, could judge the correctness of our course and reassure ourselves. Dr Eissler's paper held out the promise of the development of that confidence. For better or worse, advances in psychoanalysis have stilled that hope. In place of the clear, straightforward, somewhat unidimensional model that Dr Eissler wrote of, we are today wrestling with multiple perspectives and multiple theories, none of them either entirely satisfactory or easily disposable. I don't mean to distort our field by comparing it to physics, but our situations are similar – too many pieces of new data don't fit any of our simpler models and we must make do with messy partial theories in the place of the beauty of a single encompassing theory.

It was as a part of his attempt to make the presentation scientific that Eissler attempted to discuss analytic technique while omitting two of the three variables that he said entered into technique – he would include only the patient's disorder and personality, and would omit the patient's life circumstances, and the analyst's personality. Eissler's conception of the analyst's role was such that he could imagine an ideal analyst (one whose personality is entirely favorable to the analytic process) and an ideal ego (one not modified by defenses). Eissler implied that we can conceptualize an ego distinct from its defense mechanisms. Today, I think we would all agree that the ego is its defenses plus other dimensions, and that we cannot conceptualize it in any other way. Similarly, we cannot conceive of an analyst not engaged in interactions that arise because of the analyst's failures of understanding, and we regard these as integral to the process, not as interferences or deviations from an ideal.

Where once Eissler could claim that analysis is a process in which the analyst conducts only two activities – interpretations and questions – and everything else constitutes a departure from analytic technique, that is, a parameter requiring correction, today we accept that the analyst is carrying on a large number of essential psychoanalytic functions simultaneously. Interpretation, surely vital, can no longer be considered the sole analytic process. Rather, analysis, and surely psychotherapy, unavoidably and desirably include at one or another moment such previously disavowed analytic experiences and activities as new and corrective emotional experience, cognitive reeducation, suggestion, acting out and acting in, role modeling, maintenance of hope, concern for our patient's external reality, etc. The work of Loewald, as I have written elsewhere (see 'Our changing views of the therapeutic action of psychoanalysis: Comparing Strachey and Loewald' (Cooper 1988e)), particularly highlights the discontinuity between therapeutic paradigms that place interpretation at the center and those, which Loewald considers critical, that permit a new and growth-enhancing interactive experience with a new object, assisted by interpretation. What we require is a theory or theories that *permit* us, even *encourage* us to engage psychoanalytically in these non-interpretive activities with our patients; without the sanction of theory we do these things badly, inappropriately or grudgingly.

My purpose in this paper is to stress that in the modern psychoanalytic world we not only have multiple theories, a generally accepted proposition, but that we use multiple techniques and these techniques have received too little attention and have not been given an adequate place in our theories.

One word of warning: I will, both deliberately and accidentally, mix up my use of the terms analysis and psychotherapy, often intending both meanings under either heading.

As one example of our many unspecified actions, I will briefly discuss the provision of a sense of safety as a therapeutic activity. All of our contemporary schemas acknowledge the significance of the environment of safety and predictability that the analyst provides through the specific elements of the therapeutic situation. We all consider that an analytic task is to provide an analytic setting, i.e. an environment of holding, or facilitation, or safety with its peculiarly analytic mixture of abstinence and gratification and intimacy and distance, and the forms of interpretations and understanding that follow from our analytic theories. However, we will define these safety conditions very differently with different patients, not hesitating to be quite confrontational with some patients at some times, supportive with others at other times, skeptical, sympathetic, probing, or accepting. We may be more or less withholding of our words, or of our presence, or of information about ourselves in ways that frustrate or gratify, creating more or less anxiety or satisfaction. Any of these actions may fall within a definition of a safe setting, attuned to the patient, following from our empathy and our theory and not at all involving role-playing. Within some limit set by our theories, we will appropriately, consciously and unconsciously, respond differently to different patients. An aggressively narcissistic–masochistic man will, although initially angry, actually feel safer if he feels that his analyst is not cowed by his aggressive façade and does not hesitate to call into question actions that the patient knows are self-destructive but cannot stop. On the other hand, a timid, fragile, narcissistic individual, challenged early in the treatment, would experience this as a blow to his self-esteem, a humiliation by a superior figure, and might be unable to continue the treatment with any comfort. Safety then does not designate a steady state; it designates a goal of the analyst's responsiveness to the patient, attuned to his patient's needs as seen through the lens of our theories. Technical neutrality is not passive equidistance among the mental agencies. It requires the analyst's active role to assure that each agency will receive a fair analytic hearing.

Consider a 35-year-old woman who is in a first treatment, has a sense that she has never before been listened to and has never been able to listen to herself. The quietness of the therapeutic setting, the analyst's slowness in response, his questions about her ways of feeling and their sources and connections, his labeling or relabeling of feelings and perceptions that she has kept out of awareness, attunes her to a different mode of listening, and levels of sadness and old memories of loneliness begin to emerge that were never available to her before in the noisy life that she has led. She experiences this on the one hand as safe enough so that she can have these new experiences. On the other hand, she has a certain dread before each session because she has a sense of surprise and perhaps doom as she realizes how unhappy her childhood was, far more so than she has ever imagined. With this she begins to be aware of a level of anger greater than she has ever acknowledged, and she begins to form a picture of herself as a child who was isolated, sad, and lonely, a picture that she has never before allowed to surface. The background of safety therefore is relative: safe enough for her to recapture an old self that she has spent a lifetime trying to deny, but those recollections themselves create a dangerous situation. She forgets appointments, attributes this to her busy schedule, dismissing the idea that it may in any way connect to feelings of anger or fear towards the analyst or the therapeutic situation. She is simultaneously safe and unsafe, just as her prior adaptive arrangement of denial, identification with aggressors, and counter-phobic action made her differently safe and not safe.

In this setting she experiences the therapist as an enigma, kindly but somehow manipulative, someone she cannot figure out, 'The Doctor' – bland, blank, remembering everything, contributing nothing – non-human. After a summer vacation break, she says, 'thank God you're back,' and then says 'I don't know why I said that.' She feels the therapist could do more than he is doing to help her and is angry that he withholds. At the same she finds herself interrupting whenever he begins to attempt an interpretation, fearful that he will tell her more than she wants to hear. It seems to me that my job in this situation requires doing at least two different things simultaneously. I want to be able to adopt a stance of freely hovering attention that will enable me to become aware of the elements in her story that suggest new connections or that clearly fail to connect as the patient wishes they would. I also need to attend specifically to her anger and fear in the therapeutic situation, her lack of safety, because I sense a fragility of her attachment to me – not because she has no involvement, but because she is desperately afraid of the intensity of dependence she brings to the treatment, and she cannot bear too quickly to know how needy she feels. Feeling her ambivalence towards me and the treatment, I carefully monitor myself for evidences that I am seducing her into treatment, or that I am too fearful of telling her what she doesn't want to hear.

Furthermore, I am concerned that against this background of safety she is acting out and I feel responsible and unable to bring it to awareness, let alone prevent it. Shortly after beginning treatment, she decided she was unhappy with her job and quickly decided to quit, and when thwarted in that by her boss's angry insistence that she stay, she began a negotiation marked by an assertiveness that she had never experienced before. I see this new capacity both as a release of inhibitions related to new insights into her lifelong denials of her childhood unhappiness and anger towards her parents, and a totally uninsightful regressive effort to prove that she has no need of me and that she can defeat an authority figure who denies her instant gratification. During a session in which she has fallen silent, I say she seems sad and she bursts into tears, sobbing uncontrollably, explaining that nothing like this has ever happened to her before, both relieved and chagrined at this turn of events. The next session, she says, 'I suppose you want to know the latest in my business life' and proceeds to tell me of her negotiation. When I ask why she thinks I would be more interested in her business life than in her tears of the last session, she ignores the question and continues on the topic of her business. While I know what she is avoiding, it is true that I am interested in her external reality since I worry that she will act out in a damaging way and, in fact, I believe that I have several times saved her from potentially self-destructive moves by pointing to the possible effects of some contemplated actions and by raising questions about her intentions and the sources of her motivations. At the same time she is, with a mixture of motives, and in the context of feeling safe with me, succeeding in doing what she wants to do in the world, and I fear – perhaps excessively – that I can derail her with a questioning attitude that she will interpret as the kind of vote of no confidence that she has been used to at home. The situation is not made simpler by my perception that she is one of those people who sporadically, intermittently and not entirely predictably – at least by me – is capable either of extraordinary psychological insight or startling psychological stupidity and naivety as one or the other suits her resistances and defensive needs. I have described matters from the point of view of the background of safety, and the many activities and delicate balances required to maintain it, although that is not all that is going on. At this point in her therapy, I believed that we would go on to convert this treatment into an analysis dealing with issues of the inhibited capacities for intimacy and sexuality. I was mistaken. Shortly after the successful conclusion of her business negotiation, she told me she was feeling good and wanted to stop, and did so shortly after.

Somewhat in contrast, I now want to describe a difficult, although not too atypical, case to emphasize the variety of measures, in addition to interpretation, that we may bring to bear when treating patients with psychotherapy or analysis at the present time. Mrs C. was a 25-year-old business woman, married to a nice, rather removed, passive man, who came to treatment because she was becoming increasingly anxious and depressed as her workload increased, her situation at work became more competitive, her husband's pressure to have children aroused her fears that she was unfit to be a mother. She was a pleasant-looking woman, rather plainly dressed, appearing a bit shy, fearful, and a little remote. She was aware of some longstanding minor inhibitions and phobias. She was afraid to dance, could not invite people to her house, was afraid to drive a car, and could not swim. Exhibitionistic conflicts were readily apparent. She knew of me by reputation, had heard mostly good things and expressed some concern over whether I would want to treat her. I liked her but I was aware, I think from the start, that I felt not quite in touch with her. She had had a brief psychotherapy a few years earlier and while this had been helpful, she now wanted analysis, and I thought that was the appropriate treatment. Because at that moment I didn't have enough time and she didn't have job flexibility we agreed to start a psychotherapy twice a week that we converted to a four times a week analysis a year later.

Mrs C was the oldest of three girls in a family with a violently ill-tempered alcoholic father who threatened the children verbally and was also sexually seductive, perhaps abusing them. The mother was described as an anxious, disorganized, distant, self-involved woman unable to provide any consistent sense of warmth, protection, or calm, unable to express, or perhaps even to experience, loving feelings. The patient recalls being in the backyard, falling down and hurting herself, crying, and seeing her mother come to the window to look without making any further effort to comfort her.

The patient had always perceived herself as different from the other children, physically uncoordinated, and more intelligent. She had one or two close friends, described herself as a rather isolated child, but she did usually find a teacher who appreciated her and to whom she felt close, and she had good social skills. As far back as she could recall, she believed that her body was somehow not made right. She could not run, jump, skip, or throw a ball as the other children could and she felt clumsy. Interestingly, I always saw her as graceful. Once, when leaving the office she tripped against a chair that was out of its usual position and said, 'You see how clumsy I am,' when it seemed obvious to me that she had not been at fault. It became a characteristic of the treatment that my perception of her seemed unreliable. When I thought I knew or understood something about her I quickly or eventually discovered, or was told, that I had misperceived her, or I was given contradictory information.

As a child she was easily startled by sounds, reading a book would so excite her that she had to pace for hours, she had to shut herself in her room so as not to hear the voices of the household, etc. Primal scene fantasies seemed clear, but the heightened stimulus sensitivity was probably an independent biological phenomenon. Most importantly, she remembered her childhood as one of constant anxiety focused around the idea that she must save her younger sisters from destruction by her parents. She remembered herself from age five on as the most mature member of the household, believing that she was the only one who could provide any order and organization to the family. This narcissistic fantasy was justified to herself by her conviction that her parents were in every way incompetent, and that the household was mortally dangerous; she and her sisters could, literally, be killed by her father or mother if she didn't take protective measures. In fact, those protective measures seemed confined to anxious watching. This sense of living in great danger was immediately apparent in the transference. At the beginning of every session she would quickly scan my face and assess my mood, my friendliness, attentiveness, and availability. From about age 15 on she had a boyfriend who, she felt, loved and protected her from her family. He, incidentally, found her home to be so oppressive and unpleasant that he would never enter her house; years later her husband had the same attitude. Her sisters never left the small Midwestern community in which they were raised, and achieved little.

She left home to go to college on a full scholarship and described herself as both carefree and chronically anxious. She had another boyfriend in college, enjoyed some casual girlfriends, was overtly amiable and well-liked but felt disconnected and unhappy. She met, pursued, and shortly after college graduation, married her husband-to-be. Academically successful in school and later in graduate school, she nonetheless was unable to rid herself of feelings of impostership – that she was faking her life and making believe she was a person. However, if I attempted to probe this, she would then tell me that her sexual pleasures were real and she was truly close to her friends.

We began psychotherapy and she quickly formed a seemingly gratifying dependent bond with me, while I continued to be aware of a feeling of something missing. The sessions were taken up with her mounting anxiety over problems at work, and I tried to focus on her barely hidden ferocious competitiveness, her capacity to turn the admiration of others into disappointment, and her need to deny any successful performance. All of these issues were prominent in her relationship to me, although my attempts to explore were turned away, either ignored or denied, and my interpretations were perceived as humiliating and controlling. For instance, the patient complained bitterly that she worked harder than anyone else in her company and that she was on the brink of exhaustion. When I suggested that we might look at why that was, she impatiently said I misunderstood – she really didn't work hard at all and that wasn't the problem. I was puzzled, often felt helpless, and I thought I understood it as a projection of the chaotic unaffirming world of her childhood; neither parent ever admitted a difficulty or clarified a confusion. It was only years later that I realized fully that she was not interested in being understood or helped; she wanted only to know that I fully appreciated, affirmed, shared, empathized, or sympathized with her experience in a way that allowed her to feel merged or fused with me. Understanding was already a two-person system and a threat.

A certain blandness in sessions alternated with what seemed to me to be suppressed rage beneath the surface of her pleasantness. I tried to bring to awareness her difficulty in feeling free with me, her barely hidden struggle for control of the sessions, her fear of allowing someone else to know her, her conviction that she was evil and unlovable, and her sense that what she enjoyed about me were aspects of me that she took, rather than were given by me. I didn't know if we were making progress but her blandness in sessions did begin to give way to greater distress and increasing concern over whether I would abandon her. There were frequent images in her dreams of torn, bleeding, mutilated children, usually in a context of bland surroundings. No one noticed or was bothered. Interpreting her conviction that I was insensitive to her suffering seemed to elicit vague affirmation but no change.

It wasn't until years later that she was able to tell me how much she dreaded lying on the couch. She believed that to tell me that at the time would prove that she was so abnormal that I would give up on her immediately. From the start, the analytic situation oscillated between fantasies that she had at last found a safe haven with me and therefore needed me with her every minute, and the opposite feeling of being constantly endangered by me, either by my not being available on weekends, or by my canceling an appointment, or by my efforts at interpretation, all indications of my profound lack of connection to her. At times she had overt sexual fantasies about me, reporting cheerfully and without embarrassment that she had spent a weekend fantasizing making love with me, which had a soothing effect on her. She became furious if I made any effort to inquire further about these fantasies, convinced that I hated her and didn't even want to be in her thoughts. Interpretive or reconstructive efforts were seen as malignant intrusions. Often when I thought I was reflecting back what she had just told me, she would lapse into angry silence, convinced that I had misunderstood her and criticized her, and we were unable to clarify our difficulty. With unconscious ironic intent, every statement of mine was recast by her in all-or-none terms, all ambiguity and modulation were removed and every question or suggestion or attempt at amplification or clarification was misconstrued as an order or a criticism. She suffered intensely, and I felt I was being made a prisoner of her emotional demands; she was inducing in me the same feelings of danger and unpredictability that she had experienced. I found myself feeling confused and helpless and angry. There was also an untouchable pseudo-idealization of me as perfect, someone she could love, but who could never love her. She was convinced I would spoil anything she showed me, that if she had a positive feeling, I would bring up the negative. Splitting was rampant.

Her requirement that I be a non-presence in her presence, the archetypal narcissistic demand, created obvious, if not unusual, therapeutic dilemmas. I could exist, in effect, only if she had the safety of total control over me. Thus, the moment the patient lay on the couch, unable to incorporate and control me with her eyes, she felt in mortal danger, and that I would use my control against her, perhaps killing her. She complained that my distance from her, the actual number of inches between my chair and the couch, was intolerable, that I was determined to flee from her, and that something about her made me hate her. She gradually developed increasing anxiety, with panics and agoraphobia, expressing the view that I really hated her, that she was in danger of dying as a result of the analysis, and she began expressing suicidal thoughts, while her barely concealed hatred was aggressively disavowed. At the same time she also wanted to be a small girl under my loving care, with numerous fantasies of being held by me and feeling that whenever she was in distress a look at a photograph of me would instantly calm and relieve her. Without my actual presence, she could construct her own fantasy of a loving, wonderful, androgynous parent who could perform all functions for her and would protect her from all harm. In effect, the only good parent was a dead one, or one that had never existed.

It was clear that the treatment, by provoking closeness to a person whom she could not control, was making her worse, and that the negative thera-peutic reaction totally dominated the treatment situation. My problem was compounded by my increasing uncertainty that I understood her and by my difficulty in maintaining my own benign feelings. Should I move my chair closer when she asked? Undoubtedly I often did and more often I did not. The capacity of severely regressed narcissistic–masochistic patients to induce sadism and boredom in the therapist cannot be overestimated.

Because this patient functioned so successfully and at such a high level in so many work and social situations, I was slow to appreciate that initially in therapy she could only tolerate an affirmation of her existing self and object repre-sentations, in a slightly safer environment. She had spent her entire childhood consciously trying to be entirely 'good' and suppressing all emotional display, so that neither parent could ever criticize or doubt her, thereby maintaining her grandiose and masochistic fantasies of perfect martyrdom, and the massive emotional expression that began to emerge in the analysis represented, among other things, a revenge against controlling dangerous objects, an ego defense that effectively disarmed and disorganized those around her and a masochistic perpetuation of the sense that she was damaged and beyond understanding. Her emotional life had been a private preserve into which her parents could not intrude, and I was threatening that safety barrier. The idea that feeling could be understood interrupted her masochistically gratifying fantasies of an isolated child perpetually misunderstood by cruel, self-centered parents.

I was perceived as a restrictive constraining parent, interfering with soiling and wetting and masturbatory fantasies. A frequent fantasy of hers on the couch was that she would somehow soil it, that she would leave a puddle behind, either of sweat or feces or urine or vaginal discharge, and that I found her disgusting. Feeling empty, unaccomplished, lacking confidence in her ego skills, her dramatic self-portrayal sustained a very fragile self-esteem. As she oscillated between malignant murderous rage and fairytale feelings of loving care, she induced in me the feeling of always 'walking on eggs.' Every step was likely to be greeted with an unpredictable emotional storm; no word or movement of mine elicited a predictable response and I was in the position she had been in as a child. Attempts to work with this simply led to a role reversal in which she, rather than I, was now the threatened infant. Unlike the typical borderline patient, there was never a question of her quitting and she was never late for an appointment, paid her bills instantly, and missed a session only under extreme necessity. Splitting was a characteristic mode of her relating, but object constancy was maintained so that I existed in her eyes as dangerously unpredictable but still the person to whom she was tied. The tie never broke as it does in the usual borderline patient. Attempts to explore these aspects of the transference elicited little relief.

I, mistakenly in retrospect, tried to steer a middle course that would provide the unintrusive holding that Mrs C seemed to need, while allowing some interpretive work that would indicate both that she could be understood and that she need not fear that her rage would destroy me. However, her work situation deteriorated and I became alarmed as her depression, anxiety and suicidal feeling increased beyond a level that either of us could tolerate. She developed clear evidence of an atypical depression and suicide now seemed to me a significant danger. Two years after the analysis began I insisted that she should both sit up and have a trial of medication. On a combination of chlomipramine and clonazepan, administered by a psychopharmacologist, the patient showed a rapid, dramatic change – so rapid that placebo effect could not be ruled out. She said she felt better than she could ever remember feeling in her life, less anxious and less depressed, calmer. Her relationship to me changed dramatically. She felt able to be with me with much less sense of threat, and she began to be able to consider interpretations of her emotional states. Medication, and/or sitting up, damping her dysphoria and restoring voyeuristic control, allowed her to begin to take in new information and to experience herself and her objects differently. It was also the case, as we discovered later, that her dramatic improvement was her vengeful way of informing me of how brutally she had been victimized by being on the couch. However, after a year, the patient decided that she wanted to become pregnant and stopped her medication. She became more depressed and anxious and she was again more intolerant of any independent activity on my part. She also now endlessly blamed me for the terror and humiliation she had suffered when she was on the couch, most of which I had not known of before. I felt we were stalemated. After considerable urging she agreed to a consultation with another analyst. He spoke to her openly about her paranoia, which she knew but could not accept from me, and she felt relieved to hear that a change of therapists was not recommended. We continued, both of us reassured.

The therapeutic task was slow and difficult and I will not attempt a full account of the treatment. Only after she felt that I had fully experienced her as the defective and deprived and abused person she perceived herself to be, and accepted her as that, that I was not trying to tame her and make her into the good girl she felt she had had to be to survive and be victorious in her battle with her parents, was she able to begin to tolerate the idea that she might begin to live in my world as she had made me live in hers. She required prolonged evidence that I could permit her the narcissistic pleasures of soiling, farting, masturbating and being naughty that had never been permitted her as a child, and that I would love her anyway. The enormous hatred and envy that fueled her masochistic, paranoid, malignant object-representations could not be approached until I had indicated that I fully understood her side of the story as victim, with no reservations, i.e. without interpretation. These narcissistic needs could not be bypassed. I think it was also necessary that I suffer enough to gratify some of her need for vengeance against her parents, or at least enough to prove to herself that she was capable of hurting but not killing another person, who would not kill her for having such desires. At the same time there was a sweetness and goodness that emerged when she was not feeling too dysphoric, and a genuine concern that I should know that even at her most paranoid she also knew that I was a potentially benign figure. In time, she gradually began to recapture some of the hidden positive feelings she had kept about her mother, and began to show the modulation of affect that accompanied the increasingly benign internal representations that were developing. She not only became available to interpretation but revealed how much she had absorbed of inter-pretations that she had previously rejected. She began to show a quite dramatic improvement in every area, although with frequent brief dramatic relapses. It also became clear, after several trials, that anti-depressant medication was a necessary part of her treatment.

I have deliberately chosen a difficult case that I handled poorly, one that many would say has little to do with analysis, in order to stress my current convictions concerning the mode of therapeutic action. I want to emphasize two points: (1) we will do better analysis by accepting the need for multiple theoretical per-spectives, and (2) we will do better analysis if we give specific focus to the many non-interpretive activities that are *inherent* in psychoanalysis. Both sequentially and simultaneously, a variety of psychotherapeutic strategies and techniques were brought to bear in the treatment of Mrs C. While every therapeutic action can probably be uncomfortably squeezed within the confines of any single theoretical point of view, I think it is more useful not to attempt to distort our theories and techniques to achieve a false theoretical neatness. Rather, at this time in the development of psychoanalytic theory, treating the range of patients we see under the umbrella of the widening scope of psychoanalysis – or psychotherapy – we will do better if we recognize the need for familiarity with more than one point of view, prepared to use a range of strategies and techniques that stem from a variety of theories. While interpretation is a part of all of our theories of therapeutic action, it is best viewed as a necessary but not sufficient source of therapeutic effect. However, most important for my purpose in this paper is that the case I have described brings into sharp relief some of the many other actions we are engaged in with all our patients, including our analytic cases, with whom our non-interpretive and supportive activities are far more subtle, but always and necessarily there as part of the relationship of analyst and patient. I am, therefore, deemphasizing the interpretive strategies required for this patient. I will mention just a few of these non-interpretive actions, as examples, indicating to which theoretical framework they may be most comfortably ascribed.

(1) *Listening*: We do not often think of listening as a technical element in therapeutic action. It was, of course, Breuer's great technical discovery that if the doctor listened to his patient – an extraordinary idea a hundred years ago – he and the patient could learn what neither of them had previously known. Schwaber has written eloquently on this topic, but I will emphasize that we always listen through a theoretical filter and that what we hear our patients saying is one of the great ongoing disputes in every case discussion. Analytic or psychotherapeutic listening is unlike any other form of listening, but at this time we have no agreed-upon lexicon of listening strategies that can assure a concordance of what is heard. We have many different ways of listening. To listen in a state of freely hovering attention is only one of our skills. Therapists, at different times, listen to our patients the way we listen to music, or to instructions, or to children in various states of hurt or play, or to riddles of resistance, or to a storyteller and so on. Some of us listen better in one mode than in another, but we *should* be able to listen in all of these modes, and more, and we can cultivate our capacities to do that. It would also be nice if we knew better when to listen in which mode or modes. I believe that for this patient, Kohut's views on listening to severely narcissistically disordered patients can help to elucidate some of what I for a long time missed – her need for empathic registration of her efforts at idealization and control of me as a mirroring object only, without interpretation. My usual strategy of early interpretation of hidden rage in severe narcissistic characters was ineffective and probably harmful in this instance, engendering negative therapeutic reactions that were unavailable to interpretation. I might also have heard her demand for explicit closeness as a concrete need requiring some action before its other meanings could be understood.

(2) *Manipulation of the setting*: Her treatment posture – lying or sitting – and frequency were important variables in helping her to be able to tolerate transference regression. Alexander's old and usually denigrated ideas are relevant to this issue, but we lack an adequate theoretical base for conceptualizing the setting as a variable rather than as the constant against which we understand the fluctuations in transference. Just as we have abandoned the idea of the analyst as a screen or mirror or neutral figure, so we might alter our view of the setting as constant or neutral. Rather, the setting is interactive with the patient's changing experience of safety and the nature of the internalized object-relationship that dominates at a particular moment. A facilitating environment, to be that, must be responsive to the patient's changing needs and state of regression. We assume this to be true for children and it is unlikely to be different for analytic patients.

(3) *Empathy*: Since Kohut we are all in agreement that we are attuned and empathic. However, there is more to it than that. While each of the prevailing dynamic points of view can accommodate the kinds of transference reactions that this patient displayed, and the countertransferences that they elicit, a focus

240

on the self concept and the development of the self as we understand it through infant research, not necessarily including Kohut's theory of the bipolar self, can help in appreciating the patient's experience in these very regressed states.

(4) *Control of regression*: While during important phases of the treatment her transference regression was out of control, she would also not have been treatable without an at least near psychotic regression, including positive oceanic feelings of engulfment and radiant love and unity, as well as her feelings of primitive paranoid rage and perverse fantasy. Structural theory, certainly including a theory of shame, ego ideal and superego function, combined with some version of object-relations helps one to navigate through these stormy seas. A contemporary concept of splitting, and perhaps of projective identification, is essential in understanding regression of this type.

(5) *Interpersonal interactions*: We tend to take for granted as aspects of transference–countertransference responses the continuing actual interpersonal relationship of therapist and patient. This patient was exquisitely alert to my moods, responsiveness, state of well-being or fatigue, etc., and it was essential for the treatment that I be able to acknowledge – gratify, if you wish – her need for an actual vivid presence (someone not like her mother). It was also essential that I be willing to discuss her perceptions of my perceptions, and our agreement or discordance. The actions we take, overt and subtle, to maintain hope, convey an underlying loving attitude, transmit respect for the patient, and our sense of a future, etc., are usually taken for granted, but in cases like the one I have described, they move from background to foreground. The humanity and decency of the analyst and the ways that they are conveyed to the patient have been assumed as an unremarkable portion of the setting. They are, in fact, vital and variable activities and we should take greater care to note and specify their characteristics. The interpersonal point of view, long kept in the background of analytic theory, can best help us to conceptualize this essential part of the treatment.

(6) *Consultations*: We have moved far from the period when consultation was considered a violation of the transference that could not be repaired. We still consult too little, and understand too little about the role of consultation in analysis and psychotherapy. In this case the consultant was vital, providing a necessary infusion of reality into an increasingly psychotic transference and enabling the treatment to continue. The dynamics of this were crucial.

(7) *Medication*: Not only are we more aware of our many forms of interventions, but therapists today have a heightened awareness that our patients have a biology and that while every depression or every panic has a meaning, meaning may not be the totality of the event. We may be constitutionally or temperamentally predisposed towards a certain stance towards our feelings and our objects, and our adaptations occur within these limits. Also, certain psychological maladaptations, even those formed out of defensive responses to meaning, can become so fixed that behavioral or cognitive techniques may be

desirable to help the patient to overcome them, or at least to begin to be freer. In selected instances, the need for medication or even a round of behavioral therapy is necessary to facilitate the therapeutic actions of dynamic psychotherapy and psychoanalysis.

I believe this patient required medication both for regulation of affect and for help with a subtle thought disorder that was consonant with the primitive quality of her splitting and her object-relations generally. There is almost no information, neither for this individual patient nor for the group of patients requiring medication with psychotherapy, as to whether they can then continue without medication after psychotherapeutic alteration of their intra-psychic state. A theoretical view that sees personality as an expression of, and interactive with, biological, psychological and social pressures is essential if we are to use medication appropriately and adequately, rather than grudgingly and ineffectively. Psychoanalysts should welcome those pharmacologic discoveries that may provide an additional measure of plasticity to relatively fixed affective and relational patterns.

Clearly there are many more components to therapy and more complex theoretical considerations than I have elaborated. My aim has been to establish, as a matter of principle, the need to conceptualize therapeutic action to include *all* of our activities rather than prematurely labeling one or another as *the* effective element. This offers us the best opportunity to study what it is that we do and to reconceptualize the complex activities of conducting psychoanalysis and psychotherapy. To do this at the present time probably requires the use of several different theoretical points of view. The desire for a grand unified, overarching theory is irresistible in every science but we should not let that wish fog our vision of our current theoretical difficulties. We are so far unable to predict with any success which patients at which times will be analyzable nor can we predict the extent of responsiveness to psychotherapy. I am afraid an analysis or a psychotherapy is still a bit like a work of art – we may know when it has been done well or badly, we can specify many of the evolving elements, but we cannot fully describe the process. It seems to me that this is the current state of affairs. We know that although we know a lot, we don't know much. That gives us a wonderful opportunity to learn more.

FORMULATIONS TO THE PATIENT

Explicit and implicit*

Analysts have, until recently, been far more interested in theory than in technique, perhaps following the example of Freud, whose technical papers are a small portion of his corpus. In recent years, significant efforts have been made to repair this gap, on the one hand by actual recording of analytic sessions, as Horowitz (1991) and Dahl *et al.* (1988) have urged, and on the other by detailed reporting of the events of the session, as Jacobs (1991), Schwaber (1992) and others have done now for a number of years. Since Freud's experience with Dora (1905a) we have known of the danger inherent in our being excessively devoted to our own theoretical formulations, while giving shorter shrift to the patient's communications to us. As long ago as 1923, Ferenczi and Rank, in their monograph *The Development of Psycho-Analysis*, complained that analysts were so caught up in their theory that they neglected basic technique and knowledge of the transference, and thought it sufficient to have demonstrated that the patient had an Oedipus complex and to explain this to the patient, even though this highly intellectualized process had little therapeutic efficacy.

Gill (1994) has reminded us that though residues of the old concepts of the analyst as 'neutral' or 'a blank screen' and an authoritative source of information to the analysand are still with us, our modernist view of interpretation and our current emphasis on intersubjectivity place a premium on identifying and understanding the interactions that occur between analyst and patient, and how they are to be understood in terms of unconscious fantasy and desire. The analytic task is to assist in the development of a setting that fosters the joint creation, discovery and formulation of the psychological matter that we may claim are clinical facts. The setting itself with its privacy, regularity and reliability

* This paper was presented on a panel at the 75th Anniversary Celebration Conference in honor of the *International Journal of Psychoanalysis* in Sao Paulo, Brazil in 1995. It was published as Cooper (1994b); reproduced with permission of *International Journal of Psychoanalysis*.

and the analytic attitude that Schafer (1983) has described are significant clinical facts that we communicate in every session, and that inform all of our more active interventions.

However, we should not exaggerate the democracy of the analytic setting. The analyst, eager to understand his patient, comes armed with a theory or theories that will consistently guide his behavior. He also comes with what might be termed a moral conception of 'good' – namely, the value of unbounded curiosity about one's inner self – with a clear idea of how to manage the relationship of patient and analyst, an odd sort of relationship like no other in the world, and he will, throughout the conduct of the analysis, attempt to maintain these underlying attitudes in all his dealings with his patient. While the relationship clearly is not symmetrical, nonetheless we know that our hypotheses and ideas are not meaningful communications – i.e. clinical facts – until they have been woven into the fabric of the analysis, i.e. are sufficiently a part of the patient's thinking, not only of the analyst's, so that their expression will arouse a meaningful response. A meaningful response is a change, no matter how minute, in the patient's thinking or behavior, in or outside of the analysis.

I will not attempt to review the literature on interpretation. We would all probably agree that we intend that our expressions to the patient, large or small, formal or informal, should be affectively and cognitively available; they should address unconscious fantasies and beliefs and intrapsychic conflicts that are at the moment activated and are generating some intensity of affect; they should open avenues for previously unavailable thoughts and feelings, perhaps opening the path to new integrations; and, most often, they should be framed within the context of the transference. Clearly, few, if any, single utterances of analysts meet this prescription. Rather, what one hopes is that the multiple interactions, verbal and nonverbal, of analyst and patient will over time achieve these aims.

As Shapiro (1970) has pointed out, one essence of interpretation is naming, and our more formal and complete formulations to the patient are often the final naming of knowledge that has been gestating over a long period of time. It gives a sense of act completion to a process that is far more complex, and messier, than merely naming implies. In effect, the baby exists before he has a name, but once named, that word assumes almost magical powers, instantaneously calling up all the attributes of the object, as well as helping to shape new developmental events. Similarly, some of our interpretations serve as shorthand summaries of complex narratives of prior experiences and the beginnings of new chains of experience. However, most of what we formulate to the patient does not lie in our carefully prepared statements, but rather resides in the complex minutiae of our moment-to-moment interactions with the patient, and the multiple affects that are aroused by these interactions in both patient and analyst. In this paper I shall attempt to focus on these difficult-to-describe aspects of analytic formulation. I am aware that a certain amount of blur is built into the topic.

Many of our important communications to the patient are intended as trial balloons to see which way the psychic wind is blowing; an exposure to the patient of our current hypothesis, so that we may begin to understand how the patient perceives notions that either may seem self-evident to us or about which we are quite uncertain, and that the patient's response will help us to evaluate. From the patient's responses we may begin to help the patient and ourselves to develop clinical facts concerning the forms and layers of resistance and unconscious fantasies. Although I am not suggesting that every analysis is a research project, we are following good research methodology when we begin with an hypothesis, and proceed to test it with an experimental procedure – what I am calling a trial balloon. If I say to a patient, 'It seems to me that you are very angry at me and frightened to let me know it,' or 'You're embarrassed to let me know how proud you feel,' or 'You're shy about speaking of things that you feel are defects of yours,' etc., I am floating trial balloons, with the aim of initiating a discourse.

Behind each of these mild, close-to-observational comments, which might be made by any discerning friend, lies a mountain of analytic theory. When I talk of my patient's fear of his anger, I have already formed a theory of his internal fantasy relationships with his parental figures of infancy and childhood that are suffused with hatred and cripple his life. I think my other patient's rather charming embarrassment over his experience of pride is part of a large narcissistic system of aggressive and grandiose fantasy, but that is nothing that can be discussed at this point. When I mention to another patient his shyness about his defects, I am also entertaining the idea – more accurately, the conviction – that this man has a tremendous terror and shame over his profound belief that his body and tiny penis are entirely inadequate. In each instance, I believe that my comments to the patient are based on observations of behaviors and interactions that are on, or close to, the surface of our interactions and have been observed by both of us, and I have little doubt of their correctness.

However, while even these seemingly objective observations require con-firmation of some sort, it is even more important that the patient's response to these observations will inform us and the patient about the state of his relationship to our inquiry. Are we joined in an attempt to understand more, or am I arousing fierce opposition? When the patient to whom I suggested that he is frightened of his anger replies, 'I don't know whether I am so angry and frightened. It's much more that it makes me feel so guilty if I feel any anger towards you. I know that you are doing your best, so what right do I have to be angry at you? It must be my own fault that I am not getting better faster, and so I stop being angry,' he is making an important emendation and elaboration of my communication that will lead me both to see him somewhat differently and to formulate his underlying difficulty more distinctly. The focus on his guilt (this patient once described his mother as being the Queen of Guilt) is a crucial intermediary step that I had bypassed, and I now have a better appreciation of how he processes anger. He has also enjoyed the experience of correcting me rather than passively accepting my formulation, an important experience for this timid man.

On the other hand, I shall describe a different response to my intervention with a patient who feels that for the first time in her life, she is now truly in love with an 'adorable man.' While it does seem to be the case that she has never enjoyed this kind of emotional involvement before, I am struck with how she alternates between describing her great disappointment that his erections are not entirely hard and her uncertainty that she can live with that, or else what an extraordinary lover he is and no one before has ever excited her so much and the size of his erection doesn't matter, or telling me that the problem is over and he now has the hardest erections she has ever experienced and she is completely happy. These descriptions succeed each other within days, each with total conviction. I am impressed by the totality of each emotional state and her seeming inability to bring any of her previous attitudes to bear on the most recent one. I have a lot of previous evidence for her splitting and intolerance of ambivalence or ambiguity. I decide to take this extra-transferential opportunity to try again to show this to her. I say to her, 'Each of your responses is so total and overwhelming. Your disappointment one day seems to overwhelm any optimism of the previous day, and a single good experience abolishes the caution you had felt only a short while earlier. I think that being on this emotional roller-coaster interferes with your getting to know your lover and your self better.' She rebuffs my observation and asks, 'Isn't it normal to be concerned over our sex life?' I hear the irony, but I try to tell her that I am not talking of any abnormality, but am calling attention to her inability to sustain an integrated, reasonably constant picture of her lover. I suggest again that this interferes with her capacity to develop greater depth in the relationship, note how this has characterized our relationship, and remind her how similar her behavior is to what she has experienced all her life with her mother.

Perhaps because of her abrupt brush-off of my 'insight' I am saying more than is desirable. I have a large but rather straightforward formulation in mind. Her relationship with her lover mirrors rather precisely her relationship with her mother – every event carried maximal emotional weight, representing either total disaster or total salvation; she was either the best girl in the world, or intolerably evil and ungrateful. Throughout her life she had been masochistically tied to her mother and enraged with her. By imitating her mother she is maintaining her closeness to her mother and simultaneously demonstrating the cruelty and emptiness of her mother's attitude towards her. She is, I believe, frightened of sensing genuine security either with her lover or with me, since that would threaten her intensely masochistic relationship with her mother, and require a kind of tenderness that she is uncertain she can ever develop. (Early in her treatment she told me that she loved her little dog more than anything in the world, but would episodically throw him against the wall, with a feeling of power, unaware of any rage.) I also think that erections have a special meaning for her, because she harbors strong feelings of deprivation over being a woman.

However, I did not say all these things to her at that moment. To my comment about her emotional swings and maintaining her emotional distance, she replied, 'You're being very crusty. I don't know why you can't be more supportive of me.' One could say she was carrying on with her program of maintaining emotional distance, and I certainly felt that. She then brought up my declining an invitation to a party in her honor, saying: 'You're just like my mother. You think because we have a good enough relationship here, you don't have to do anything else to let me know how you feel about me. She isn't going to that party either. She says she doesn't have to go to a party in order for me to know how she feels about me. Yes, I know you think that I am a bottomless pit, and no amount of reassurance makes any difference to me. I know that's true, but why shouldn't you give me more?'

In this instance, my attempt to explore what seemed to me to be surface traits of my patient – her splitting, her lack of modulation, her emotional distance, her intolerance of a degree of constructive ambivalence – led to a powerful feeling of my lack of appreciation of her, experienced by her as my being just like her mother, with the accusation that I could not tolerate her attempt to be closer to me. I felt that she had enacted my interpretation, but her feeling that she was being attacked limited our ability to explore the idea at this moment. However, I also felt that her connecting me so directly with her mother would yet provide opportunities to help both of us to know what she was experiencing in her intimate relationships. Our trial balloons have served their purpose if in response we learn something of the patient's psychic state.

In floating trial balloons, one need not be discouraged by stormy weather. Some analysts have maintained that no interpretation should be made until the patient is so ready to receive it that it is as if it were 'on the tip of his tongue,' and the interpretation will seem completely familiar when it is finally uttered. Others, of whom I am one, hold that there are many times in the course of an analysis when the presentation of consciously unacceptable interpretations is essential if the patient is ever to come to grips with certain painful clinical facts of his mental life. As Bergler (1952) pointed out, the analytic process mobilizes the superego on the side of the analyst's interpretations, not because of any inherent tendency to be helpful, but because aspects of the analysis provide one more opportunity for inner torture. For example, the patient who pleads his guilt rather than his fear in relation to his anger is not only correcting me; he is engaged in an inner dialogue with his punitive conscience, which says to him, 'Go ahead and admit finally what an angry, hating, murderous, ungrateful and frightened baby you are. You know he has found you out.' The patient, in his effort to plea-bargain with his conscience, replies, 'It may be true that I'm a little bit angry, but I am full of gratitude, surely not guilty of hate, and I accept that I should feel terribly guilty for the little bit of anger that I feel.' For many patients, helping them toward an acceptance of inner feelings and thoughts requires the process of repeated expression to the patient of not yet acceptable ideas – an important aspect of working through – during which initially too-painful unconscious fantasies are detoxified, become more familiar and lose some of their danger through the gradual alteration of internal objects, modification of the superego, and the relative strengthening of the ego that occurs through the relationship to the analyst.

For example, my repeatedly and insistently discussing with a patient the possibility that his parents were rather unusually insensitive and self-involved, quite unable to perceive or respond to his needs and dedicated to making him into an image of themselves, had a powerful mutative effect, not just because it was probably an accurate playback of his projected representations, i.e. it seemed likely to me that this was how the patient himself had perceived his parents during development. Rather, it was effective because it represented an attack on his parents by someone he could not easily dismiss as crazy, which he could never imagine doing himself. My lack of fear of his parents and the fact that a bolt of lightning did not strike me dead were very important new data – analytic facts – for him to consider. They were significant at this point in his treatment not because they were the true facts of his development, although I believed them to be so; rather, they were important because they demonstrated that his frightening introjected parental imago was not as powerful as he imagined, and could be challenged without retribution. This interaction between us, which provided him with an ally against a ferocious inner conscience, was a necessary step before he could confront the more detailed unconscious fantasies. The more complete formulation would have referred to his fear of attacking his parents, convinced that any attack upon them would reflect the full degree of his hatred and totally destroy them, leaving him guilty and helpless, and simultaneously that they would retaliate with such power that he would be destroyed.

Clearly, as is always the case in an interaction of this kind, the analyst's countertransference responses play a role. My 'attack' on his parents, for example, derived from many sources, and another analyst might have responded differently. Perhaps related in part to his sensitivity to my countertransference, I was also aware that not only was he revising his conception of the power of his superego, but he was probably elevating me to a position of greater or equal power, as I became the increasingly harsh and critical authority to whom he was required to give grudging passive–aggressive obedience. One aspect of this quickly became apparent when the patient developed a regular pattern of arriving five or ten minutes late to every session – replacing his earlier more sporadic lateness. When I tried to discuss this, he at first claimed fearful embarrassment and reassured me that he would stop. As I made clear that I was not asking him to stop, but thought we should try to know why he was late, he told me that his parents had always told him that he should keep himself a bit above his friends because he was better than them. He should always be late so that they should wait for him and he should never wait for them, which would be insulting to him. As he felt a bit more comfortable internally, the overt power struggle between us escalated.

One other aspect of our mode of communication to patients may be worth noting. As psychoanalysts, we are amazingly persistent in our insistence on curiosity as an activity of highest value. In one sense every one of our communications to our patients is in the service of deepening the spirit of inquiry, and assuring our patients that it is worthwhile for two people to try to know each other. The knowledge of this clinical fact is created and communicated in every successful analysis. The analyst's doggedness and his values, at least at this level, are always communicated and the patient's ability to participate in the analytic process is partly dependent on his willingness to share some of this world-view.

The non-interpretive influence of the analyst is explicit in Loewald's description of the analytic task. He says that an analyst:

> requires an objectivity and neutrality the essence of which is love and respect for the individual and for individual development. This love and respect represent that counterpart in 'reality,' in interaction with which the organization and reorganization of ego and psychic apparatus take place.
>
> The parent–child relationship can serve as a model here. The parent ideally is in an empathic relationship of understanding the child's particular stage in development, yet ahead in his vision of the child's future and mediating this vision to the child in his dealing with him. This vision, informed by the parent's own experience and knowledge of growth and future, is, ideally, a more articulate and more integrated version of the core of being that the child presents to the parent. This 'more' that the parent sees and knows, he mediates to the child so that the child in identification with it can grow. The child, by internalizing aspects of the parent, also internalizes the parent's image of the child – an image that is mediated to the child in the thousand different ways of being handled, bodily and emotionally . . . The bodily handling of and concern with the child, the manner in which the child is fed, touched, cleaned, the way it is looked at, talked to, called by name, recognized and re-recognized – all these and many other ways of communicating with the child, and communicating to him his identity, sameness, unity, and individuality, shape and mould him so that he can begin to identify himself, to feel and recognize himself as one and as separate from others yet with others . . . In analysis, if it is to be a process leading to structural changes, interactions of a comparable nature have to take place.
>
> (Loewald 1960: 229–230)

This is the language of human interaction, far from metapsychology. It is of a piece with this view that interpretations are referred to as forms of poetry expressing the ineffable. I have previously published a vignette (Cooper 1987c) to illustrate how clinical facts may be represented by the patient and analyst in subtle and complex ways reflecting the nature of their relationship and are only formulated as an interpretation much later.

A large variety of our clinical actions, the entirety of the analytic setting and perhaps the bulk of our communications are devoted to encouraging the patient's capacities for psychological curiosity and self-exploration, often through altered forms of intrapsychic conflict. The safety that is required for the patient to join the analyst in this quest is an obvious first step in probing unconscious fantasy, enabling the patient to construct new internal structures and representations that may include the possibility of self-analysis both during and after the formal analytic process. The analyst's relative tolerance, his devotion to attempting to understand the patient, the atmosphere of stability and safety inculcated through the peculiar imbalance of the analytic setting, can be conceived of as the conveyance of an analytic fact to the patient – the fact that it is possible to relate to an object that will not conform to the objects of his inner world nor to the projection of that inner world on to objects in the outer world. This analytic fact, formulated through our attitude, is often weightier than the content of our formulation at any given moment. This may account for the fact that so many different interpretations from different systems of analytic theory seem to be effective, according to clinical reports. No matter how conceived – and we have multiple theories for framing our conceptions – our actual behavior in the analytic setting presents the patient with facts that are as significant as those that we are also formulating in every transference interpretation. For example, silence can in various ways convey skepticism, acceptance, mutuality, the demand for more from the patient, withholding by the analyst, anger, and so forth.

Alternatively, we may choose to make or find ourselves making our formulations not through a formal utterance but in the course of a conversation with the patient. While hardly a Socratic dialogue with the patient, we are nonetheless engaged in an effort to help the patient to see something that we think we have seen and that we believe he is ready to see. These conversations may be part of an interaction designed to help the patient to see the nature of our relationship or how that relationship is being influenced by each of us towards play, acceptance, irritation, etc. When my patient and I sometimes engage in a spirited exchange, with his opposing an idea of mine, or vice versa, the fact that we keep our relationship intact and sustain a friendly attitude toward each other, and that I remain warmly disposed toward him, is a most important communication to him of the fact, quite surprising to him, of being able to love someone while fighting.

In one fashion or another, we are helping the patient to see how we think he sees us, and how we see ourselves grossly or slightly differently. The affective and cognitive dissonance that we create between the patient's experience

250

with us and his unconscious object representations is a consequence of our confronting the patient with the analytic fact of our analytic presence through the totality of our relationship. When I say to a patient who is bewildered by his children's coldness towards him, 'Did you never wonder about your children's reaction to your divorcing your wife and living in a different town?,' I am conveying to the patient that I think our relationship is now firm enough that I can suggest that he was insensitive, narcissistically preoccupied and rather spectacularly unempathic to his children's needs. When he responds, with tears in his eyes, 'You mean they feel I have abandoned them,' I think that he has understood me, and of much greater significance, he has begun to understand something about relating to his children. My question, framed probably with a slight tone of disbelief and surprise, and perhaps even disapproval, has provided him with a very precise formulation. We are all aware these days of how much information we convey to the patient through our subtle behaviors, intended or not, that contribute significantly to opening or closing pathways to communication. Interpretations that are mutative may be quite inexact, but effective because they are part of the analytic attitude. To try to demonstrate further the points I am making, I will present a brief account of the attempt to begin an analytic process. I shall give an overview of the first year of an analysis, and describe several sessions occurring early in the second year.

A highly intelligent, socially and professionally successful woman had become deeply depressed in her late forties and had begun psychotherapy. The depression was clearly related to her growing conviction of the emptiness of her 20-year marriage, the feeling that her career was at a dead end, and she was aware of her growing isolation − she had few friends, and a growing list of enemies. Her psychotherapy had not been as effective as she had hoped, and after two years she and her therapist thought analysis was indicated and she was referred to me. The patient's first aim in analysis, of course, was to diminish the continuing painful depression by any means possible. A mixture of fluoxetine and the stabilizing relationship with the analyst succeeded in somewhat diminishing the depression within several months, but she remained significantly depressed during the first year of her four-times-weekly analysis. It quickly became apparent that an important second aim of hers was to provide herself with an adequate rebuttal to her inner accusations that she had badly damaged herself, had realized little of her intellectual promise, had few pleasures and had irreparably spoiled her life. Her response to these inner accusations took two forms: (a) none of it was her fault; her husband misled her, friends mistreated her; there was nothing wrong with her that would not be cured by a bit of kind and decent treatment, and her analyst was now responsible for providing that; (b) the damage to herself was, in fact, not significant and could immediately be repaired. To prove this she was engaging in frantic counterproductive efforts at pseudo-repair. She was determined to get an immediate divorce, or to establish a new career, or to sell her possessions and totally change her way of life, but her actions were all ineffective, without planning or reflection. Despite having entered analysis, she was ferociously determined to maintain her lifelong avoidance of self-examination, which would inevitably lead her towards recognition of intolerable inner feelings and the realization of the extent of her own self-defeating behaviors. She felt she could not bear the shame of such revelations.

Early on it became obvious that this analysis would not be typical, because I felt that I had to play an active role to discourage her desire for immediate action, and to help her to see that her frantic efforts at immediate repair were compounding her feelings of helplessness and defeat and were aimed at providing a cover-up of her behavior before we had a chance to examine it. The prospect of being still and allowing time for reflection to begin to understand herself filled her with dread and loathing, reflecting the inner, denigrated picture of herself that she desperately tried to avoid acknowledging by her outer narcissistic display. I found myself, rather atypically, making speeches about the importance of our having the chance to find out what her life was all about, and how a divorce or house-moving was going to make that impossible. Although she understood this, she also interpreted this as proof that I was a social conservative, like her mother, trying to prevent her from having an adventurous life and finding her true self. To further confuse matters, her previous therapist had, according to her, urged her to stop being so timid and to take some bold actions to prove her independence.

As I got to know her I learned that all her life she had believed that she was different from her peers and her family, brighter and more intellectual, or more moral, or more adventurous and ambitious, and that socially and interpersonally she established herself as a 'special' person, witty or naughty or glamorous or specially accomplished, and she now bent her efforts to recruiting me as a new part of that superior world that would respond to her specialness. By and large I declined to enter this game, indicating that the great social and intellectual world that so entranced her was largely unknown to me and not of great interest. She mostly didn't believe me, but since her job as she saw it was to please me so that I would please her, she would do it my way if that is what it took, and reluctantly delayed, or at least pursued with less vigor, the huge actions she had been contemplating, giving us a chance to talk without a crisis hanging over us.

A part of this initial calm also represented her making her analysis the new special aspect of her life. I often got the feeling that she was creating an atmosphere of our being a 'special couple,' carrying on a secret, conspiratorial life, superior to others, and that the two of us could ignore the 'outside world.' It showed in knowing and ironic smiles that she would often give me at the beginning and end of sessions or turning around to smile at me during a session, or making elliptical statements whose meaning eluded me, and when I asked for clarification, she usually didn't bother to answer, as if she knew I really had

252

understood her. I was at times made uncomfortable by this behavior, feeling invaded and controlled and uneasy, and aware that I was in danger of distancing myself, as she undoubtedly wanted me to. I understood this as reflecting her own sense of never having had any privacy and her resenting my intrusion into her. Often, when I told her that I did not understand her and was not party to her musings, I was aware of being more than usually worried about being rude to her, a signal of the uneasiness of our relationship. I felt caught in a narcissistic battle to test which of us would dominate, but wasn't sure how to avoid it. Bit by bit, it was becoming clear to her that however 'special' she was, I thought we had an important job to do, and I was interested in how we could get on with our work and understand our relationship, and little else. She felt this as both a rebuff and a relief. Of course, the fact that I have chosen her as a patient to write about surely marks her as 'special.' While there were many subtle denigrations of me, as I have described, there were also unrealistic idealizations of me as a person of total understanding and wisdom, which made me uncomfortable, at least in part, because they seemed to me ironic – she was too sophisticated and subtly masochistically cynical (although she did not know it) to think of me or anyone else in such glowing terms except for the purpose of being disappointed later. The idealizations were also projections on to me of her own narcissistic strivings, without which she could not have begun to trust me; she tried to see me as an improved version of herself. Kohut has urged that these idealizations be permitted to develop without interference early in the analysis of narcissistic patients. My own technique is to bring them to the patient's attention without attempting to demolish them. I felt I was steering a cautious path between allowing her to engulf me sufficiently so that she felt able to continue to work with me, and maintaining enough differentiation so that work could be done. The alternate side of those idealizations would reveal itself periodically in the peremptory way in which the patient would sometimes say, 'I don't want to hear what you're saying now. You have to listen to me.' Or, 'What I'm going to tell you now is really important and you have to understand it.' Or at the end of the session, 'We can't stop at this minute, you have to let me tell you something else,' etc.

Very early in the treatment, I was struck by the patient's constant reference to some version of authority as justification for any thought or action of hers, whether major or minor. For example, in discussing her feelings about furnishing her house, she spoke entirely in terms of how her neighbors expected her to behave and what her friends would think if she furnished it one way or another, implying that she would not be permitted to gratify her own highly developed tastes. She was also writing fiction, but was paralyzed by her constant concern over what one or another of the great contemporary writers, who served as her models, would have done with the scene or the character that interested her. Her own imagination withered as she tried to envision what her models would do. Similarly, in relation to me, she would frequently turn around on the couch to see my response to whatever it was she had just said, usually with a smile of expectant hopefulness, followed by disappointment if I had no comment. She would, however, then apply her own logic to my behavior and say, 'Of course, you are unable to comment because your Freudian rules don't allow it.' It was clearly a source of great narcissistic satisfaction to her that the authorities commanding her, and me, were all figures of great stature. It was also apparent, and I often so commented, that she deprived both of us of any freedom of action. We were both prisoners of more powerful parents, not letting us do what we wanted. Ultimately, I was as denigrated and helpless a figure as she.

Her speech was often hesitant, with many unfinished thoughts. A portion of this derived from her fantasy that I magically knew all her unfinished and unspoken thoughts, and another portion derived from her inner denigration of all her ideas, as if whenever she began a thought she felt she must have a better idea than that. But I was also convinced that she was doing her best to censor her communications to me, uncertain of what I would approve. She was unwilling to begin a train of thought that might be in mid-passage at the end of the session, when my cutting her off might leave her bereft and humiliated. She felt that she had to control me so that I would know what to do to help her. Not infrequently, when I told her that I thought she was feeling afraid, not sure that she could allow herself to show herself to me, she would cry or say she felt like crying, but could not explain why. I assumed that her tears were in part a bitter reflection of her conviction that she had never before experienced kindness, a way of informing me of her deprived life. While her early life had been quite barren emotionally, I also was convinced that this was part of her defensive position of claiming that she was prepared to be cured by kindness alone, without the painful self-examination of the extent of her masochistic pursuit of unloving figures – male and female – with whom she had surrounded herself.

At the same time her depression remained a significant factor. Afraid to bore or discourage me, she often did not tell me about the extent of her depression, which would then be revealed in a burst of sobs or a wrenching description of how wretched she had been between sessions. During this time, I was often uneasy, aware of the actuality of her depression, the depth of her sense of injury, and the power of her feeling that I was the last resort and that she couldn't allow herself to be aware of fighting with me; but I also felt impatient and controlled. Perhaps sharing her view that she was special, I felt there was a rich psychological lode that we could mine, and that was blocked off from us. I wanted to say to her, 'For God's sake, stop being or pretending to be such an obedient little girl and tell me what you really think, not what you think you're supposed to think,' quite aware that my impatience reflected her bitter, hating response of ironic obedience to a parent unconcerned for her desires; and I did say a variety of watered-down versions of that to her. Or alternatively, 'Where are you in the story of your life? All I hear about is what you're supposed to be doing or what people are demanding that you do, most of which you don't like. What are your own desires?'

In effect, I was buffeted between her provocation and her genuinely sad plight. In suggesting she might stop being obedient and give credence to her own needs, I was of course enacting the role of yet one more person making demands of her, a vicious circle. The depth of her despair and the continuing threat of her acting out in some dramatic fashion were powerful spurs to my interventions. I was caught up, as she was, in a set of contradictory demands and desires, leaving me uncertain and unsatisfied with whatever I did. I did not say this to her at that time, feeling that it would be too discouraging if in any way I indicated that she was damaging or destroying me, but I am sure she had some awareness of these feelings in both of us.

My own dynamic formulation of the state of affairs included several elements, of which I list a few.

(1) The patient's oversized narcissistic defensive grandiosity did not permit her to imagine herself doing anything 'ordinary.' She could only act as a great person, while deeply ashamed of her feelings of inadequacy. Lacking her own inner construct as a great person, she tried to borrow the strength of others who were known to be great persons. At the moment she hoped that I would fill that role.

(2) The child of a cold, demanding, socially ambitious mother, and a frivolous, self-preoccupied, charming father, she had worked out a complex unconscious, extremely masochistic scheme designed to reproach her parents for their lack of concern for her. Unconsciously, in her slavish devotion to official style, she was making a public display of her parents' total lack of interest in any of her individual qualities, saying, in effect, 'This is how you treated me as a piece of social matter. I'm doing what you wanted me to, and you are responsible for my misery, and you are unconcerned.' Within the analysis this appeared in her 'girlish charm' as she turned around on the couch after almost every communication to me with a look of 'Is that right? Am I on the right track? Am I doing what you want?' She looked pleading and vulnerable, clearly shifting responsibility for her welfare on to me.

(3) She was also demonstrating that this attitude of others was extremely damaging to her, depriving her of the ability to choose anything for the sake of her own happiness, forced to sacrifice her own desires and needs for the scraps of love obtainable through official, social approval. A large portion of our relationship revolved around her feelings that she now had to do my bidding because she had failed on her own, and I would not lead her towards pleasure and independence, but towards my own version of conformity.

(4) This woman from a religious background was enormously guilty over the amount of anger and bitterness she harbored, and which leaked out in provocations toward those around her. She attempted to dispel her guilt by dividing the world into those she could hate, and those who received her total

love and admiration. This splitting broke down in any relationship of depth or intensity, leaving her anxious and directionless, but more determined than ever to find something to which she could give total devotion and thus prove to her inner attackers that she was a 'good' person. Each of these objects of devotion in time disappointed her.

Under these circumstances, it was clear to me that any utterance of mine that sounded like an 'interpretation' would immediately be categorized by her as the word of authority, a religious edict, consciously respected and admired, unconsciously ironically mocked. Similarly, a silence on my part was construed by her either as evidence of my deep wisdom, my complex thought processes for the preparation of the grand oracular statement that would solve all her problems, or as a humiliating rebuff of her attempt to join her ideas to mine. Partly through conscious choice, and partly through her successful communication of her vulnerability, I therefore found myself carefully avoiding either of these courses, and my interventions took the form much more of questions about her missing inner life, indicating that I was puzzled by her apparent obeisance to authority, and I wondered what she hoped to gain, or was it all bitter irony. I was also letting her know that I thought we were in for a long haul, that I did not expect any rapid change, and that her lively interest in my thoughts, opinions and attitudes served both to hide her own and to confirm her conviction that no one, not even I, was really interested in her. But, of course, she construed this as evidence of my saintliness and superb use of analytic skill and tactics, avoiding a direct response to me. Gradually, however, she gave up her intention to engage in some grand action, and focused more on how she was the innocent victim of the insensitivity, competitiveness, lack of appreciation, and malice of those around her, and how she was not the organizer of her life.

Through the first year of analysis she reported no dreams. When I asked about her dreams, she would tell me she didn't remember having dreamt, or she might say that she had had a dream and had written it down, but had lost the notes, or vaguely indicate that she had had a dream, but it didn't seem as important to her as other things she wanted to talk about. I explained to her that she was doing her best to convince me that there was no point in looking at her inner life for the answer to her difficulties, since she was merely the innocent victim of external forces. Finally, I said to her, certainly not for the first time, but perhaps more forcefully, 'This hostile environment that you blame for your plight is your alibi. I think that you hope that your analysis will also be part of your alibi. You can claim you have left no stone unturned. How about looking at why you have selected the people and the life you claim not be able to stand. How about looking at how your own provocations make so much of the difficulty.' The patient was simultaneously angrily indignant and reassured: 'You think I'm making alibis. You think I'm not really trying to explore myself. It is terrifying to imagine shaking up my whole life now. In fact, I don't know how I would do it. I have no support. I have so isolated myself that I can't change my life. Maybe I should recognize that I'm my problem.'

During the following weeks she would conclude every remark to me with a rueful smile, and say 'Is that an alibi, too?' or, 'Was that a provocation?' when she knew it was not an example of her provocation. I told her I thought I had hurt her feelings and she was teasing me. I also felt that we were much closer to each other – we were talking more directly, and she could let me know how she felt. Her communicative pattern of trying to tell me half a dozen things at the same time, unfinished thoughts, pauses that were clearly part of decisions not to say things, became less marked. We parted for the summer break with both of us feeling encouraged. At the end of the second week after the summer break, which had passed quietly, beginning the second year of treatment, she began a session by telling me that she had had some dreams earlier in the week and also a dream last night. She then went on to mention that women suffered from shame, an affect that was unknown to men, and in a manner very different from her usual speech pattern proceeded to give me a very clear chronological account of her relations with men during the years before her marriage. The theme that emerged was her unfailing selection of manipulative, self-centered men, who were careless of her needs. She said how ashamed she was about this. She mentioned that she had, during the past week, developed a sense of direction in her writing, and felt that she was no longer so jumbled with thoughts tumbling on top of each other, without a capacity to select among them, and she felt more confident that her narrative would develop. As the session was nearing an end, I said that she hadn't yet told me her dream. She had dreamt that she was with me at a swimming pool. She decided to jump in and swim and it was very pleasant and refreshing. When she came out I was sitting at the end of the pool looking very benign, but she noticed that I was sitting on a platform that was made of live boa constrictors. The snakes weren't threatening me, but she found it very scary. She then said that this was the second part of the dream; the earlier part concerned being with her daughter and their going riding together.

The session was now over, and I was not going to see her for four days. I told her that I thought she had enacted the dream in the session. She had, in this session, jumped in and begun to talk about herself with a new interest in trying to let me know her. She was terribly worried that I was looking on as a man like all the men she had known – immune to shame, involved with my penis, threatening an attack and not really interested in her. But she had taken the plunge. It was all we had time for, and she left looking thoughtful. I noted to myself that the session was 'backwards,' as was the dream. She gave me her associations before telling the dream, and told the second part of the dream before the first.

When I next saw her, four days later, I was dressed in a dark suit and she looked at me and said 'you're going to a funeral, aren't you? In my world a white shirt and dark suit meant a funeral.' I asked her to tell me more and she said 'maybe it's a dinner, but I think it is a funeral.' I said it was troubling to her not to know more about me and I wondered if she was worried about me. She didn't respond to this, but then told me that she was euphoric after the last session, experiencing a sense of relief that she could rarely recall ever having had before. It had lasted over the weekend. I was puzzled over what had been so relieving, assuming it had to do with her beginning to tell me a coherent life story, and finding it less shameful than she had imagined. She didn't know why she had been so relieved, told me that she had dreamt over the weekend, but didn't tell me the dreams, and proceeded in a very calm and quiet way to elaborate and enlarge her description of her life during her twenties – describing in more detail the series of unsuitable men with whom she had had romances that came to naught, but left her feeling empty. In her late twenties, in despair of restoring order to her life, she had turned to religion, and married a co-religionist. The session was calm and quiet, but at the end of the session she gave me one of her ironic smiles, indicating, I thought, that she was feeling cheated. She had not got enough out of the session, and expected something more from me.

I began the next session by asking her about her feelings at the end of the previous session. She replied that she had been absolutely miserable over the previous 24 hours, although her writing was going well. She despaired that there was any repair for her loneliness, and she had been reading *The Scarlet Letter* and found it terrifying. Puzzled, I asked what was terrifying. She began to sob soundlessly. I felt I had been clumsy in some way and suggested that to her. After a long silence, she began to tell me Bible stories, how moved she was by the psalms, how the Bible taught forgiveness, sobbing the entire time. I told her that I did not understand why she was sobbing, and how it related to *The Scarlet Letter*. She told me that she felt for Hester Prynne, so persecuted and misunderstood by the Puritans, and how she felt there was so little forgiveness in the world, which distressed her deeply.

In a burst of relief and disbelief, I said, 'Are you telling me at this point in your life that you are surprised that the world is not filled with kindness? Having had your mother and father you are telling me you are amazed to discover that people aren't filled with love. And what an odd reading of Hawthorne! Hester is obviously a triumphant figure, who ends up beloved and respected within her community, sees her daughter happily married to a nobleman, and achieves contentment. Aren't you attributing to Hester all the bitterness that you feel towards those around you, and aren't you doing your damnedest to blame everyone but yourself for the fix you're in?'

She stopped crying, laughed, and told me that she was being pursued by former colleagues to write for various publications, but she knew they didn't want to have what she would write for them. She then described an offer to do an article, which she had declined because she wanted to say provocative things.

I pointed out that she wished she were perfectly capable of writing that article and saying exactly what she wanted without being excessively provocative, but she preferred to see herself – and Hester Prynne – as totally rejected and abandoned. She said she couldn't stand the way she was living, and needed a remedy. I said once again that I understood that she was miserable, but unfortunately there was no immediate repair available to her, and I believed she now knew this.

Our time was up. Getting up off the couch, she said with animation, 'I'm arranging my whole life around coming here. It's a very large task.' She was telling me as openly as possible that she had committed herself to her analysis, but also letting me know that I too was turning out to be a let-down, and she was not sure she could stand the idea that she had to take responsibility for her own life. Refusing to join her in her version of her life, I too was turning into one more philistine who lacked the capacity to understand her. But I also felt that this was a rearguard action, and she had already begun the self-scrutiny she had spent her life desperately avoiding. We now had the possibility of her being able to examine her viewing me both as the perfect understanding person of her fantasy and as the philistine who represented the entire universe of people who did not sympathize with her. I felt our bond was strong enough that she could not discard me and would have to deal with her profound splitting.

The following day she said, 'I was in awe of how you treated me yesterday. With humor and sympathy you were able to disagree with me and show me that an attitude of mine was destructive. If anyone else had done that I would have felt as if the skin had been flayed off of me.' Although all her splitting tendencies are still visible in this remark, there has been a beginning of integration and a significant shift in the analytic climate.

I shall end this account at this point. A year of analysis had produced a change in the character of the analytic process, with a deepening of trust and curiosity that enabled the patient to begin to tell me – and herself – about herself. I believe that very little of what I communicated to the patient would come under the heading of an interpretation, i.e. restatement of the meanings of current behaviors in terms of past conflicts and early repressed wishes and fears. Rather, the major portion of our work together consisted of myriad attempts to arouse her curiosity, to indicate that actions had meanings, to try to understand with her her conviction of lack of agency, to indicate the ways in which one might go about thinking of one's self as an agent, etc., so much of what transpired occurred within the context of our actual behaviors with each other. Interpretations were largely ineffective and inappropriate with this woman who was by some definitions in the pre-stages of analysis, but by contemporary standards was at the beginnings of a difficult analysis. Our attitudes to the patient, our questions, and our steadfastness are for many patients, for a significant portion of their analyses, far more important than interpretation.

ARNOLD M. COOPER
BIBLIOGRAPHY

Auchincloss, E. and Cooper, A. (1994) 'A conversation with Arnold M. Cooper', *The American Psychoanalyst*, 28: 17–22.

Busch, F., Cooper, A.M., Klerman, G.L., Penzer, R.J., Shapiro, T. and Shear, M.K. (1991) 'Neurophysiological, cognitive–behavioral, and psychoanalytic approaches to panic disorder: toward an integration', *Psychoanalytic Inquiry*, 11: 315–322.

Busch, F., Milrod, B., Cooper, A. and Shapiro, T. (1995) 'Psychodynamic approaches to panic disorder', *Journal of Psychotherapy Practice and Research*, 5: 73–83.

Busch, F.N., Shear, M.K., Cooper, A.M., Shapiro, T. and Leon, A.C. (1995) 'An empirical study of defense mechanisms in panic disorders', *The Journal of Nervous and Mental Disease*, 18: 299–303.

Cooper, A.M. (1969) Review of *The Two Faces of Medicine* by C. Binger, *Psychoanalytic Quarterly*, 38: 143–144.

—— (1972) 'Value systems and ego integration', *Psychiatric Quarterly*, 46: 556–562.

—— (1973) 'Value systems and ego integration', in *Progress in Psychiatric Research and Education*. New York: Psychiatric Quarterly Press.

—— (1977) Review of *Caring* by W. Gaylin, *American Journal of Psychiatry*, 134: 1056–1057.

—— (1980a) Review of *The Interface Between the Psychodynamic and Behavioral Therapies*, eds J. Marmor and S.M. Woods, *American Journal of Psychiatry*, 137: 1634–1635.

—— (1980b) Review of *Homosexuality in Perspective* by W.H. Masters and V.E. Johnson, in *Women, Sex and Sexuality*, eds C.R. Stimpson and E.S. Person. Chicago, IL: University of Chicago Press.

—— (1981a) 'Narcissism', in *American Handbook of Psychiatry*, Vol. VII, eds A. Silvano, H. Keith and H. Brodie. New York: Basic Books.

—— (1981b) 'Masochism and long distance running', in *Psychology of Running*, eds M.H. Sacks and M.L. Sachs. Champaign, IL: Human Kinetics Publishers.

—— (1981c) 'Research in applied analysis', *Bulletin of the Association for Psychoanalytic Medicine*, 20: 37–48.

—— (1982a) 'Narcissistic disorders within psychoanalytic theory', in *The American Psychiatric Association Annual Review*, Vol. 1, ed. L. Grinspoon. Washington, DC: American Psychiatric Press, pp. 487–498.

261

—— (1982b) 'Notes on the ethics and dynamics of fund raising among former patients', *Bulletin of the Association for Psychoanalytic Medicine*, 21: 60–64.

—— (1982c) 'Some persistent issues in psychoanalytic literary criticism', *Psychoanalysis and Contemporary Thought*, 5: 45–53.

—— (1982d) 'Discussion: problems of technique in character analysis', *Bulletin of the Association for Psychoanalytic Medicine*, 21: 110–118.

—— (1983a) 'The place of self psychology in the history of depth psychology', in *The Future of Psychoanalysis*, ed. A. Goldberg. New York: International Universities Press, pp. 3–17.

—— (1983b) 'Psychoanalytic inquiry and new knowledge', in *Reflections on Self Psychology*, eds J.D. Lichtenberg and S. Kaplan. Hillsdale, NJ: The Analytic Press, pp. 19–34.

—— (1983c) 'Some suggestions for the education of psychoanalysts', presented at a joint meeting of the Department of Psychiatry, University of Colorado School of Medicine, Colorado Psychiatric Society, and Denver Psychoanalytic Institute to celebrate the 30th anniversary of Herbert S. Gaskill's arrival in Colorado.

—— (1984a) 'Narcissism in normal development', in *Character Pathology, Theory and Treatment*, ed. M. Zales. New York: Brunner/Mazel, pp. 39–56.

—— (1984b) 'The unusually painful analysis: a group of narcissistic–masochistic characters', in *Psychoanalysis: The Vital Issues*, Vol. II, eds J.E. Gedo and G.H. Pollack. Madison, CT: International Universities Press, pp. 45–67.

—— (1984c) 'Psychoanalysis at one hundred: beginnings of maturity', *Journal of the American Psychoanalytic Association*, 32: 245–267.

—— (1984d) Review of *Dire Mastery – Discipleship from Freud to Lacan* by Francois Roustang, *American Journal of Psychiatry*, 141: 599–600.

—— (1985a) 'A historical review of psychoanalytic paradigms', in *Models of the Mind: Their Relationships to Clinical Work*, Monograph 1, ed. Arnold Rothstein. New York: International Universities Press, pp. 5–20.

—— (1985b) 'Will neurobiology influence psychoanalysis?', *American Journal of Psychiatry*, 142: 1395–1402.

—— (1985c) 'Difficulties in beginning the candidate's first analytic case', *Contemporary Psychoanalysis*, 2: 143–150.

—— (1985d) Review of *The Annual of Psychoanalysis*, Vol. 10, ed. Chicago Institute for Psychoanalysis, *American Journal of Psychiatry*, 142: 978–979.

—— (1985e) Review of *The Search for the Self: Selected Writings of Heinz Kohut, 1950–1978*, ed. Paul Ornstein, *American Journal of Psychiatry*, 142: 976–977.

—— (1986a) 'Some limitations on therapeutic effectiveness: the "burnout syndrome" in psychoanalysts', *Psychoanalytic Quarterly*, 55: 576–598.

—— (ed.) (1986b) *The Termination of the Training Analysis: Process, Expectations, Achievements*, IPA Monograph No. 5. New York: International Universities Press.

—— (1986c) 'What men fear: the façade of castration anxiety', in *The Psychology of Men*, eds G. Fogel, F.M. Lane and R. Liebert. New York: Basic Books, pp. 113–130.

—— (1986d) 'Preface', 'Introduction' and 'Summary', in *The Termination of the Training Analysis: Process, Expectations, Achievements*, International Psychoanalytic Association Monograph Series No. 5. New York: International Universities Press.

—— (1986e) 'The concept of psychic trauma: an attempt at clarification', in *The*

Reconstruction of Trauma: Its Significance to Clinical Work, No. 2, Workshop Series, American Psychoanalytic Association. New York: International Universities Press.

—— (1986f) 'Toward a limited definition of psychic trauma', in *A Reconstruction of Trauma: Its Significance in Clinical Work*, American Psychoanalytic Association Monograph No. 2, ed. A. Rothstein. New York: International Universities Press, pp. 41–56.

—— (1986g) 'Narcissism', in *Essential Papers on Narcissism*, ed. A. P. Morrison. New York: New York University Press, pp. 113–143.

—— (1986h) Review of *The Medical Value of Psychoanalysis* (1931) by Franz Alexander, *American Journal of Psychiatry*, 143: 929–930.

—— (1986i) 'Psychoanalysis today: New wine in old bottles or the hidden revolution in psychoanalysis', presented as the Distinguished Psychiatrist Lecture at the Annual Meeting of the APA, Washington, DC.

—— (1987a) 'Histrionic, narcissistic, and compulsive personality disorders', in *Diagnosis and Classification in Psychiatry: A Critical Appraisal of DSM–III*, ed. G.L. Tischler. Cambridge and New York: Cambridge University Press, pp. 290–299.

—— (1987b) 'The role of the residency review committee: general principles for residency programs', in *Training Psychiatrists for the '90s*, eds C.C. Nadelson and C.B. Robinowitz. Washington, DC: American Psychiatric Press.

—— (1987c) 'Changes in psychoanalytic ideas: transference interpretation', *Journal of the American Psychoanalytic Association*, 35: 77–98.

—— (1987d) 'The changing culture of psychoanalysis', *Journal of the American Academy of Psychoanalysis*, 15: 283–291.

—— (1987e) 'The transference neurosis: a concept ready for retirement', *Psychoanalytic Inquiry*, 7: 569–585.

—— (1987f) Discussion of 'The interpersonal and the intrapsychic: conflict or harmony?', *Contemporary Psychoanalysis*, 23: 382–391.

—— (1987g) Review of *Making Contact: Uses of Language in Psychotherapy* (1986) by Leston Havens, *American Journal of Psychiatry*, 144: 1088.

—— (1987h) Review of *Freud and His Father* by M. Krull, *American Journal of Psychiatry*, 144: 1614–1615.

—— (1987i) 'Comments on Freud's "Analysis terminable and interminable"', in *On Freud's 'Analysis Terminable and Interminable'*, ed. J. Sandler. London: IPA Educational Monographs.

—— (1988a) 'The narcissistic–masochistic character', in *Masochism: Current Psychoanalytic Perspectives*, eds R.A. Glick and D.I. Meyers. Hillsdale, NJ: Analytic Press, pp. 117–138.

—— (1988b) 'House call perils, serious and silly', in *Psychiatric House Calls*, eds J. Talbott and A. Manevitz. Washington, DC: American Psychiatric Press, pp. 7–8.

—— (1988c) 'The intrapsychic and the interpersonal dimensions: an unresolved dilemma', *Psychoanalytic Inquiry*, 8: 593–597.

—— (1988d) 'Commentary: what is psychoanalysis?', *Psychoanalytic Inquiry*, 8: 593–597.

—— (1988e) 'Our changing views of the therapeutic action of psychoanalysis: comparing Strachey and Loewald', *Psychoanalytic Quarterly*, 57: 15–27.

—— (1989a) 'Narcissism and masochism: the narcissistic–masochistic character', *Psychiatric Clinics of North America*, 12: 541–552.

—— (1989b) 'Concepts of therapeutic effectiveness in psychoanalysis: a historical review', *Psychoanalytic Inquiry* 9: 4–25.

—— (1989c) 'The teacher: an endangered species?', *Academic Psychiatry*, 13: 13–23.

—— (1989d) 'The narcissistic–masochistic character', in *Essential Papers on Character Neurosis and Treatment*, ed. R.F. Lax. New York: New York University Press, pp. 288–309.

—— (1989e) 'Some limitations on therapeutic effectiveness: the "burnout syndrome" in psychoanalysts', in *Essential Papers on Character Neurosis and Treatment*, ed. R.F. Lax. New York: New York University Press, pp. 435–449.

—— (1989f) 'Infant research and adult psychoanalysis', in *The Significance of Infant Observational Research for Clinical Work with Children, Adolescents, and Adults*, eds S. Dowling and A. Rothstein. Madison, CT: International Universities Press, pp. 79–89.

—— (1989g) 'Will neurobiology influence psychoanalysis?', in *Psychoanalysis: Toward the Second Century*, eds A.M. Cooper, O.F. Kernberg and E.S. Person. New Haven, CT: Yale University Press, pp. 202–218.

—— (1989h) Review of *Projection, Identification, Projective Identification*, ed. J. Sandler, *American Journal of Psychiatry*, 146: 540–541.

—— (1989i) Review of *The Role of Psychoanalysis in Psychiatric Education: Past, Present, and Future*, eds H. Weissman and R.J. Thurnblad, *International Review of Psycho-Analysis*, 16: 391–393.

—— (1990a) 'The future of psychoanalysis: challenges and opportunities', *Psychoanalytic Quarterly*, 59: 177–196.

—— (1990b) 'Changes in psychoanalytic ideas: transference interpretation', in *Essential Papers on Transference*, ed. A.H. Esman. New York: New York University Press, pp. 511–528.

—— (1991a) 'Psychoanalysis: the past decade', *Psychoanalytic Inquiry*, 11: 107–122.

—— (1991b) 'The unconscious core of perversion', in *Perversions and Near-Perversions in Clinical Practice: New Psychoanalytic Perspectives*, eds G.I. Fogel and W.A. Myers. New Haven, CT: Yale University Press, pp. 17–35.

—— (1991c) 'Our changing views of the therapeutic action of psychoanalysis', in *The Work of Hans Loewald: An Introduction and Commentary*, ed. G.I. Fogel. Northvale, NJ: Jason Aronson, pp. 61–76.

—— (1991d) 'On metapsychology and termination', in *On Freud's 'Analysis Terminable and Interminable'*, ed. J. Sandler. New Haven, CT: Yale University Press, pp. 106–123.

—— (1991e) Review of *Freud: A Life for Our Time* by P. Gay, *American Journal of Psychiatry*, 148: 258–259.

—— (1991f) Review of *Tragic Drama and the Family: Psycho-Analytic Studies from Aeschylus to Beckett*, by Bennett Simon, *Psychoanalytic Quarterly*, 60: 499–504.

—— (1992a) 'Psychic change: development in the theory of psychoanalytic techniques: 37th IPA Congress Overview', *International Journal of Psychoanalysis*, 73: 245–250.

—— (1992b) 'Psychiatric education in the United States', *Psychiatria Hungarica* (Journal of the Hungarian Psychiatric Association), 7: 547–557.

—— (1992c) Review of *Producers and Consumers of Psychotherapy Research Ideas* by W.B. Stiles, *Journal of Psychotherapy Practice & Research*, 1: 309–310.

—— (1993a) 'Psychotherapeutic approaches to masochism', *Journal of Psychotherapy Practice & Research*, 2: 51–63.

—— (1993b) 'Paranoia: a part of most analyses', *Journal of the American Psychoanalytic Association*, 41: 423–442.

—— (1993c) 'Psychotherapeutic approaches to masochism', in *Clinical Challenges in Psychiatry*, eds W.H. Sledge and A. Tasman. Washington, DC: American Psychiatric Press, pp. 157–179.

—— (1993d) 'Discussion on empirical research', *Journal of the American Psychoanalytic Association*, 41S: 381–392.

—— (1994a) 'Paranoia: a part of every analysis', in *Paranoia: New Psychoanalytic Perspectives*, eds J.M. Oldham and S. Bone. Madison, CT: International Universities Press, pp. 133–150.

—— (1994b) 'Formulations to the patient: explicit and implicit', *International Journal of Psychoanalysis, Special 75th Anniversary Edition*, 75: 1107–1120.

—— (1994c) 'Theodore Shapiro, M.D.: an appreciation', *Journal of the American Psychoanalytic Association*, 42: 11–14.

—— (1994d) Review of *Forty-Two Lives in Therapy: A Study of Psychoanalysis and Psychotherapy*, by R.S. Wallerstein, *Journal of the American Psychoanalytic Association*, 42: 264–267.

—— (1995) 'Discussion: on empirical research', in *Research in Psychoanalysis: Process, Development, Outcome*, eds T. Shapiro and R.N. Emde. Madison, CT: International Universities Press, pp. 381–391.

—— (1998a) 'Psychoanalytic education: past, present and future', *Samiksa*, 52: 27–37.

—— (1998b) 'Further developments in the clinical diagnosis of narcissistic personality disorder', in *Disorders of Narcissism: Diagnostic, Clinical and Empirical Implications*, ed. E.F. Ronningstam. Washington, DC: American Psychiatric Press, pp. 53–74.

—— (1998c) 'The impact on clinical work of the analyst's idealizations and identifications', presented at 87th Annual Meeting of the APA, Toronto.

—— (1999) 'Psychoanalytic technique – diversity or chaos? Commentary on paper by Lewis Aron', *Psychoanalytic Dialogues*, 9: 31–40.

—— (2000) 'Judith S. Schachter, M.D.', *Journal of the American Psychoanalytic Association*, 47: 671–673.

——, Eckhardt, R.D., Faloon, W.W. and Davidson, C.D. (1950) 'Investigation of the aminoaciduria in Wilson's disease (hepatolenticular degeneration): demonstration in renal function', *Journal of Clinical Investigation*, 29: 265–278.

—— and Fischer, N. (1981) 'Masochism: current concepts', *Journal of American Psychoanalytic Association*, 29: 673–688.

——, Frances, A. and Sacks, M. (1985) 'The psychoanalytic model', in *Psychiatry*, eds R. Michels, J.O. Cavenar, H.K.H. Brodie, A.M. Cooper, S.B. Guze, L.L. Judd, G.L. Klerman and A.J. Solnit. Philadelphia, PA: Lippincott.

——, Frances, A.J. and Sacks, M.H. (eds) (1986) *The Personality Disorders and Neuroses*. New York: Basic Books; Philadelphia, PA: Lippincott.

——, Karush, A., Easser, B.R. and Swerdloff, B. (1966) 'The adaptive balance profile and prediction of early treatment behavior', in G. Goldman and D. Shapiro (eds), *Developments in Psychoanalysis at Columbia University*. New York: Hafner, pp. 183–214.

——, Kernberg, O.F. and Person, E.S. (eds) (1989) *Psychoanalysis: Toward the Second Century*. New Haven, CT: Yale University Press.

—— and Michels, R. (1978a) 'The future of psychoanalysis', in *Controversy in Psychiatry*, eds J.P. Brady and H.K.H. Brodie. Philadelphia, PA: Saunders.

—— and Michels, R. (1978b) 'Psychoanalysis and future growth', in *American Psychoanalysis: Origins and Developments*, eds J.M. Quen and E.T. Carlson. New York: Brunner/Mazel.

—— and Michels, R. (1981) Review of *American Psychiatric Association: Diagnostic and Statistical Manual of Mental Disorders*, 3rd edn, *American Journal of Psychiatry*, 138: 128–129.

—— and Michels, R. (1988) Review of *Diagnostic and Statistical Manual of Mental Disorders,* 3rd edn, rev. (DSM-III-R), *American Journal of Psychiatry*, 145: 1300–1301.

—— and Ronningstam, E. (1992) 'Narcissistic personality disorder', in *Review of Psychiatry*, Vol. 11, eds A. Tasman and M. Riba. Washington, DC: American Psychiatric Press, pp. 80–97.

——, Schomer, J. and Swan, S. (1994) The ethics of fund-raising in psychiatry, *Journal of Psychotherapy Practice and Research*, 3: 68–82.

—— and Shamoian, C. (1979) 'Depression as seen by the psychiatrist', *Disease-A-Month*, 25: 1–64.

Eckhardt, R.D., Cooper, A.M., Faloon, W.W. and Davidson, C.S. (1948) 'The urinary excretion of amino acids in man, *Transactions of the New York Academy of Science*, 10 (series 2): 284–290.

Faloon, W.W., Eckhardt, R.D., Cooper, A.M. and Davidson, C.S. (1949a) 'The effects of human serum albumin, mercurial diuretics and a low sodium excretion in patients with cirrhosis of the liver', *Journal of Clinical Investigation*, 28: 595–602.

Faloon, W.W., Eckhardt, R.D., Murphy, T.L., Cooper, A.M. and Davidson, C.S. (1949b) 'An evaluation of human serum albumin in the treatment of cirrhosis of the liver', *Journal of Clinical Investigation* 28: 583–594.

Fonagy, P. and Cooper, A.M. (1999) 'Joseph Sandler's intellectual contributions to theoretical and clinical psychoanalysis', in *Psychoanalysis on the Move: The Work of Joseph Sandler*, eds P. Fonagy and A.M. Cooper. London and New York: Routledge, pp. 1–29.

Fonagy, P., Cooper, A.M. and Wallerstein, R.S. (eds) (1999) *Psychoanalysis on the Move: The Work of Joseph Sandler*. London and New York: Routledge.

Frances, A. and Cooper, A.M. (1980) 'The DSM-III controversy: a psychoanalytic perspective', *Bulletin of the Association for Psychoanalytic Medicine*, 19: 37–43.

—— and Cooper, A.M. (1981) 'Descriptive and dynamic psychiatry: a perspective on DSM-III', *American Journal of Psychiatry*, 138(9): 1198–1202.

Granet, R. and Cooper, A.M. (1990) 'Career choices in psychiatry: the evolution from resident to practitioner', *Comprehensive Psychiatry*, 31: 540–548.

Jacobson, W. and Cooper, A.M. (1993) 'Psychodynamic diagnosis in the era of the current DSM', in *Psychodynamic Treatment Research: A Handbook for Clinical Practice*, eds N.E. Miller, L. Luborsky, J.P. Barber and J.P. Docherty. New York: Basic Books, pp. 109–126.

Karush, A., Easser, R.B., Cooper, A.M. and Swerdloff, B. (1964) 'Evaluation of ego strength I: a profile of adaptive balance', *Journal of Nervous and Mental Disease*, 139(4): 332–349.

Kaufman, E., Shader, R., Cooper, A.M. and Sarles, R. (1989) 'The future of clinical psychiatry', in *Future Directions for Psychiatry*, ed. J. Talbott. Washington, DC: American Psychiatric Press, pp. 121–130.

Kelly, K. and Cooper, A.M. (1989) 'Intrapsychic models', in *Models of Depressive Disorders*, ed. J. Mann. New York: Plenum, pp. 79–91.

Koenigsberg, H.W., Kaplan, R.D., Gilmore, M.M. and Cooper, A.M. (1985) 'The relationship between syndrome and personality disorder in DSM-III: experience with 2,462 patients', *American Journal of Psychiatry*, 142: 207–212.

Lister, E.G., Auchincloss, E.L. and Cooper, A.M. (1995) 'The psychodynamic formulation', in *Psychodynamic Concepts in General Psychiatry*, eds H.J. Schwartz, E. Bleiberg and S.H. Weissman. Washington, DC: American Psychiatric Press, pp. 13–25.

Milrod, B., Busch, F.N., Cooper, A.M. and Shapiro, T. (1997) *Manual of Panic-Focused Psychodynamic Psychotherapy*. Washington, DC: American Psychiatric Press.

Nickerson, A., Burns, T. and Cooper, A.M. (1946) 'Effect of anti-reticular cytotoxic serum (ACS) on the healing of experimental wounds in rats', *Federation Proceedings*, 5(1): 196.

Offenkrantz, W., Altschul, S., Cooper, A., Frances, A., Michels, R., Rosenblatt, A., Schimel, J., Tobin, A. and Zaphiropoulos, M. (1982) 'Treatment planning and psychodynamic psychiatry', in *Treatment Planning In Psychiatry*, eds J. Lewis and G. Usdin. Washington, DC: American Psychiatric Association.

Olds, D. and Cooper, A.M. (1997) 'Dialogue with other sciences: opportunities for mutual gain – guest editorial', *International Journal of Psychoanalysis*, 78: 219–225.

Pauker, S.L. and Cooper, A.M. (1990) 'Paradoxical patient reactions to psychiatric life support: clinical and ethical considerations', *American Journal of Psychiatry*, 147: 488–491.

Perry, S., Cooper, A.M. and Michels, R. (1987) 'The psychodynamic formulation: its purpose, structure and clinical application', *American Journal of Psychiatry*, 144: 543–550.

Sacks, M.H., Karasu, S., Cooper, A.M. and Kaplan, R.D. (1983) 'Medical student's perspective of psychiatry residency selection procedures', *American Journal of Psychiatry*, 140: 781–783.

Shear, M.K., Cooper, A.M., Busch, F.N. and Shapiro, T. (1994) 'Dr. Shear and colleagues reply', *American Journal of Psychiatry*, 151: 788.

Shear, M.K., Cooper, A.M., Klerman, G.L., Busch, F.N. and Shapiro, T. (1993) 'A psychodynamic model of panic disorder', *American Journal of Psychiatry*, 150: 859–866.

Stern, G. and Cooper, A.M. (1995) 'Una psicoterapia como comienzo del analisis', *Revista de Psioanalisis*, 3: 225–247.

Tamminga, C.A., Medoff, D.R. and Cooper, A.M. (2002) 'Diseases of the mind and brain: overview', *American Journal of Psychiatry*, 159: 917.

See also

Sandler, J., Michels, R. and Fonagy, P. (2000) *Changing Ideas in a Changing World: The Revolution in Psychoanalysis: Essays in Honour of Arnold Cooper*. London and New York: Karnac.

REFERENCES

Ackerknecht, E.H. (1955) *A Short History of Medicine.* New York: Rolling Press.

Akiskal, H.S. (1983) 'Dysthymic disorder: psychopathology of proposed chronic depressive subtypes', *American Journal of Psychiatry*, 140: 11–20.

Alexander, F. and Selesnick, S.T. (1965) 'Freud–Bleuler correspondence', *Archives of General Psychiatry*, 12: 1–9.

American Psychiatric Association (1980) *Diagnostic and Statistical Manual of Mental Disorders III.* Washington, DC: APA.

American Psychiatric Association (1987) *Diagnostic and Statistical Manual of Mental Disorders III*, revised edn. Washington, DC: APA.

Arlow, J. (1971) 'Character perversion', in *Currents in Psychoanalysis*, ed. I. Marcus. New York: International Universities Press, pp. 317–336.

Auchincloss, L. (1950) *The Injustice Collectors.* Boston, MA: Houghton Mifflin.

Bachrach, H. (1993) 'The Columbia Records Project and the evolution of psychoanalytic outcome research', *Journal of the American Psychoanalytic Association*, 41S: 279–297.

Benjamin, L.S. (1974) 'Structural analysis of social behavior', *Psychological Review*, 81: 392–425.

Bergler, E. (1949) *The Basic Neurosis: Oral Regression and Psychic Masochism.* New York: Grune & Stratton.

—— (1952) *The Superego.* New York: Grune & Stratton.

—— (1961) *Curable and Incurable Neurotics.* New York: Liveright.

—— (1969) *Selected Papers of Edmund Bergler, M.D. 1933–1961.* New York: Grune & Stratton.

Bion, W.R. (1966) Review of *Medical Orthodoxy and the Future of Psychoanalysis* by K.R. Eissler, *International Journal of Psychoanalysis*, 47: 578–579.

Blatt, S. (1992) 'Differential effect of psychotherapy and psychoanalysis with anaclitic and introjective patients: the Menninger Psychotherapy Research Project revisited', *Journal of the American Psychoanalytic Association*, 40: 691–724.

Bloom, H. (1973) *The Anxiety of Influence.* New York: Oxford University Press.

Bloom, H. (1986) 'Freud, the greatest modern writer', *The New York Times Book Review*, 23 March.

Bowlby, J. (1969) *Attachment and Loss.* Vol. 1, *Attachment.* New York: Basic Books.

—— (1988) 'Developmental psychiatry comes of age', *American Journal of Psychiatry*, 145: 1–10.

Brenner, C. (1959) 'The masochistic character: genesis and treatment', *Journal of the American Psychoanalytic Association*, 7: 197–226.

—— (1982) *The Mind in Conflict*. New York: International Universities Press.

Breuer, J. and Freud, S. (1893–1895) *Studies on Hysteria*. The Standard Edition (S.E.) of the *Complete Psychological Works of Sigmund Freud*. London: Hogarth Press (1950–1974), vol. 2.

Brody, J. (1996) 'Personal health – changing thinking to change emotions', *The New York Times*, 21 August, p. C9.

Brown, N.O. (1959) *Life Against Death*. Middletown, CT: Wesleyan University Press.

Buckley, P. (ed.) (1986) *Essential Papers on Object Relations*. New York: International Universities Press.

—— (1997) 'Analysts in romantic rebellion', *Journal of the American Psychoanalytic Association*, 45: 577–582.

Chasseguet–Smirgel, J. (1984) *Creativity and Perversion*. New York: W.W. Norton.

Coen, S. (1997) Review of *Fantasy and Reality in History*, by J. Loewenberg, *The International Journal of Psychoanalysis*, 78: 199–202.

Cooper, L.N. (1980) 'Source and limits of human intellect', *Daedalus*, Spring, 1–18.

Crowe, R., Pauls, D., Kerber, R. and Noyes, R. (1981) 'Panic and mitral valve prolapse', in *Anxiety: New Research and Changing Concepts*, eds D.F. Klein and J. Rabkin. New York: Raven Press, pp. 103–116.

Curtis, H.C. (1980) 'The concept of therapeutic alliance: implications for the 'widening scope', in *Psychoanalytic Explorations of Technique*, ed. H. Blum. New York: International Universities Press, pp. 159–192.

Dahl, H., Kachele, H. and Thoma, H. (eds) (1988) *Psychoanalytic Process Research Strategies*. Heidelberg and New York: Springer-Verlag.

Davanloo, H. (1980) *Short Term Dynamic Psychotherapy*. New York: Aronson.

de Saussure, F. (1915) *Course in General Linguistics*, trans. from the French by W. Baskin. New York: Philosophical Library.

Dizmang, L. and Cheatham, C. (1970) 'The Lesch–Nyhan Syndrome', *American Journal of Psychiatry*, 127: 671–677.

Eissler, K.R. (1953) 'The effect of the structure of the ego on psychoanalytic technique', *Journal of the American Psychoanalytic Association*, 1: 104–143.

—— (1969) 'Irreverent remarks about the present and the future of psychoanalysis', *International Journal of Psychoanalysis*, 50: 461–471.

Emde, R.N. (1981) 'Changing models of infancy and the nature of early development: remodeling the foundation', *Journal of the American Psychoanalytic Association*, 29: 179–219.

—— (1988) 'Development terminable and interminable. 1. Innate and motivational factors from infancy', *International Journal of Psychoanalysis*, 69: 23–42.

Emde, R.N. and Harmon, R.J. (eds) (1984) *Continuities and Discontinuities in Development*. New York and London: Plenum Press.

Engel, G. (1953) *Maternal Deprivation in Young Children*. Film produced by J. Aubry. Distributed by New York University.

Engel, G., Reichsman, F., Haway, V. and Hess, D. (1985) 'Monica: infant-feeding behavior of a mother gastric fistula-fed as infant: a 30-year longitudinal study of enduring effects', in *Parental Influences in Health and Disease*, eds E. Anthony and G. Pollock. Boston, MA: Little, Brown.

Erikson, E. (1963) *Childhood and Society*. New York: W.W. Norton.

Erle, J.B. and Goldberg, D.A. (1984) 'Observations on assessment of analyzability by experienced analysts', *Journal of the American Psychoanalytic Association*, 32: 715–737.

Fairbairn, W.R.D. (1941) 'A revised psychopathology of the psychoses and psychoneuroses', in *Essential Papers on Object Relations* (1986), ed. P. Buckley. New York: International Universities Press, pp. 71–101.

—— (1958) 'On the nature and aims of psychoanalytic treatment', *International Journal of Psychoanalysis*, 39: 374–385.

Fenichel, O. (1945) *The Psychoanalytic Theory of Neurosis*. New York: W.W. Norton.

Ferenczi, S. (1988) *The Clinical Diary of Sandor Ferenczi*, ed. J. Dupont. Cambridge, MA: Harvard University Press.

Ferenczi, S. and Rank, O. (1923) *The Development of Psycho-Analysis*. New York: Dover Publications.

Fogel, G., Lane, M. and Liebert, R.S. (eds) (1986) *The Psychology of Men: New Psychoanalytic Perspectives*. New York: Basic Books.

Fonagy, P. (ed.) (1999) *An Open Door Review of Outcome Studies in Psychoanalysis*. London: International Psychoanalytical Association.

Freud, A. (1946) *The Ego and the Mechanisms of Defense*. New York: International Universities Press.

—— (1966) 'The ideal psychoanalytic institute: a utopia', *The Writings of Anna Freud*, Vol. 7, 1966–1970. New York: International Universities Press, pp. 73–93.

Freud, S. (1905a) 'Fragment of an analysis of a case of hysteria' Chapter IV: Postscript, S.E. 7: 112–122.

—— (1905b) 'Three essays on the theory of sexuality', S.E. 7: 226 (Footnote 1, added 1920).

—— (1908) '"Civilized" sexual morality and modern nervous illness', S.E. 9: 181–204.

—— (1909) 'Analysis of a phobia in a five-year-old boy', S.E. 10: 3–147.

—— (1911) 'Psycho-analytic notes on an autobiographical account of a case of paranoia (dementia paranoides)', S.E. 12: 3–82.

—— (1912a) 'The dynamics of transference', S.E. 12: 97–108.

—— (1912b) 'Recommendations to physicians practising psycho-analysis', S.E. 12: 111–120.

—— (1914) 'On the history of the psychoanalytic movement', S.E. 14: 7–66.

—— (1920a) 'Beyond the pleasure principle', S.E. 18: 3–66.

—— (1920b) 'The psychogenesis of a case of homosexuality in a woman', S.E. 18: 145–172.

—— (1923a) 'The ego and the id', S.E. 19: 3–66.

—— (1923b) 'Two encyclopaedia articles', S.E. 18: 235–259.

—— (1926a) 'Inhibitions, symptoms and anxieties', S.E. 20: 77–178.

—— (1926b) 'The question of lay analysis', S.E. 20: 179–258.

—— (1931) 'Female sexuality', S.E. 21: 225–243.

—— (1933a) 'New introductory lectures', S.E. 22: 5–182.

—— (1933b) 'Revision of the theory of dreams', S.E. 22: 7–30.

—— (1937a) 'Analysis terminable and interminable', S.E. 23: 209–254.

—— (1937b) 'Constructions in analysis', S.E. 23: 255–270.

—— (1938) 'An outline of psycho-analysis', S.E. 23: 141–208.

—— (1939) 'Moses and monotheism', S.E. 23: 3–140.

Gardner, R.M. (1983) *Self Inquiry*. New York: Little, Brown.

Gifford, S. (1978) 'Psychoanalysis in Boston: innocence and experience', in *Psychoanalysis, Psychotherapy and the New England Medical Scene, 1894–1944*, ed. G.E. Gifford. New York: Science History Publications.

Gill, M.M. (1982) *Analysis of Transference*, Vol. 1: *Theory and Technique*. New York: International Universities Press.

—— (1984) 'Psychoanalysis and psychotherapy: a revision', *International Review of Psycho-Analysis*, 11: 161–180.

—— (1994) *Psychoanalysis in Transition: A Personal View*. Hillsdale, NJ: Analytic Press.

Glover, E. (1955) *The Technique of Psychoanalysis*. New York: International Universities Press.

Goldberg, A. (ed.) (1978) *The Psychology of the Self: A Casebook*. New York: International Universities Press.

Goodman, S. (ed.) (1977) *Psychoanalytic Education and Research*. New York: International Universities Press.

Greenacre, P. (1960) 'Regression and fixation: considerations concerning the development of the ego', *Journal of the American Psychoanalytic Association*, 8: 703–723.

Grossman, W.I. (1986) 'Notes on masochism: a discussion of the history and development of a psychoanalysis concept', *Psychoanalytic Quarterly*, 54: 379–413.

Harlow, H. (1960) *Mother Love* (film). Produced by CBS; distribution by Pennsylvania Cinema Register at Pennsylvania State University.

Hartmann, H. (1937) *Ego Psychology and The Problem of Adaptation*. New York: International Universities Press, 1958.

—— (1960) *Psychoanalysis and Moral Values*. New York: International Universities Press.

Hartmann, H. and Loewenstein, R.M. (1962) 'Notes on the superego', *Psychoanalytic Study of the Child*, 17: 42–81.

Heimann, P. (1956) 'Dynamics of transference interpretation', *International Journal of Psychoanalysis*, 37: 303–310.

Hermann, I. (1976) 'Clinging – going in search – a contrasting pair of instincts and their relation to sadism and masochism', *Psychoanalytic Quarterly*, 44: 5–36.

Hofer, M.A. (1981) *The Roots of Human Behavior*. San Francisco, CA: W.H. Freeman.

Horney, K. (1950) *Neurosis and Human Growth: The Struggle Towards Self-Realization*. New York: W.W. Norton.

Horowitz, M.J. (ed.) (1991) *Person Schemas and Maladaptive Interpersonal Patterns*. Chicago, IL: Chicago University Press.

Huxster, H., Lower, R. and Escoll, P. (1975) 'Some pitfalls in the assessment of analyzability in a psychoanalytic clinic', *Journal of the American Psychoanalytic Association*, 23: 90–106.

Hyman, S. (1996) 'Melding mind and brain', *Psychiatric News*, 31(8), April.

Imperato-McGinley, J., Peterson, R.E., Gautier, T. and Sturla, E. (1979) 'Androgens and the evolution of male gender identity among male pseudohermaphrodites with 5-2-reductose deficiency', *New England Journal of Medicine*, 300: 1233–1237.

Jacobs, T. (1991) *The Use of the Self: Countertransference and Communication in the Analytic Situation*. New York: International Universities Press.

Jacobson, E. (1959) 'The "exceptions": an elaboration of Freud's character study', *Psychoanalytic Study of the Child*, 14: 135–154.

—— (1964) *The Self and the Object World*. New York: International Universities Press.

Jelinek, E. (1983/1988) *The Piano Teacher*. New York: Weidenfeld and Nicolson. English translation.

Jones, E. (1946) 'A valedictory address', *International Journal of Psychoanalysis*, 27: 7–12.

—— (1957) *The Life and Work of Sigmund Freud*, Vol. 3. New York: Basic Books.

Kafka, F. (1923) 'The burrow', in *The Complete Stories*. New York: Schocken, pp. 325–359 (1971).

Kandel, E.R. (1979) 'Psychotherapy and the single synapse. The impact of psychiatric thought on neurobiologic research', *New England Journal of Medicine*, 30: 1028–1037.

—— (1983) 'From metapsychology to molecular biology: explorations into the nature of anxiety', *American Journal of Psychiatry*, 140: 1277–1293.

Kantrowitz, J. (1993) 'Outcome research in psychoanalysis', *Journal of the American Psychoanalytic Association*, 41S: 313–329.

Kardiner, A. (1939) *The Individual and His Society: The Psychodynamics of Primitive Social Organization*. New York: Columbia University Press.

—— (1945) *The Psychological Frontiers of Society*. New York: Columbia University Press.

Keiser, S. (1969) 'Psychoanalysis – taught, learned, and experienced', *Journal of the American Psychoanalytic Association*, 17: 238–267.

Kermode, F. (1972) *The Art of Telling*. Cambridge, MA: Harvard University Press.

—— (1985) 'Freud and interpretation', *International Journal of Psychoanalysis*, 12: 3–12.

Kernberg, O.F. (1975) *Borderline Conditions and Pathological Narcissism*. New York: Aronson.

—— (1984) *Severe Personality Disorders: Psychotherapeutic Strategies*. New Haven, CT: Yale University Press.

—— (1986) 'Institutional problems of psychoanalytic education', *Journal of the American Psychoanalytic Association*, 34: 799–834.

Khan, M.M.R. (1979) *Alienation in Perversions*. New York: International Universities Press.

Kinsey, A.C., Pomeroy, W.B. and Clyde, E.M. (1948) *Structural Behavior and the Human Male*. Philadelphia, PA: W.B. Saunders.

Klein, D. and Fink, M. (1962) 'Psychiatric reaction patterns to imipramine', *American Journal of Psychiatry*, 119: 432–438.

Klein, M. (1932) *The Psychoanalysis of Children*. New York: Grove Press (1960).

—— (1935) 'A contribution to the psychogenesis of manic-depressive states', in *Essential Papers on Object Relations*, ed. P. Buckley. New York: International Universities Press (1986), pp. 40–70.

—— (1957) *Envy and Gratitude*. London: Tavistock.

Knight, R. (1953) 'The present status of organized psychoanalysis in the United States', *Journal of the American Psychoanalytic Association*, 1: 197–221.

Kohut, H. (1959) 'Introspection, empathy, and psychoanalysis: an examination of the relationship between mode of observation and theory', in P. Ornstein (ed.) *The Search for the Self*, Vol. 1 (1978). New York: International Universities Press, pp. 205–232.

—— (1970) 'Scientific activities of the American Psychoanalytic Association – an inquiry', *Journal of the American Psychoanalytic Association*, 18: 462–484.

273

—— (1971) *The Analysis of the Self.* New York: International Universities Press.

—— (1972) 'Thoughts on narcissism and narcissistic rage', *Psychoanalytic Study of the Child*, 27: 360–400.

—— (1976) 'Creativeness, charisma, group psychology: reflections on the self-analysis of Freud', in *Search for the Self*, Vol. 2, ed. P. Ornstein. New York: International Universities Press.

—— (1977) *Restoration of the Self.* New York: International Universities Press.

—— (1980) 'Summarizing reflections', in *Advances in Self Psychology*, ed. A. Goldberg. New York: International Universities, pp. 473–554.

—— (1984) *How Does Analysis Cure?* Chicago: University of Chicago Press.

—— and Wolf, E.S. (1978) The disorders of the self and their treatment: an outline. *International Journal of Psychoanalysis*, 59: 413–426.

Krafft-Ebing, R.F. (1895) *Psychopathia Sexualis*. London: F.A. Davis.

Laplanche, J. and Pontalis, J.-B. (1973) *The Language of Psychoanalysis*. New York: W.W. Norton. English translation.

Levenkron, H., Schaffer, A. and Kispit, J. interview of 'A Conversation with Theodore Jacobs', *The American Psychoanalyst*, 30(2).

Lewin, B. (1950) *Psychoanalysis of Elation*. New York: W.W. Norton.

Lichtenberg, J.D. and Kaplan, S. (eds) (1983) *Reflection on Self Psychology*. Hillsdale, NJ: The Analytic Press.

Lipton, S. (1977) 'The advantages of Freud's technique as shown in his analysis of the Rat Man', *International Journal of Psychoanalysis*, 58: 255–274.

Loewald, H. (1960) 'On the therapeutic action of psychoanalysis', *International Journal of Psychoanalysis*, 41: 16–33.

—— (1970) 'Psychoanalytic theory and the psychoanalytic process', *Psychoanalytic Study of the Child*, 25: 45–68.

Loewenstein, R. (1957) 'A contribution to the psychoanalytic theory of masochism', *Journal of the American Psychoanalytic Association*, 5: 197–234.

Luborsky, L. and Crits-Cristoph, P. (1990) *Understanding Transference: The Core Conflictual Relationship Theme Method*. New York: Basic Books.

Luborsky, L. and Luborsky, E. (1993) 'The era of measures of transference: the CCRT and other measures', *Journal of the American Psychoanalytic Association*, 41S: 329–351.

McDougall, J. (1984) 'The significance of the reconstruction of trauma in clinical work', paper presented at the American Psychoanalytic Association Workshop for Mental Health Professionals, New York, November.

—— (1985) *Theaters of the Mind: Illusion and Truth on the Psychoanalytic Stage*. New York: Basic Books.

McLaughlin, F. (1978) 'Some perspectives on psychoanalysis today', *Journal of the American Psychoanalytic Association*, 26: 3–20.

Mahler, M. (1972) 'Rapprochement subphase of the separation–individuation process', *Psychoanalytic Quarterly*, 44: 487–506.

Mahler, M., Pine, F. and Bergmann, A. (1975) *The Psychological Birth of the Human Infant*. New York: Basic Books.

Maleson, F. (1984) 'The multiple meanings of masochism in psychoanalytic discourse', *Journal of the American Psychoanalytic Association*, 32: 325–356.

Meissner, W.W. (1978) *The Paranoid Process*. New York: Aronson.

—— (1986) *Psychotherapy and the Paranoid Process*. Northvale, NJ: Aronson.

Michels, R. (1988) 'The future of psychoanalysis', *Psychoanalytic Quarterly*, 57: 167–185.

Miller, I. (1975) 'A critical assessment of the future of psychoanalysis: a view from outside', *Journal of the American Psychoanalytic Association*, 23: 587–602.

Money, J. and Ehrhardt, A. (1972) *Man and Woman, Boy and Girl: Differentiation and Dimorphism of Gender Identity from Conception to Maturity*. Baltimore, MD: Johns Hopkins University Press.

Mother Love (video recording) (1960) New York: Carousel Film and Video, CBS Television Network, produced by Michael Sklar, directed by Harold Mayer; written by S.S. Schweitzer; records the experiments of H.F. Harlow.

The Nature and Development of Affection (video cassette) (1959) University Park, PA: University Division of Media and Learning Resources, The Pennsylvania State University; produced by University of Wisconsin at Madison, studies conducted by H.F. Harlow and R. Zimmerman.

Panel (1992) 'Classics revisited: Eissler's "The effect of the structure of the ego on psychoanalytic technique".' L. Friedman, chair. Presented at Fall Meeting of American Psychoanalytic Association, New York.

Penzias, A. (1979) 'The origin of the elements', *Science*, 205: 549–554.

Person, E. (1986) 'Male sexuality and power', *Psychoanalytic Inquiry*, 6: 3–25.

Person, E. and Ovesey, L. (1976) 'Transvestism: a disorder of the sense of self', *International Journal of Psychoanalytic Psychotherapy*, 5: 219–236.

—— (1983) 'Psychoanalytic theories of gender identity', *Journal of the American Academy of Psychoanalysis*, 11: 203–226.

Rado, S. (1956) *Psychoanalysis of Behavior: The Collected Papers of Sandor Rado*, Vol. I. New York: Grune & Stratton.

—— (1962) *Psychoanalysis of Behavior: The Collected Papers of Sandor Rado*, Vol. II. New York: Grune & Stratton.

—— (1969) *Adaptational Psychodynamics*. New York: Science House.

Richards, A.D. (reporter) (1984) 'Panel report: The relations between psychoanalytic theory and psychoanalytic technique', *Journal of the American Psychiatric Association*, 32(3): 587–602.

Ricoeur, P. (1970) *Freud and Philosophy, an Essay on Interpretation*. New Haven, CT: Yale University Press.

Robertson, J. and Robertson, J. (1952) *A Two-Year-Old Goes to the Hospital* (16mm film, b&w, sound, 45- and 30-minute versions; English/French; guide booklet). London: Tavistock Child Development Research Unit; New York: New York University Film Library; produced by James Robertson and Joyce Robertson.

Roiphe, H. and Galenson, E. (1981) *Infantile Origins of Sexual Identity*. New York: International Universities Press.

Rothgeb, C.L. (ed.) (1971) 'Fragment of an analysis of a case of hysteria', Chapter IV: Postscript. In *Abstracts of the Standard Edition of the Complete Psychological Works of Sigmund Freud*. Rockville, MD: U.S. Department of Health, Education and Welfare, p. 45.

Roustang, F. (1982) *Dire Mastery*. Baltimore, MD: Johns Hopkins University Press.

Sacher-Masoch, L. von (1870) *Sacher-Masoch: An Interpretation* by G. Deleuze, together with the entire text of *Venus in Furs*, trans. J.M. McNeil. London: Faber and Faber.

Sandler, J. (1983) 'Reflections on some relations between psychoanalytic concept and psychoanalytic practice', *International Journal of Psychoanalysis*, 64: 1–11.

—— (1987) *From Safety to Superego*. New York: Guilford Press; London: Karnac.

—— (1991) *On Freud's 'Analysis Terminable and Interminable'*. New Haven, CT: Yale University Press.

—— and Joffe, W.G. (1969) 'Towards a basic psychoanalytic model', *International Journal of Psychoanalysis*, 50: 79–90.

—— and Sandler, A.-M. (1987) 'Past unconscious, present unconscious, and vicissitudes of guilt', *International Journal of Psychoanalysis*, 68: 331–342.

Schafer, R. (1976) *A New Language for Psychoanalysis*. New Haven, CT: Yale University Press.

—— (1981) *Narrative Actions in Psychoanalysis*. Worcester, MA: Clark University Press.

—— (1983) *The Analytic Attitude*. New York: Basic Books.

—— (1985) 'Wild analysis', *Journal of the American Psychoanalytic Association*, 33: 275–299.

Schwaber, E.A. (1983) 'Psychoanalytic listening and psychic reality', *International Review of Psycho-Analysis*, 10: 379–392.

—— (1992) 'Countertransference: the analyst's retreat from the patient's vantage point', *International Journal of Psychoanalysis*, 73: 349–362.

Shapiro, D. (1965) *Neurotic Styles*. New York: Basic Books.

Shapiro, D. (ed.) (1981) 'Survey of psychoanalytical practice: a summation', distributed to members of the American Psychoanalytic Association.

Shapiro, T. (1970) 'Interpretation and naming', *Journal of the American Psychoanalytic Association*, 18: 399–421.

Simons, R.C. (1981) 'Contemporary problems of psychoanalytic technique', *Journal of the American Psychoanalytic Association*, 29: 654–655.

Smith, M.L., Glass, G.V. and Miller, T.I. (1980) *The Benefits of Psychotherapy*. Baltimore, MD: Johns Hopkins University Press.

Spence, D.P. (1982) *Narrative Truth and Historical Truth*. New York: W.W. Norton.

Stade, G. (1984) 'Men, boys and wimps', *New York Times Book Review*, 89, 12 August, 1.

Starke, O. (1973) 'Castration complex', in *The Language of Psychoanalysis*, eds J. Laplanche and J.-B. Pontalis. New York: W.W. Norton, pp. 56–60.

Stein, G. (1935) 'How writing is written', in *The Previously Uncollected Writings of Gertrude Stein*, ed. R.B. Haas. Santa Barbara, CA: Black Sparrow Press, Vol. 2, 1974, pp. 111–160.

Stein, M. (1979) Review of *The Restoration of the Self*, by H. Kohut, *Journal of the American Psychoanalytic Association*, 27: 665–680.

—— (1981) 'The unobjectionable part of the transference', *Journal of the American Psychoanalytic Association*, 29: 869–892.

Stern, D.N. (1985) *The Interpersonal World of the Infant*. New York: Basic Books.

Stoller, R.J. (1974) 'Hostility and mystery in perversion', *International Journal of Psychoanalysis*, 55: 425–434.

—— (1975) *Perversion: The Erotic Form of Hatred*. New York: Pantheon.

Stolorow, R.D. (1975) 'The narcissistic function of masochism and sadism', *International Journal of Psychoanalysis*, 56: 441–448.

Stone, L. (1961) *The Psychoanalytic Situation*. New York: International Universities Press.

Strachey, J. (1934) 'The nature of the therapeutic action of psychoanalysis', *International Journal of Psychoanalysis*, 15: 127–159.

Sullivan, H.S. (1953) *The Interpersonal Theory of Psychiatry*. New York: W.W. Norton.

—— (1956) *Clinical Studies in Psychiatry*, eds H.S. Perry, M.L. Gawel and M. Gibbon. New York: W.W. Norton.

Tanizaki, J. (1982) *The Secret History of the Lord of Musashi*. Putnam, NY: Wideview/Perigee.

Thomas, A., Chess, S. and Birch, H. (1968) *Temperament and Behavior Disorders in Children*. New York: New York University Press.

Trilling, L. (1963) *Beyond Culture*. New York: Viking Press.

Waelder, R. (1960) *Basic Theory of Psychoanalysis*. New York: International Universities Press.

Wallerstein, R. (1986) *42 Lives in Treatment: A Study of Psychoanalysis and Psychotherapy*. New York: Guilford.

—— (1993) 'The effectiveness of psychotherapy and psychoanalysis: conceptual issues and empirical work', *Journal of the American Psychoanalytic Association*, 41S: 299–312.

Westen, D. (1990) 'Towards a revised theory of borderline object relations: contributions of empirical research', *International Journal of Psychoanalysis*, 71: 661–694.

Winnicott, D.W. (1960) 'Ego distortion in terms of true and false self', in *Maturational Processes and the Facilitating Environment*. New York: International Universities Press, 1965, pp. 140–152.

—— (1965a) *The Family and Individual Development*. London: Associated Book Publishers.

—— (1965b) *The Maturational Processes and the Facilitating Environment*. New York: International Universities Press.

—— (1971) *Playing and Reality*. New York: Basic Books.

Wolff, P. (1996) 'The irrelevance of infant observations for psychoanalysis', *Journal of the American Psychoanalytic Association*, 44: 387–473.

Zuger, B. (1984) 'Early effeminate behavior in boys: outcome and significance for homosexuality', *Journal of Nervous Mental Disorders*, 172: 90–97.